Augmentative and Assistive Communication with Children

This practical resource is designed to help the families and professionals who support children who use augmentative and assistive communication (AAC) to interact with the world around them. The research-based *Hear Me into Voice* protocol, presented at the American Speech-Language-Hearing Association Annual Convention in 2018, the California Speech-Language Hearing Association Annual Convention in 2017, and the International Society for Augmentative and Alternative Communication Conference in 2016, provides communication partners with a functional knowledge of the child's communication skills and provides a practical intervention plan to carry forward. Through this protocol and intervention plan, communication partners can engage with the child's personal voice, through their varying multimodal forms of communication; the child is given the space to grow into a competent and confident communicator.

Key features include:

- Photocopiable and downloadable resources, including the *Hear Me into Voice* protocol, an AAC report shell template, an AAC report teaching template, and tools including how to make a communication wallet, and a *Let's Chat* communication partner tip card template
- Guidance for offering AAC intervention sessions, including an intervention plan supported by case studies
- Practical activities that can be used to engage children with complex communication profiles

Engaging and easy to follow, this resource is not only essential for professionals and students looking to support children with complex language needs, but also families looking to understand their child's unique communication style.

Lesley E. Mayne, Ph.D., CCC-SLP

Lesley E. Mayne is Assistant Professor at the University of Wisconsin-Eau Claire (Fall 2020) after completing five productive years with California Baptist University. Her interests include augmentative and assistive communication (AAC) and pedagogy. Dr. Mayne has taught as an adjunct faculty member at California State University, Fullerton and worked in the public school, charter, and private settings for 20 years. She has presented at local, state, national, and international events and conferences including the California Speech-Language Hearing Association, American Speech-Language-Hearing Association, and International Society for Augmentative and Alternative Communication. Dr. Mayne participates in special education trans-disciplinary diagnostic and treatment teams, lectures and writes on topics such as AAC, social skills, accommodations and modifications in the mainstream academic setting. She received an award for Outstanding Achievement at the 2013 California Speech-Language Hearing Association State Conference. In 2013, she co-presented a five-hour Ablenet University webinar series with Dr. Sharon Rogers titled *AAC: Developing Participation* that reached an international audience. She is the author of *Let's Talk Social Skills*, 2nd edition (Speechmark, 2019).

Sharon M. Rogers, Ph.D., CCC-SLP

Sharon M. Rogers served as Assistant Professor in Teacher Education at Claremont Graduate University and as an adjunct faculty member in the Department of Communication Sciences and Disorders at California State University, Fullerton, where she taught the seminar and practicum in Augmentative and Alternative Communication (AAC). Dr. Rogers was awarded for Outstanding Achievement by the California Speech-Language Hearing Association in 2010. As a speech-language pathologist (SLP) in public schools in California and Kentucky, she found her real passion was in assessing and developing communication of children with complex physical and communication profiles. She continues as a consultant with students as they participate using AAC. She published an article, *Two Perspectives on Technology for Children with Special Needs*, co-written with Dr. Suzi Hoge, that included viewpoints of both parents and speech-language pathologists. Her writing with Mary Poplin has appeared in the *Learning Disabilities Quarterly*. She is a presenter at the California Speech-Language Hearing Association, the American Speech-Language-Hearing Association, and the International Society of Augmentative and Alternative Communication (ISAAC) conferences in the United States, Ireland, Denmark, and Spain.

Augmentative and Assistive Communication with Children

A Protocol and Intervention Plan to Support Children with Complex Communication Profiles

LESLEY E. MAYNE AND SHARON M. ROGERS

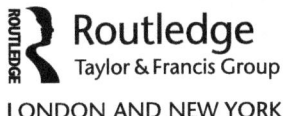

Taylor & Francis Group

LONDON AND NEW YORK

First published 2020
by Routledge
2 Park Square, Milton Park, Abingdon, Oxon OX14 4RN

and by Routledge
52 Vanderbilt Avenue, New York, NY 10017

Routledge is an imprint of the Taylor & Francis Group, an informa business

© 2020 Lesley E. Mayne and Sharon M. Rogers

British Library Cataloguing-in-Publication Data
A catalogue record for this book is available from the British Library

Library of Congress Cataloging-in-Publication Data
A catalog record has been requested for this book

ISBN: 978-0-367-33055-2 (pbk)
ISBN: 978-0-429-31777-4 (ebk)

Typeset in Vectora LH
by Swales & Willis, Exeter, Devon, UK

Visit the companion website: www.routledge.com/cw/speechmark

Dedication

To every AAC user, facilitator, and communication partner who achieve participation and to each family who inspired our 25-year journey of learning, joy, and perseverance.

–Lesley and Sharon

Contents

Acknowledgments

What do you know about AAC? Dr. Sharon Rogers' marvelous first words, uttered with complete enthusiasm, started a 25-year journey of friendship, mentorship, and scholarship. I met the indomitable Dr. Rogers, coined by our DynaVox representative as the Guru of AAC for Southern California, at California State University, Fullerton (CSUF) in the Fall of 1995 at the public-school practicum placement meeting. My nervous response to her palpable energy sailed across the field like a lame duck pass at a football game. *I took a class?* My fleeting confidence was bolstered that day and every day since thanks to Dr. Rogers. This book started as a poster. Why nobody was interested in a 4x5 foot sheet of paper with 10-point font with negligible margins and no pictures packed with information on AAC was baffling. A little much? We realized we may have failed at making a poster, but we succeeded in outlining a book.

Collecting best friends is a worthy gift that brings richness and add to foundational strength that served as a significant support during the writing of this book. Thank you, Lisa, for being my friend for over four decades, for still mailing handwritten letters with stunning script, and keeping us both honest in maintaining life's balance. To Jamie: You make friendship family. An expert in everything from administration, special day class support for medically fragile children, to nursing, cooking, dog care, and plumbing (yes, even plumbing). To Elaine: The ties that bind like five-hour IEPs and lunch no matter what, your support keeps *our* goals on target. Lucy: Never a stronger competitor have I met. Named one of the most powerful women in business by Harvard Business School, you are a formidable champion, an inspiration to be better, and always a text away, no matter what, wherever you are in the world. To Sharon C.: Thank you for sharing your life's adventures. Friendship crosses life's chapters.

Are you on to the next chapter yet? Rich, my app, before apps were apps. Thank you for the instant calculations, the word spellings, and the daily newspaper word scrambles. Thank you, Riley for the example of what it means to forge your own intellectual life path and for sharing your photography prowess including the photo shoots, the edits, and the re-shoots. Jordan, your pictures bring a special heart to the book through your journey to us as a family and the gift you bring others through your daily perseverance with verbal apraxia. Finally thank you to CT for the *Let's do lunch* breaks. You work and play for the team, bring strengths together, and support needs that shapes everyone's success. None of this adventure happens without my parents Tom and Edna who support my every venture.

–LEM

My passion to help children communicate started as an undergraduate at the University of Nebraska and then deepened while doing a master's degree at the University of Pittsburgh where we were encouraged to develop our own theories and practices.

For more than six decades, my late and much loved husband Jack, cheered me on and provided a foundation of faith and love. Together we parented three sons, Matthew, John Mark, and Toby who broadened our understanding of the world through their interactions with us and with other cultures.

As our children got older, I became a speech-language pathologist in the public schools in Pasadena, California and then in Louisville, Kentucky. I knew I needed new tools and strategies when I first met with Anthony, a nonverbal student with the diagnosis of autism. So together with another speech language teacher we figured out how to install an adaptive firmware card in an early Apple computer with a Muppet keyboard. Within minutes Anthony showed me language by changing animals, colors, numbers, and actions on the display. Early conferences such as Technology and Persons with Disabilities opened my eyes to the range of new tools being developed and utilized to provide augmentative and assistive communication.

Judy Montgomery persuaded me to earn a Ph.D. at Claremont Graduate University. The chair of my committee, Mary Poplin, taught me to explore new paradigms of teaching and learning, introduced me to qualitative research, and encouraged me to embrace the messiness and nuance the truths of conflicting observations, for which I am eternally grateful. I listened and observed in the homes of seven children with complex communication and physical profiles; interviewed their parents, educators, and speech-language pathologists; sifted through the interviews to write the case studies; and finally designed the protocol *Hear Me into Voice*. Li-Rong Lilly Cheng emphasized the importance of culture and encouraged me to keep writing.

I am exceedingly grateful for the vital insights of the children Diego, Moses, Alexa, Jada, and Joy and their amazing families (names have been changed to protect their identities) whose real lives are the basis for the case studies. Individual case experiences were changed to reflect the evolution of technology and vocabulary decision making in AAC.

When I met the incredibly talented Lesley Mayne, she was preparing to run in the 800-meter track race at the Olympic Trials in Atlanta, Georgia. We formed a new partnership for a deepening AAC emphasis. She has contributed abundant creativity, dedication, faith, collegiality, and skills.

I am grateful to David Beukelman for transforming the field through his emphasis on seeing communication from the perspective of the learner. I also learned from other pioneers in AAC including Sarah Blackstone, Mats Granlund, Janice Light, Stephen von Tetzchner (who introduced me to the writings of Lev Vygotsky), and the International Society of Augmentative and Alternative Communication.

Friends and family supported me personally and professionally: Carol Brainerd, Corinne McNamara, Jack Brickson, Joni Eyler, Stephen and Maggie Mangold, Lisa Quinn, Marilyn Brydolf, and Margaret McConnell. Susan Simmons and I worked together to implement AAC more widely in the schools.

My hope is that this book will be a resource for parents, speech-language pathologists, and educators to support the full participation of children in all aspects of society. Hearing the compelling and enthusiastic communication of these children and their families made it essential that Lesley and I write this book.

–SMR

From Sharon and Lesley to all of our friends and colleagues, especially Candace Vickers and Bryan Ness at California Baptist University and the iBook Club of Pasadena, we thank you for your support. Ashley Murtha and Tori Strobel-Sabatino shared their skillful talents in artistry and writing. We thank them for donating their time to be a part of this book. To our students past, present, and future, let your voices, like all of our AAC users' voices, be heard.

–LEM & SMR

Permissions acknowledgments

A gracious thank you to the following people and companies for granting permissions to include photos and content that bring ideas and concepts to life in this book. Your work changes lives of people with complex communication profiles.

1 Ablenet: Joe Volp for the images of AAC tools and devices
2 Expanding Expression Tool: Sarah Smith for EET that supports AAC expression
3 MindWing: Sheila Moreau and Bill Noss for Story Grammar Marker images and content

PART I
Hear Me into Voice

Beginnings

Why the protocol *Hear Me into Voice*, the case studies, and the intervention plan matter

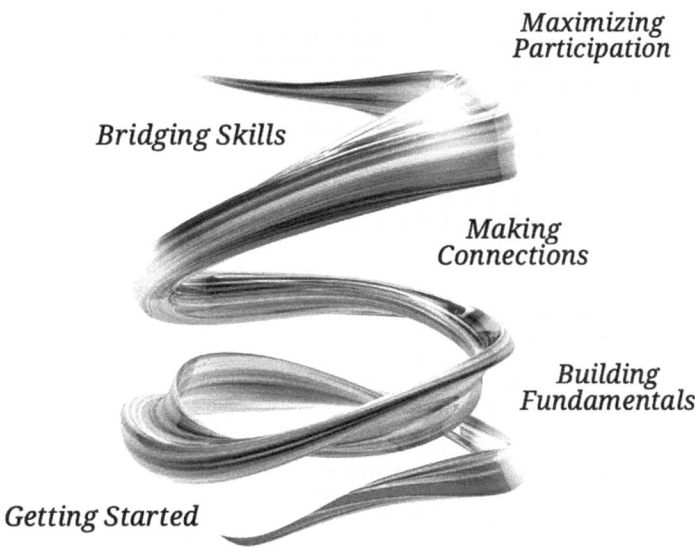

Maximizing Participation

Bridging Skills

Making Connections

Building Fundamentals

Getting Started

My child is there, in a greater sense, than what the diagnosis tells me.

Parent (Rogers, 1999)

We believe that children with complex communication profiles (CCP) express their unique identity each with individual thoughts, feelings and emotions, and a depth of understanding that impacts participation with others across environments. Children with complex communication profiles want to learn and communicate with other children, siblings, parents, teachers, coaches, and anyone ready to listen in the participation of life's activities. Our goal then is to hear each child's voice by augmenting and assisting communication vital to their participation across cultures. We aim to enable children in a variety of interactions and participate in activities of their choice (Beukelman & Mirenda, 2013). Prizant and Fields-Meyer (2015, p. 214) note that human development is a lifelong process – and that priorities shift. The authors go on to state that when a child becomes a competent and confident communicator, regardless of how he or she is communicating, the child is more available for learning and engaging (p. 234). This engagement includes a family centered approach that will build confidence and trust as each team member contributes to decisions about AAC in the best interests of the child, an idea that is supported by Mandak and Light (2018).

Children's communication grows as each child participates in activities with others. Our priorities change when we see communication like a dance, with each communication partner synchronizing with the other by moving our eyes, gestures, smiles, voices, and forms of technology. Children and their communication partners are stating, *I share my meaning in unique sounds, gestures, and tools. My body may work differently than yours, but I see that we are sharing what matters to both of us.* We aim to demystify forms of augmentative and assistive technology (AAC) by unifying perspectives of family and professionals as communication partners with children that use AAC. Helen Keller wrote in her book *Optimism* (1903) that she came to know finger spelling as a form of living and belonging, no longer isolating.

> *Once I only knew darkness and stillness . . . my life was without past or future, but a little word from the fingers of another fell into my hand that clutched at emptiness and my heart leaped to the rapture of living . . . With the first word I used intelligently, I learned to live, to think, to hope.*
>
> (pp. 10–11)

The purpose of our book is to detail how the focus on participation drives vital learning and engagement for children that use AAC through case studies and practical intervention strategies.

Augmentative and Assistive Communication: A Protocol and Intervention for Children with Complex Communication Profiles offers families and interventionists a functional protocol titled *Hear Me into Voice* that identifies communication behaviors, and provides intervention strategies including case studies for children that use AAC and their communication partners who support communication and participation. McNaughton et al. (2019) state that the use of case studies can provide students with clinical context for new information and introduce them to the wide range of goals and strategies. *Students*, in this book refers to you, the reader.

The primary chapters cover stages of AAC including *Getting Started, Building Fundamentals, Making Connections, Bridging Skills*, and *Maximizing Communication*. Each chapter provides the reader with a case study and a six-section intervention plan including social awareness, communication activities, facilitator tips, vocabulary, literacy, and tools and access. The authors recognize and invite you to recognize that a child may be interacting and communicating at different stages. For example, a child may be in the stage of *Making Connections* with communication activities and in the *Getting Started* stage of literacy. Progress across stages as appropriate for each individual child. At the end of each chapter we offer a section of functional tips and resources titled, *Before we go*. Investigate how the tips and resources support your child's communication and participation today and plan for every tomorrow.

Defining augmentative and assistive communication (AAC)

Augmentative and assistive communication is defined in this book as all forms of communication, both physical and technological, that children and adults with limited-verbal or nonverbal abilities use to learn, comprehend, and express themselves with communication partners across environments. All communicators augment their communication with nonverbal gestures, facial expression, and body positions. Similarly, most communicators access technology for work, school, and social purposes. When the use of technology is required for access to life functions, that includes communication, the term is called assistive technology. AAC technologies fall under the umbrella term of assistive technology. For a person with a complex communication profile who is limited-verbal or nonverbal, the use of assistive technology or augmentative communication for expression is often not an alternative but rather a primary way to communicate. Therefore, the term used throughout this book is augmentative and assistive communication.

The protocol rationale

Interventionists and families alike will find completing the protocol, *Hear Me into Voice*, to be an exciting step in the journey of discovering communication with children who use AAC and their communication partners. It is a valuable tool to use in the AAC assessment repertoire for children with complex communication profiles. The protocol items are based upon meaningful nonverbal and verbal interactions observed between children that use AAC and communication partners (e.g. peers, parents, siblings, interventionists, educators) in their homes, schools, and communities. The statements in the protocol use an active voice from the child's point of view about topics such as activities, literacy, and emotions, such as, *I laugh when . . . (e.g. I watch cartoons. I hear a joke. I hear other people laughing.)*. The protocol takes account of the importance of emotional competency, an important developmental area recognized by researchers Na, Wilkinson, Karny, Blackstone and Stifter (2016). The information collected serves as insight into the logical next steps into communication and participation. Identifying children's strengths and needs rather than deficits is an opportunity for success (Owens, 2014, p. 6). Through the protocol child's preferences, feelings, social graces, vocabulary, and tools are compiled and available to be tied to communication and participation. The findings from the protocol as a part of a complete AAC assessment yield a multimodal communication plan including nonverbal, vocal, verbal, low technology communication boards and tools, and high technology speech generating devices that nurtures communication and participation development between a child with a complex communication profile and known, familiar, and unknown communication partners across environments.

The case studies rationale

○ Case study theoretical development

The development of the case studies included at the beginning of each stage of the intervention plan is based on the qualitative research through the observation and interaction with seven children with complex communication and physical profiles and their families. The case studies are inspired by authentic interactions over three days, but not verbatim accounts, from Dr. Rogers's research in the homes, at school, and in the community. All names in the case studies have been changed to protect identities. International researchers in communication and socialization use ethnographic methods and case studies (Boavida, Aguiar & McWilliam, 2014; Damico & Ball, 2010). Substantive literature emphasizes the importance of expanding our knowledge base by examining case studies (Hammer, 2011). Dr. Rogers was influenced by the question of how the lives of families, communities, and classrooms influenced language development (Bronfenbrenner, 1986; Heath, 1983). Her task was to become acquainted with the communication, topics, and methods children and their communication partners learned and taught in everyday activities at home and at school as they went about daily routines (Moll, 1990). She saw families with a deeply loving understanding of children's communication across a broad range of communicative functions in everyday relationships and environments, as reflected through a poem by a sister of a child with a complex communication profile.

My Silent Angel
My silent angel watches before me,
So near, yet so obtuse,
His angelic face holds the mysteries of God,
Will the key, ever be unlocked
*To give my **silent guardian** a voice.*
By C. M. (Rogers, 1999)

Dr. Rogers was convinced she had to create a protocol reflecting the multiple forms of communication with the parents and interventionists as experts. The theoretical constructs that shaped the case studies include Bruner's culture and quest for meaning (1990, p. 20), Piaget's developmental stages (Ginsburg & Opper, 1988, p. 26), Gardner's multiple intelligences (1993, pp. 73–77), Delpit's culturally adapted teaching methods (1995, p. 49), Poplin (1988a, 1988b), and Vygotsky's linguistic and social cultural activity (Moll, 1990, p. 1). She saw how children with complex communication profiles were especially attentive to written language (Stone, Silliman, Ehren & Apel, 2004; Wallach, 2018). The protocol and case studies developed for this book are also a result of key global perspectives taken by the World Health Organization (World Health Organization, ICF-CY, 2007), the UN General Assembly Convention on Rights of

Persons with Disabilities, Article 30 (2007), and Universal Design for Learning (Rose & Meyer, 2002; CAST, 2018). The protocol, *Hear Me into Voice*, honors the contributions that children with complex communication and physical profiles make as individuals. The goal is to advance the most effective service delivery by addressing the child's strengths and needs in communication as the team seeks, provides, and uses assistive technology for communication (McLeod, 2018). Dr. Rogers's work along with works by researchers Fried-Oken and Granlund (2012), and Granlund, Björck-Åkesson, Wilder and Ylven (2008), supports the belief that families' lifestyles and priorities need to match AAC service delivery strategies and outcomes that are sensitive to children and their cultural communities.

The intervention plan

O Developing participation: describing five stages

The intervention stages include *Getting Started* with communication for nonverbal or limited verbal children just beginning with communication and participation, *Building Fundamentals* for the emerging communicator, *Making Connections* with friendships and other relationships through extended listening, speaking, reading, and writing, *Bridging Skills* to increase communication independence, and *Maximizing Participation* to expand children's communication opportunities and contributions across environments. Everyone needs resources and support to participate as full members of the family and society. The stages are designed to facilitate growth experienced by children using AAC. They are reminders that our goal of using AAC is for the children to participate with purposeful communication across environments and communication partners with necessary supports. The plan to develop purposeful communication is based in two key concepts developed by Janice Light that include the purposes of communication and the AAC competencies (Light, 1988, 1989; Light & McNaughton, 2014). Investigate the intervention stages and begin working within or across stages as appropriate for your child's communication and participation. Each child is unique. Communication and participation, regardless of the stage, is success.

The six sections of developing participation

Within each of the five stages of AAC development there are six sections that guide interventionists and practitioners with intervention. We are continually reminded that to be human is to be unique (Prizant & Fields-Meyer, 2015). Vygotsky (1986) and Bruner (1990) applied social interaction as an essential component to children's learning. We must each listen for the everyday communication of the whole person and their communication partners and others who are social supporters (Duchan, 2004, p. 181; Holland, 2007; Travis & Worrall, 2004). The information from the protocol and examples from each case study establish a context for the sections for developing participation.

○ Section 1: Social interaction

Social interaction, the first section, emphasizes what matters most in using AAC: participation of the children, their families, and all communication partners. In each chapter perspectives on how to foster social interaction are offered. Social interaction is kick started in *Getting Started*, with a focus on the critical skill of developing joint attention. In *Building Fundamentals*, the social interaction focus is on supporting participation across environments, celebrating successes, and fostering multiple purposes of why and what children that use AAC communicate. As you progress through *Making Connections*, the social interaction emphasis is placed on expressing feelings and emotions, using language to contribute to others' lives across cultures, understanding implications, following directions, and developing friendships. The growth in social interaction is exponential. In *Bridging Skills*, we look into understanding the multifaceted aspects of inclusion, psycholinguistics, behavior, language learning, and feature matching of AAC tools. An important addition to this chapter is tools for facilitators to aid children that use AAC as they bridge skills. Children *Maximizing Participation* with AAC are using all forms of communication to meet their social and academic needs across the family, cultures, school, and community environments.

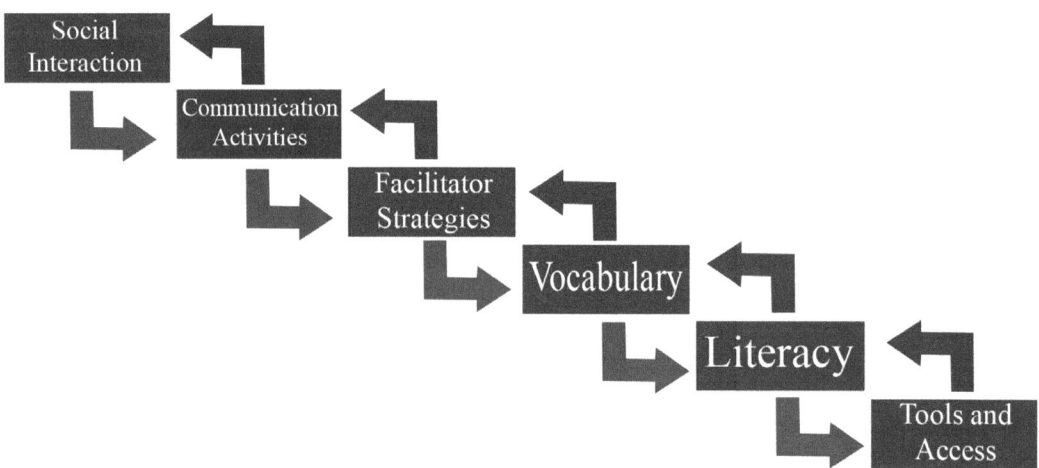

Figure 1.2   AAC Intervention Plan Intersections

○ Section 2: Communication skills and activities

Investigate the numerous activities across the five chapters offered in *Communication Skills and Activities*. The activities explore skill development for each person through conceptual ideas and language that support participation. Explore communication on a walk about the environment. Learn to increase independence in sequencing daily routines in the home and school. Act out and tell stories. Engage in pretend play. Get creative with art activities. Play with toys. Participation with others involves active involvement such as negotiating likes and dislikes, listening to peers with interest, cheering on sports teams, ordering food, and completing puzzles. Children can report on one, or many, activities of their day, identify a new challenge, consider change in the future, and talk and comment on a friendship or actions of others. These skills foster the expectation that children as AAC users participate in discussions, become community helpers, and show leadership as AAC users.

○ Section 3: Facilitator strategies

AAC facilitators can explore a number of ideas in their own *Coaches Corner Grab and Go* section to support children that use AAC. Facilitators are keen observers, intuitive partners, and connect children that use AAC to communication partners. A facilitator will notice how a child's eyes search a room, what the child means when she raises her eyebrows, rolls her eyes, and/or raises a finger. Communication partners will bring their own interpretation and ways to interact with the child that uses AAC and the facilitator can bring rich meaning to the interaction. Look to the *Coaches Corner* for recommendations for fostering fun in play, literacy and language, tips for building communication boards or page sets for speech generating devices, and advanced topics like safety, emergency preparedness, and social negotiation to name a few.

○ Section 4: Literacy

Literacy, the ability to read and write, is a critical skill most people depend on to connect globally. Literacy skills or the lack thereof play into the child's competency perceived by others. We respect the knowledge children gain as they broaden their perspective through knowing other people, situations, information, and opinions. They express their own understanding and identity through reading and writing. Literacy learning is driven by the individual's interest and communication needs (Light, McNaughton & Caron, 2019). In most cultures, we typically think of children speaking before reading and writing, but children with complex communication profiles may learn to read and write before speaking (Light & McNaughton, 2009; Snow, Burns, & Griffith, 1998; Yoder, 2001). Learning to read and write allows the AAC user to increase participation and access to the world. Explore the guidance offered in each stage of the chapters. Infusing literacy into participation opportunities puts spoken words into written words thus moving the heard language from an auditory world into the visual world (Westby, 2019). For the visually impaired child, the channel for literacy becomes tactile and kinesthetic. Parents, interventionists, and children using AAC will use their strengths and work with needs to learn skills to become reader, writers, and knowers (Thomas & Oldfather, 1997). Charts and strategies from *Getting Started* to *Maximizing Participation* are offered to build literacy skills of children that use AAC.

O Section 5: Vocabulary

One word, one concept, expressed via any modality is success. Children that use AAC need to experience vocabulary that allows them to thrive as they use images with words to name objects and concepts, combine nouns with actions, and identify locations and times that may be difficult to identify nonverbally. Manipulating vocabulary to build phrases that become sentences influences participation through rich language including feelings and emotions across communicative purposes. Children that use AAC see new ideas and form concepts through vocabulary and language. Developing participation requires words that spark conceptual language. Children that use AAC have their own identities and are learning to use communication tools and strategies to express their own understanding and ideas through vocabulary. Use the vocabulary recommendations listed in each chapter as a springboard of ideas to new vocabulary that is specific to your child. The lists of words and recommended combinations for quick phrases are based on or inspired from published lists by lead researchers in speech-language pathology. Use the words, adapt the lists, and sculpt the complexity of vocabulary based on each child's linguistic needs, cultural identity, curriculum topics, and personal preferences.

O Section 6: Tools and access

Each chapter offers tools and access methods for children that use AAC from low technology to high technology however it is critical to know that the tools and access methods are not stage specific. A child *Getting Started* with communication may benefit from a high technology device and low technology tools. A child *Maximizing Participation* may benefit from a low technology communication board as well as speech generating devices. Just like ideas offered in *Vocabulary*, the tools and devices in each stage are a springboard of ideas. You are encouraged to look at all stages of *Tools and Access* and work with your child's team, vendor representatives, and AAC experts to make informed decisions on AAC tools and access methods for your child to generate an effective plan for today and for your child's future at home, school, and in the community.

An AAC architectural plan with purpose

The implementation of AAC requires a plan, best visualized as an architectural framework. Seminal work by Light (1988, 1989) details a framework through the four purposes of communication and four AAC competencies. Light's original work, updated in 2014 with David McNaughton, provides interventionists with an architectural plan.

○ The four purposes of communication

Light's work invites us to answer *why* we use communication. What is communication doing for us and our children that use AAC? The four main purposes of communication include expressing wants and needs, information transfer, social closeness, and social etiquette. Review the following definitions and ask these or related questions. *Is my child exposed to the four purposes of communication in enough quality and quantity so that the skills are learned and the social-emotional and linguistic impact is known? Which of the four purposes does my child already communicate? What vocabulary or nonverbal means of expression does my child use to transfer information and express wants and needs? How does my child initiate and develop social relationships? If a purpose is not represented, what is the best way to implement the communication purpose into my child's repertoire?*

1 Expression of wants and needs: The people, places, or things people want or need that help regulate internal and external states.
2 Information transfer (called sharing information in this book): The use of language to share information by commenting on a topic (e.g. the shape of a cloud, a funny joke, a sad story, current events, school subjects).
3 Social closeness: The expression of feelings and emotions both positive and negative to establish, maintain, and develop personal relationships such as, *I need a hug*, or, *Go away.*
4 Social etiquette: The understanding and use of social norms for greetings, discourse skills, appropriate topics, and closures or ending social interactions with familiar and unfamiliar partners (Light, 1988).

Light's work also asks us to answer the *What* question by examining the AAC communication competencies that include linguistic, operational, social and strategic. Familiarize yourself with the brief term definitions.

○ AAC communication competencies

1 **Linguistic**: The use of any language for comprehension and production.
2 **Operational**: The use of the body to express a message such as the fingers for sign language or the ability to control, work, activate or run features of technology.

3 **Social**: Language and pragmatic skills including discourse, knowledge of self-identity and with a range of participation opportunities and levels of interaction.

4 **Strategic**: Ways people use AAC to support themselves or support communication partners. For example, a child may hold up for fingers when saying *po* to indicate the number 4. A child may employ pointing or activating pictures, symbols, or words. A person might use a quick message that states, *Give me a minute to answer your question*, to regulate the behavior of others, or state, *That's not what I meant to say*, to repair a message. *Help me turn on my device*, may be on a tip card that informs another communication partner to set up the user's AAC technology.

Now, ask yourself how your child's communication is represented? Linguistic: *What languages need to be represented in my child's AAC multimodal plan? What vocabulary does my child already understand and express? What words are put together in sentences, used to develop narratives of characters, actions, settings, and problems to solve?* Operational: *What operational skills both through my child's body and technical skills can my child and communication partners perform on my child's behalf?* Social: *How can AAC give my child a chance to participate with culturally appropriate social strategies? What social skills does my child have and would be a good idea to work on next? What significant life experiences should be included so my child can share ideas with others?* Strategic: *What strategies would help my child and communication partners navigate social communication interactions more effectively?* Enlist the help of others including family, friends, and interventionists to help answer these and other questions.

The extraordinary contributions of Light's work are more than great theory, they are an effective, doable, architectural communication plan, that all people, whether experts in AAC or just getting started with AAC, can conceptually digest and implement for a child that uses AAC. You do not have to design or implement a multimodal plan alone. In fact, the more you work with the team of communication partners in the child's life and those partners feel like contributing members to the plan, the more effective communication will be for each person.

Terms of AAC trade

When you think of assistive technology, think access. Assistive technology (AT) is potential access for a person with *any* disability for social, academic, or work purposes. AT is an umbrella term for a tool that supports a person with a disability to improve, accommodate, and support major life functions like speaking, learning, working and many more. If a person has limited vision, the technology to enlarge the print or read the text is assistive technology. If a person cannot use their hands, they can control the screen with their eyes to create messages, generate email, and talk to their friends. Both children and adults, with and without disabilities, benefit from the extraordinary advances in technology. The following definitions offer you a *short-cut summary* of the terminology often associated with AAC.

Low tech AAC: Low technology, referred to as low tech or light tech tools, are associated with non-computer or non-tablet based AAC tools and devices. They include paper and photo or icon-based tools for **communication boards, communication wallets, binding or clasping rings, photos or image books, binders, albums**, and others. Icons may also include textures or dots and dashes for Morse Code. Low tech tools are often made of cardstock paper and best laminated for protection, with one or many symbols consisting of photos or images with words, no words, or may only be words that represent one idea or entire concepts. It requires no conventional technology to operate and allows for quick communication but inherently does not have voice output with the exception of a talking photo album. Copies of board images may be laminated and have Velcro® attached for communication exchanges with others. Communication boards may be made from downloaded copies of pages from high tech speech generating devices for special circumstances such as emergencies, special outings, planned repairs, or other needs. Users express themselves by pointing with fingers, eye gaze, head pointer, light pointers, and others. Some battery-operated speech generating devices offering easily

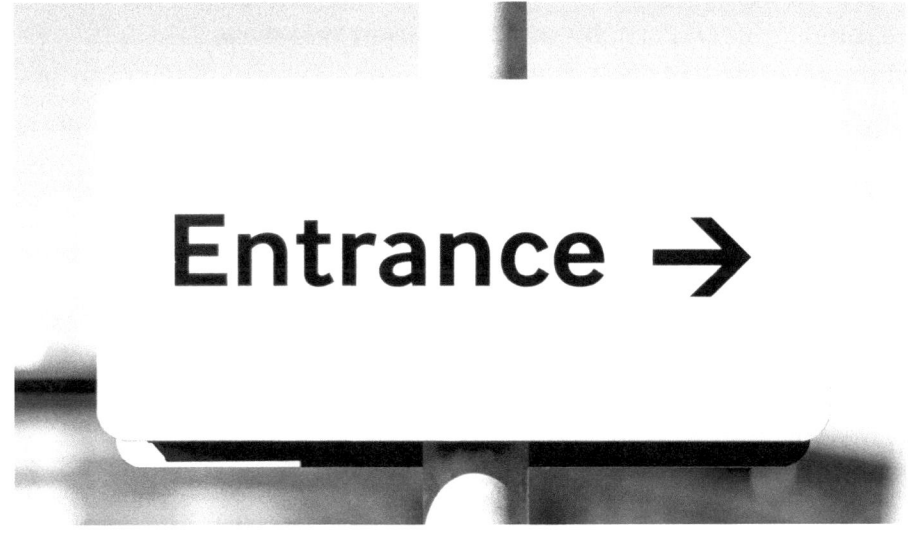

programmable speech output to record your own voice. Some people call static display battery-operated speech generating devices mid-tech.

High tech AAC: High technology tools include tablet or computer-based devices that may be a dedicated device, for communication purposes only, or non-dedicated (with additional options such as internet, educational tools, media, and etc.), and have a dynamic display that changes by accessing vocabulary within categories (e.g. pronouns, actions, locations, times, descriptive words, conjunctions) in which a user may access on multiple levels of pages, usually called folders.

Speech Generating Devices (SGD): Most SGDs allow both the AAC user and communication partner(s) to produce spoken messages. SGDs range from simple to more complex depending upon access and display options that can be low tech or high tech, static or dynamic, with digitized or synthesized speech. Fortunately, these come in many sizes, colors, and with variety of feature options.

A **static** display SGD has one, a few, or a page of multiple icons called an overlay with a message recorded by a person that is activated or played by pressing the button or plate of the device. There may be a number of levels that can be pre-programmed and typically the facilitator manually inserts or places the correct overlay on top of the programmed buttons and selects the level so the AAC user can access the messages.

A **dynamic** display, like a computer, has multiple levels of vocabulary accessed by activation of an icon that opens another level of vocabulary to produce a desired single message, a quick phrase, or a combination of icons to produce original or complex messages.

A **dedicated** SGD is a high-tech device with AAC software on a tablet or computer for the sole purpose of communication. All computer features (e.g. internet) are 'locked out' and require a 'key' or a code to unlock the features usually for a relatively small fee.

A **non-dedicated** SGD is a high-tech device with AAC communication software and often full capacities of a tablet or computer (e.g. internet, social media, email, etc.). Speech is recorded on a SGD in two ways.

Speech may be **digitized** which means a human voice is recorded or **synthesized** which means a computer-generated voice. A human voice (a digitized voice) can be synthesized to produce a closer likeness to a person's voice.

Access methods: The way a person activates a speech generating device or expresses a message on a communication board or other tool, either with direct selection with any part of the body such as pointing or using the eyes to select symbols or using an external tool (e.g. head or light pointer) or switch (e.g. Bluetooth, pillow, ribbon, or string switch) to activate or express a message.

Scanning: In the world of AAC, scanning does not mean to make a paper document electronic. Scanning in AAC means how a person uses their eyes to see things and how a high tech device shows a user which icon is active in the moment to be selected. Numerous scanning options are available for high tech AAC software programs that allow the user to use indirect scanning of 2–64 icons. Linear scanning is item by item scanning that may include the message the child hears and may highlight what the child sees for visual scanning (the outer border of the image may light up or zoom out). Other common forms of scanning include row and column scanning and group scanning. There are many more options that can be discussed given specific AAC devices including scanning controls such as inverse (holding down a switch and releasing on the desired icon), automatic (the device scans until the user activates a switch), and step scanning (the AAC user activates one switch across each icon until the desired icon is located and a different switch or side of a switch is activated to generate the desired word or message).

Symbols: A symbol can be a real object that represents an object, a partial object that represents an object, a miniature object, a photograph, a line drawing, a logo, and orthography such as letters used in writing. Check out the many options for symbols offered by Spectronics (2019) called Symbol Set Comparison at www.spectronics.com.au/article/symbol-set-comparison.

Vocabulary organization: All communication boards, tools, and devices have vocabulary that should be organized, most often in categories such as people, activities, places, questions, quick phrases, and grammatically such as pronouns, verbs, adjectives, and more. Some speech generating devices with dynamic display have vocabulary organized linguistically that includes categorical information. For example, an icon with an action word such as *Go* would have a file linked to the icon that allows a user to access places a person can go and the verb conjugations for the word *go*.

A note on visual memory and auditory memory: It is vital remember that we want to organize vocabulary well in order to limit how often vocabulary is moved, changed, or deleted. Just like your phone or tablet, when icons move, change, or heaven-forbid start shaking ready to be deleted, we panic. Our children that use AAC use visual and auditory memory to recall where buttons are located and predict when they will hear a message. Limit how often they need to reorganize their visual and auditory memory to access communication, their ideas represented in iconic language, their voice.

Forms of communication

Just as important as it is to know the technology of AAC vocabulary, the forms of communication vocabulary matter. It is within each form of communication where opportunity lies to identify existing communication, trial new forms, and consider different types in the future. For now, familiarize yourself with the forms of communication vocabulary.

Nonverbal communication: We use our body and face such as eyes, eyebrows, head, cheeks, and mouth for communication. Sometimes our nonverbal communication has intent, meaning a specific message. Other times, people infer internal states, feelings, and emotions through observation. Examples of nonverbal communication are offered in the following table.

Body Posture and Positioning	Eyes and Eyebrow Movement	Head and Face
• Shoulder shrug	• Eye roll	• Nod to say yes
• Finger pointing	• Eye blinks	• Shake the head or turn to say no
• Reach and grasp	• Eye gaze to make choices	• Tilt the head to ask questions
• Shake hands to be friends	• Look intently to express intent	• Tense cheek to access a switch or communicate intent
• Sign language	• Eyebrow(s) and forehead lift to confirm a choice	• Mouth movements: Smile to agree, pucker to reject
• Move closer to a person		

Verbalizations: Verbal. Verbalizing. Spoken communication. Oral communication. Verbalizing with a speech generating device. These terms are all represent ways words are produced with intent and follow the rules of a given language that carry meaning.

Word approximations: Words spoken with reduced intelligibility or completeness as expected from the rules of a given language yet remain understood to informed communication partners. Examples of word approximations are represented in the typical developmental articulation error of a young child saying *hello* as *hewwo* or an idiosyncratic production, words unique to the child, that carry known meaning as in *hung* for *hungry*. Some word approximations carry more than one meaning or imply a phrase, *I am all done*.

Vocalizations: Sounds from phonation, that express a state of being such as a vocal yawn, excitement or frustration, and sounds of laughter or pain are types of vocalizations. Sometimes vocalizations are sounds of purposeful intent that known communication partners can detail for others.

Interjections: *Yippee! Wooaahh!* Vocal acts, called interjections can be sounds or words that express meaning, often conveying feeling and emotion. Add to mix some intonation and the interjection *uh-huh* positively conveys the meaning of *Yes!* or negatively conveys, *Not a chance*.

Paralinguistics: Vocal changes that carry meaning include the rate of speech, intonation, loudness, pitch, stress, rhythm, and pausing.

Silence: The act of silence can be a purposeful form of communication. Known communication partners learn to read the person's silence through a lack of physical movement or the lack of any form of vocal or verbal communication (e.g. oral or speech generating devices). Silence may also represent time for processing information or formulating an idea to express.

The use of AAC supports verbal speech production

AAC is a collection of communication modalities that range from nonverbal, to vocal, to verbal using speech generating devices and for some oral speech. Many people ask, *Will using AAC keep my child from using oral speech?* Research indicates no, using AAC will not inhibit your child's production of verbal speech. Millar, Light and Schlosser (2006) completed a research review of the impact of AAC on speech production and found that of 89 percent or 24/27 cases with varying degrees of intellectual disability or autism across six studies demonstrated gains in speech, 11 percent demonstrated no gains, and none of the cases decreased their use of verbal productions with the integration of AAC tools and devices. A systematic study review by Schlosser and Wendt (2008) found AAC does not appear to impede speech production in children with autism however, speech gains were modest and families should be realistic about speech gain expectations. Romski, Sevcik, Adamson, Cheslock, Smith, Barker, and Bakeman (2010), compared toddlers using augmented and nonaugmented language intervention and concluded that using AAC with children and their parents is beneficial. Cress and Marvin (2003) state that using augmentative communication is not an indication of giving up on vocal communication, and neither parents nor interventionists should perceive it this way. Because AAC includes all forms of communication modalities, intervention should address improving viable functional vocal and verbal skills when it is the fastest and most effective form of communication, called *just in time supports, programming, or learning* and other variations by many AAC professionals.

Symbolizing relations in AAC

William James wrote a letter to Helen Keller (Lash, 1974) to describe her communication through listening, reading, writing, and speaking using her tactile sense.

> *It makes no difference in what shape the content regardless of how our verbal materials may come. In some it is more optical, in others more motor in nature. In you it is motor and tactile, but its functions are the same as ours, the relationship meant by the word symbolizing the relations existing between the things.*

> (p. 346)

So too with augmentative and assistive communication, relations exist. It is important to delineate each vocalization, word approximation, and verbalization in order to guide the selection of AAC tools and devices, vocabulary and icons, access methods and implementation. Yoder (2001, p. 5) stated that people are, 'not too anything, not too mentally retarded, not too physically impaired, not too emotionally challenged, to learn to acquire communicative competence or to learn to read and write.' Listening, speaking, reading and writing are forms of communication that we can augment and support with assistive technology for academic and social participation. Communication partners and children that use AAC participate through the purposes of expressing wants and needs, transferring information, social closeness, social etiquette (Light, 1989) and the AAC competences (i.e. linguistic, operational, social, and strategic). Together, communication partners see children competently sharing their unique identity and opportunities for participation expand.

Time to begin with *Hear Me into Voice*

It is time to complete *Hear Me into Voice*. Review the protocol items. Take time to reflect on the many ways the child communicates. Work with interventionists as a team or allow each team member to complete their own profile of the child. Generate the opportunity to meet with team members to discuss the findings. Integrate *Hear Me into Voice* as a part of a complete AAC assessment. Speech-language pathologists may use the *AAC Report Template* and *Teaching Report* to support the development of a comprehensive communication and participation plan. Use the ideas offered in the intervention plan to support your child, client, or student that uses AAC today and set a course for effective communication and participation.

Hear Me into Voice: An AAC Protocol for Children with Complex Communication Profiles

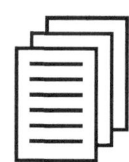

Child's Name:

Age:

Date of Birth:

Team Member Name:

Relationship to the Child:

Dates of Completion:

Language(s) Spoken Across Environments

Home: School: Community:

Directions: Complete the statements and topics to describe your child's communication. Most of the protocol items are written from your child's perspective. Let your child's voice speak through this protocol. Add as much detail as you like and clarify any items you wish. Indicate not applicable or N/A for items that do not apply to your child. Speech-language pathologists, educators, interventionists, family members, and others are each encouraged to complete a protocol to represent your child's breadth of communication across people, situations, and environments.

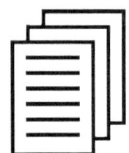

Section I: My social interaction

○ I am playful

1 I laugh when I . . . (Examples: have fun watching cartoons, hear a joke, hear other people laugh, feel someone tickling me).

2 I act silly when I . . . (Examples: know what to do, am excited, know what to do but do not want to do it, make faces).

3 I make you laugh when I . . . (Examples: tease, draw a picture, do things that surprise you).

4 I tease other people when I . . . (Examples: hide the eraser; go to Dad instead of Mom when she calls).

○ However, when I am done…

5 When I get bored I . . . (Examples: go to sleep, pretend to go to sleep, start to fuss).

6 I want you to leave me alone when I . . . (Examples: put my head down, get quiet, look away).

○ I take responsibility

7 I ask someone to pay attention when I . . . (Examples: call out, cry).

8 I ask for help when I . . . (Examples: put your hand on the candy to unwrap it, look at you until you notice, make a sign with my hand or body).

9 I want to help you when I . . . (Examples: tug on your arm, go stand beside you, look at what I want when you are not sure, smile).

10 I give and take or trade and barter with others when I . . . (Examples: offer to trade my toy with another person, give someone my turn).

11 I take responsibility when I . . . (Examples: help my mom stay awake when she is tired, get milk out when I am thirsty, feed my pet turtle, know I have to make a choice).

12 I will complete a job when . . . (Examples: I am interested, it is not too hard for me to do, I am given time to complete the task).

○ My social graces

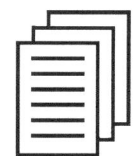

13 I say *hi* or *goodbye* when I . . . (Examples: smile and look at the person, reach out and touch a person, wave my hand).

14 I thank someone by . . . (Examples: smiling when someone praises me, saying a word approximation of *thank you* as *a-ou*).

15 I want to hear more when I . . . (Examples: keep looking at the pages or objects, smile and point, squeeze my hand).

16 I continue a conversation when I . . . (Examples: laugh, sit by you, say *again*).

17 I terminate a conversation by . . . (Examples: looking away, walking away, closing the book).

18 I say, *please* by . . . (Examples: using a 'nice' voice; smiling, using eye gaze, using sign language).

19 I say, *Let's share this by* . . . (Examples: offering you part of my snack, bringing a book to read, looking for your response with my eye gaze).

20 I show you I understand how others feel by … (Examples: sitting beside them, getting excited with others, anticipating their needs).

21 I say, *Come with me*, by … (Examples: using my hands to pull you towards me, fussing).

22 I say, *yes*, many different ways including . . . (Examples: vocal sounds, saying *uh huh*, *yes*, head nod, smile, sign language, communication board, speech generating device).

23 I take turns by . . . (Examples: looking at you, touching your game piece, pointing, using my speech generating device to say, *My turn, Your turn*).

○ My forms of negation – when things aren't quite right

24 I say *no* many different ways including . . . (Examples: shaking my head, looking away or down, low physical engagement with my body).

25 I do not like to … (Examples: touch _____ texture(s), see _____ object(s), hear _____ sounds, taste _____, or smell _____; be in large crowds; transition _____).

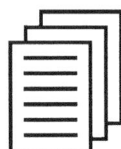

26 When I am upset, I tell you by . . . (Examples: emotionally _____ ; writing or typing an important word(s) stating my concern; taking you to or showing you the problem).

27 I protest when I . . . (Examples: vocalize angrily, close my eyes).

28 I argue when I . . . (Examples: look distressed, shake my head no, shut my body down).

○ My emotions

29 This is how I show how I feel across emotions

Joy:	Disgust:	Love:
Disappointment:	Anxiety:	Excitement:
Worry:	Surprise:	Pride:
Anger:	Fear:	Frustration:

Other emotions and ways I show how I feel . . .

Section II: My communication activities

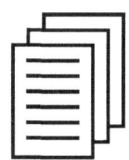

30 I am usually interested in playing with objects. I play with them a certain way. There are people I play with using the objects . . . (Examples: board games, playground games, card games, telling jokes, watching movies, group play, listening to music, playing an instrument).

Things I Play With	How I Play with Objects	Who I Play With

31 I like to be or play with other people when I . . . (Examples: look at them, smile, stand next to them, sit closely next to them).

32 I show I know the rules of a game (e.g. board or computer games) when I . . . (Examples: see the rules in pictures; learn from others' following the rules; people review the rules with me).

33 Things I like to do by myself are . . . (Examples: down time in my room, draw, play with toys, draw, play on a tablet or other form of technology).

34 I want you to stay or keep playing with me when I . . . (Examples: sign *more*, reach for your hand, smile).

35 Routines I understand are . . . (Examples: brushing teeth, riding in the car, bed time routine).

36 Routines my communication partners would like me to learn are . . .

37 I like to be or play in these places . . .

	Inside		Outside
Rooms in my home:	Therapy room:	Park:	Back or Front yard:
My School:	Community (e.g. restaurant, theater):	Playground:	Beach, Mountains, Lake, Pool:

Other places or related stories: _____

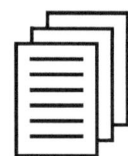

○ People I like to be with

38 People I like to be with . . . (Examples: Mom, Dad, baby sitter, friend)

  ◉ My list of people I like to be with:
  ◉ I show I like each person by . . . (Examples: smiling when she gives me as kiss, giving a hug, sitting next to the person, smiling, staying awake even when I am tired, going to him when I am upset).
  ◉ I make a difference to the people I am with when I . . . (Examples: move next to them when they are sad, listen when they talk to me)

○ I show I am thinking

39 What people that care for me say I do or contribute to them and to others?

Person: _____ says I _____

Person: _____ says I _____

Person: _____ says I _____

(Examples: give her courage, teach him to ask the right questions)

40 When something is new I … (Examples: listen, watch, push it away, feel it with my hands).

41 When someone is new I . . . (Examples: go to my room, sit by my mother, smile and watch the person).

42 When adults speak to me, I express myself by . . . (Examples: keeping quiet before I reply, responding right away).

43 When children speak to me, I express myself by . . . (Examples: smiling, laughing, vocalizing, looking at them).

44 I get my way when I . . . (Examples: look coy, state my intention, use my body or sounds).

45 Ways to get me back on track are . . . (Examples: offering sensory breaks, time breaks, touch cues, a verbal cue of _____).

46 I am just not having a good day when I . . . (Examples: am dysregulated, do not sleep well).

47 These are consequences or expectations I understand . . .
(Examples: I can watch a video after I take my medicine; I get my chocolate cake after I eat my fruit; You will finishing brushing my hair by the time you count to 10).

○ My family follows these communication rules

48 To show respect and interest I . . . (Examples: look directly at adults when they speak, repeat part or all of what the adult says using my speech generating device or my voice).

49 When someone speaks, I . . . (Examples: keep quiet, respond right away, wait for someone to ask for my opinion).

50 At home, we like to talk about . . . (Examples: my visiting grandparents, sports on tv, events that will happen during the week and weekend, something that happened at work, home or school).

51 At home I am expected to communicate about . . . (Examples: my choices, what I need, what I like to do, what happened in school each day, who I played with).

52 I say, *I don't know* when I . . . (Examples: raise my eyebrow; stop and walk away).

53 I ask you to, *Tell me another way* when I . . . (Examples: look confused; raise my eyebrow).

54 When I find I made a mistake or have a problem I … (Examples: say *oops*, *uh-oh*, ask you to give me minute to correct my message on my speech generating device).

55 I show you I remember by . . . (Examples: smiling; opening my eyes wide).

56 I say, *Yes, this is right*, or *Yes, sure*, when I . . . (Examples: smile, my body is excited, I intentionally stare).

57 I show I know what is expected when I . . . (Examples: alter my body position, smile, turn to the intended person, focus on the intended object).

58 I show I know names of people when I . . . (Examples: write people's names, look at the person whose name I just heard).

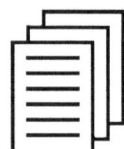

○ How I take care of myself

59 I show what is hurting me when I . . . (Examples: show you my arm or leg, rub my stomach, point to where it hurts, use my communication board or device to tell you what hurts).

60 I make choices when I . . . (Examples: look at an option a long time; open a cupboard and take out a jar, smile, my body language tells you, get excited, point to an option on my communication board or speech-generating device).

61 I say I am sleepy when I . . . (Examples: yawn, fuss, get droopy eyes, have a droopy body).

62 I dress myself when I . . . (Examples: put on my own shoes, push my arms into the sleeves).

63 I tell you I need to go to the bathroom when I . . . (Examples: tug on my pants, wiggle back and forth, have 'that look in my eye').

○ I know how my timing works best

64 I will do what you ask if you . . . (Examples: wait while I think about it, touch my arm, tell me again).

65 When I keep doing the same thing over and over, I stop when someone . . . (Examples: says *stop*, points to a different picture or word for me to attend to, touches my arm).

66 I say I am finished by . . . (Examples: signing *all done*, closing my eyes).

67 I indicate it is time to go on to the next activity when I . . . (Examples: stop scanning the current objects, items, or pages of the task; get a relaxed body).

68 I wait by . . . (Examples: sitting quietly, fussing, organizing things around me).

69 I do my work when I . . . (Examples: I have an example or model of what the finished product should look like; I am fully awake; There are few distractions).

Section III: How I express my vocabulary

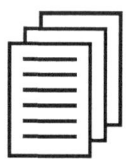

70 Sign language words I understand and use . . .

Receptive Understanding	Expressive Use

71 When I use facial expressions, I mean . . . (e.g. The facial expression *scrunchy face* means *go away*).

My facial expression _____ means _____ .

My facial expression _____ means _____ .

My facial expression _____ means _____ .

72 Words or word combinations I say using a speech generating device are . . . (Examples: more, go, stop).

73 Words I verbalize and their meaning are . . . (Example: saying *juice* when I really mean any drink).

74 My word approximations and what they mean are . . . (Example: *po* means four).

75 How well others understand me. Write in what percent of the time people understand the child:

Those closest to me understand me _____ percent of the time.

Familiar communication partners understand me _____ percent of the time.

Unfamiliar communication partners understand me _____ percent of the time.

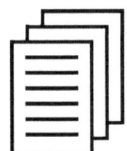

Section IV: My literacy

○ My reading

93 My favorite books to read with others are . . . (Examples: print books and magazines, e-books, audiobooks, application programs, picture books, chapter books).

94 I show you topics I am interested in reading when I . . . (Examples: bring you books, magazines, or pictures; show you images or articles on the internet).

95 I make up real or imaginary stories when I . . . (Examples: draw a picture; type a princess story; play family with my dinosaurs).

96 I engage look at books with someone (e.g. joint attention) when I . . . (Example: look at the pages, words, and pictures you are looking at, turn pages with you, sound out letters, point to words and objects, listen to you read).

97 I enjoy these books without any help from others . . . (e.g. turn pages, look at the illustrations, read).

98 I can read . . . (Examples: letters, words, phrases, simple sentences, stories).

99 My favorite forms of media entertainment and program titles are . . . (Examples: television, tablet, phone, computer, console, cartoons, movies).

100 Give me photos and I like to look at . . . (Examples: places I have been, family and friends, my favorite things to do).

101 I recognize community logos and signs for . . . (Examples: cereal, favorite restaurants, stop signs).

102 When I see my name I . . . (Examples: smile, make eye contact with you, can match it, say my letters, write my name, put my things by it).

103 When I have a book I . . . (Examples: ask someone to read, turn pages, look from front to back, read to myself, turn pages but may not attend to what is on the page).

104   When I hear a story or participate in reading I can . . . (Examples: share experiences I have with characters, setting, plot, and more; point, vocalize, arrange pictures to tell what happens first, next, and last; attend for 10 minutes, for a set number of pages, for a few books or chapters of a book).

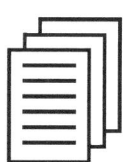

○   **My writing**

105   When I have a pencil and paper I like to . . . (Examples: scribble, trace, copy shapes, write letters).

106   My interest in writing is . . . (Examples: high but I need support; low, moderate, high depending on my self-regulation; dependent on if I am tired, hungry, the time of day).

107   When I have markers or crayons, I like to . . . (Examples: scribble, draw, color pictures).

108   When I have a key or alphabet board I . . . (Examples: touch the keys, spell my name, use a switch, spell out words with support).

109   Assistive technology tools that help me type or write are . . . (Examples: wrist guard, pencil grips, key guards).

110   People that help me type or write are . . . (e.g. parent, teacher, aide, peers, interventionists).

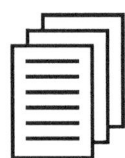

Section V: AAC options that work for me!

Directions: Talk with an AAC specialist about ways my child communicates using the head and body, low and high technology to support communication including how language is symbolized, use of auditory memory, and visual scanning.

○ **How I use my head for unaided and aided communication**

Head	Tried Indicate Yes, No, or Not Viable	Presently Used Provide Aided and Unaided Examples or No	Recommend a Trial Note Environments to be Trialed
Eyes			
Eyebrows			
Forehead			
Cheeks			
Lips/mouth			
Jaw position			
Head position			
Facial expression			
Head movement for *Yes* and *No*			
Oral production • Vocalizations • Word approximations • Verbalizations			

○ **How I use my body for unaided or aided communication**

Body	Tried Indicate Yes, No, Not Viable	Presently Used Provide Aided and Unaided Examples by Environment	Recommend a Trial Note Environments
Gestures • Fingers/thumb • Hands • Feet • Arms • Shoulders			
Sign Language • Form (e.g. finger, cued) • Idiosyncratic			
Body Positioning • Make a choice • State an opinion • State a direction			

○ Assistive technology for communication by tools and devices

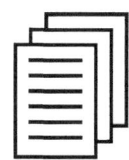

Communication Tools and Devices	Previously Tried by Environment and Noted Outcomes	Presently Used Across Environments with Measured Success	Recommend a Trial across the Following Environments
Paper, dry erase boards, and writing utensils			
Boards, book, wallet, rings			
Static single message speech generating device			
Static multiple message speech generating device			
Static sequenced message speech generating device			
Dynamic speech generating device			
Visual scenes • Static • Dynamic			
Tablet applications • Static • Dynamic			
Text to speech tools			
Other			

○ Assistive technology access methods

Access Method	Previously Tried by Environment and Outcomes	Presently Used Across Environments with Measured Success	Recommend a Trial across the Following Environments
Switches (e.g. plate, button, pillow, grasp, string, puffer, ribbon, pneumatic)			
Key guard			
Stylus			
Writing utensils			
Head pointer or mouse			
Joystick			
Mouse			
Trackball			
Eye gaze technology			
Scanning • Visual • Auditory • Types: zoom, row/column, linear, group, step inverse, auto			
Mounts on chair/table			
Other			

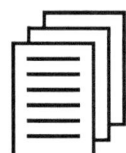

○ Symbolic communication representation

Symbolic Method	Presently Used Yes or No	Language Comprehension & Ways the Method is Used	Expressive Language & Ways the Method is Used
Tactile-texture			
Object-based			
Photographs			
Line drawings			
Symbol set			
Writing			

○ My visual scanning and auditory memory

I make choices from a visual field of . . . (Example: 2–64 or more icons)

I make choices from an auditory field of . . . (Example: 2 or more icons, auditory groups of 2–6 or more).

I make choices from a visual and auditory field of . . . (Example: 2 or more icons, auditory groups of 2–6 or more).

○ Summary of my assistive technologies for learning

Math

I access math the best when I use . . . (Examples: real objects to work on one to one correspondence, check marks or circles to draw out the numbers and then add them up, manipulatives, graph paper, calculator).

Reading

I access reading the best when I use . . . (Examples: e-books, tablets, access methods, Tar Heel Reader, Bookshare, Learning Ally).

Writing

I access writing the best when I use . . . (Examples: highlighters, dry erase boards, raised line paper, typing, have an alphabet display).

Organization

I am organized when I use . . . (Examples: folders, a countdown timer, shading on a glass clock).

Environmental control

I access items in my home by using . . . (Examples: power links to turn on and off lights and run electronics such as blenders and toys; battery interrupters to operate toys, infrared switches to run toys and devices).

Section VI: Summary of my communication

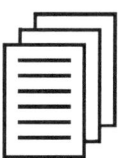

1 Who I communicate with across environments:

_____

Home   *School*   *Community*

_____

2 My most consistent modes of expression are . . . (Examples: eyes, pointing, hand squeezes, vocalizations).

_____

What I Communicate   *When I ___ This Means*   *Where I Like to Communicate*

_____

3 I am most successful with my communication when . . . (Examples: someone works with me, I have a full stomach, it's morning time, when it is quiet).

4 I am most interested in . . . (Examples: music, books, toys).

5 I would like to add to my communication by . . . (Examples: signing, picture boards, alphabet boards, electronic device).

6 My biggest communication need is to . . . (Examples: participate in discussions, choose activities, get others to understand why I am whining, address needs in a particular environment, train communication partners, add vocabulary, increase number of opportunities to speak).

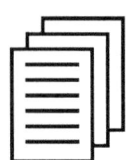

Section VII: About me . . . from people who know me best

Please let us know more about your child:

1 What are your favorite stories about your child?

2 What are your child's preferred and non-preferred foods, toys, objects, and activities?

3 What are your hopes for your child short term and long term?

4 What communication rules or expectations in your home matter the most?

5 What skills would you like your child to learn now?

6 What communication do you want help with?

7 What else would you like people to know about your child?

Thank you for making a difference.

AAC report shell template

Wonderful AAC Speech and Language Clinic
Great Department Address & Contact Information
Confidential Communication Assessment Summary Report

Child/Student: Parent(s)/Guardian:
Date of Birth: Street Address:
Age: City/State/Zip:
Date of Assessment: Phone:
Date of IEP/Meeting: Email:
School: Assessor:

   I. Purpose

  II. Background

 III. Assessment Overview

 IV. Behavior and Sensory Functioning

  V. Assessment Findings in the Area of Language

 VI. Academic Communication

VII. Seating and positioning

VIII. Nonverbal Communication: How I Use My Head and Body

 IX. Assistive Technology for Communication by Tools, Devices, and Access
     Methods

  X. Modes of Communication and Topic Choice by Partner Type

 XI. Symbolic Communication Representation

XII. Strategies Used by Communication Partners Supporting Expression

XIII. Strategies Used by Communication Partners Supporting Comprehension

XIV. Summary and Recommendations

Closing statement to the family or referral source.

_____

Name with credentials

Organizational structure name

An AAC teaching report

Wonderful AAC Speech and Language Clinic
Great Department Address and Contact Information
Confidential Communication Evaluation Summary Report

Note: Tommy Isaac, family, identifying information, and all details are fictious. The teaching report samples are adapted and used with permission from Tori Strobel-Sabatino (2019).

Child/Student: Tommy Isaac
Date of Birth: 7/5/13
Age: 5–7   Grade: Kindergarten
Date(s) of Assessment: Feb. 3–4, 2019
Date of IEP/Meeting: March 4, 2019
School: Hughes Academy

Parent(s)/Guardian: Lisa & Carl Isaac
Street Address: 123 House Street
City/State/Zip: Sierra Madre, CA 92128
Phone: (123) 456-7890
Email: TSS@HughesAcademy.org
Assessor: Tori Strobel-Sabatino, MS, CCC-SLP

For a private practice you may also need to include the following:

- ◉ Referral source:
- ◉ Supervisor of the referral source:
- ◉ Diagnostic codes:

I Purpose

The purpose of this report is to detail results of an assessment of the CHILD's present communication strengths and needs. (If the report is written in compliance with educational laws include a statement and adjust the verbiage such as: The assessment was completed in compliance with an initial/triennial individual education plan/as a part of a comprehensive psychoeducational evaluation.). The following statements/questions reflect the TEAM MEMBERS' concerns.

Note on Referral Statements or Questions: Write one or two statements or questions that reflect the team member's (e.g. parent, legal guardian, educators, medical or therapeutic interventionists) specific concerns reported during the intake and gathered from the protocol *Hear Me into Voice*. The goal of the report is to address the team members' statements or questions from a thorough assessment that justify the proposed goals, recommended instructional and assistive technology, and the intervention plan. The following questions are examples only and should be personalized for each case.

1 *Mr. & Mrs. Isaac report that Tommy becomes frustrated when he cannot express his thoughts fast enough using communication boards to communicate with friends and family members. Tommy's parents want to know if they should still be using communication boards or a different communication system that would work for him.*

2 *To what degree is Tommy's communication impacting his ability to participate socially and academically at home, school, and in the community?*

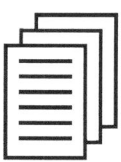

II Background

◎ Statement on child's age by year and month
◎ Denote all people who attended the assessment, the nature of the relationship, and who served as informants
◎ Present diagnosis (if known) communication concerns and strengths as reported by the family or informant
◎ Note who the child lives with
◎ Pertinent family history
◎ Ambulatory status and physical access
◎ Birth history
◎ Medical history
◎ Vision and hearing
◎ Developmental milestones
◎ Educational history
◎ Attention, memory, processing, problem solving
◎ Prior assessments
◎ Current team members
◎ Current services and goals
◎ Parent or informant report that expands on concerns
◎ Additional factors (e.g. second language, cultural background, religion, adoption, other)
◎ Child's interests
◎ Family communication rules
◎ Other information as relevant to the case

III Assessment overview

Sample list of Assessment Tools

Standardized Tests or Subtests

Note if the administration of standardized tests or subtest are not completed according to the manual (e.g. non-standardized administration); underline standardized test titles; include acronyms (as appropriate) at the end of each test name and use the test acronym in the body of the report. See the following use of WATI as an example.

Non-Standardized Tools

◎ *Hear Me into Voice*
◎ Functional Communication Profile (Kleiman, 2003)
◎ Social Networks (Blackstone & Hunt-Berg, 2003)
◎ Wisconsin Assistive Technology Initiative (WATI, 2018)

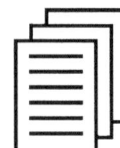

- ◉ Parent and professional interviews
- ◉ Review of records
- ◉ Observation
- ◉ Communication sample
- ◉ Oral mechanism

Provide a brief summary of each test and tool per the manual or author's information.

Sample narrative option for non-standardized administration of assessments

The assessment team agreed that a combination of dynamic assessment and informal measures would detail the communication strengths and needs of (CHILD) in order to develop goals, determine technology needs, and plan intervention. Standardized testing was not completed as the team agreed standardized testing scores would not be representative of the child's ability.

IV Behavior and sensory functioning (report each behavior as observed, reported, or elicited)

Adaptive behavior: Management of hygiene, clothing, materials, safety, responsibility, response to change, chores, self-direction, and sleep habits, and other relevant behaviors.

Example: *Parents report that Tommy currently uses visual schedules at home to aid in self-care tasks (e.g. washing his hands, brushing his teeth, getting dressed) but continues to require adult support to follow the schedule. He follows modeling from his mother or father throughout the day and is resistant to changes in routines whether at home or in the classroom. Parent and teacher both report that Tommy lacks awareness of dangerous situations and requires supervision in all environments. When frustrated, Tommy shuts down and demonstrates maladaptive behaviors such as throwing items or self-injurious behaviors (e.g. biting his hand or arm; hitting his head).*

Vision: State the current vision status and relevant history regarding acuity, field of vision, implications for visual scanning vertically, horizontally, using words, objects, or symbols, and near tasks, intermediate distance tasks up to three feet away, and far away tasks three or more feet away. Note the difference between vision acuity and how vision is used.

Example: *A review of records showed that Tommy's vision was informally assessed by the school nurse on 10/7/2018. His visual acuity and functional vision are within normal limits. Tommy demonstrates the ability to identify symbols on icons sized 1 inch by 1 inch with 100 percent accuracy. He exhibited no difficulties with visual scanning across a field of 16 icons (4x4 grid) and shows potential to advance to a 5x5 grid with smaller icons.*

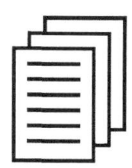

Concerns were noted with Tommy's perception of icons, however processing time may be related to novel vocabulary and not visual scanning or tracking ability.

Hearing: State the current hearing status and relevant history for attending, processing and implications for auditory scanning.

Example: *A review of records shows that Tommy's hearing was formally assessed to be within normal limits by an audiologist on 10/7/2018. He responds to sounds in his environment, but he may not identify them as a danger. He follows one-step directions and interacts with individuals who produce speech at the volume of conversational speech. His teachers report he attends to auditory information for 10 minutes. His speech-language pathologist reports he requires three seconds to process a one-step auditory direction.*

Motor: State the current status of gross and fine motor systems noting access to communication, academic tasks, play, and environmental access.

Example: *Tommy is ambulatory. He demonstrates full range of motion and control of his head and extremities. In regard to his gross motor skills, he has been observed to walk up and down the stairs of the playground equipment and run without falling. He is reported to have challenges with rapid alternative movements such as biking and swimming. In regard to his fine motor skills, he is able to stack blocks and put Lego together, as well as flip through his communication notebook and pull off Velcro® icon cards. He was observed to correctly hold a pencil or crayon during academic tasks and isolate his index finger to point to objects.*

Play behavior: In addition to observations note responses from *Hear Me into Voice.*

Example: *Based on findings from* Hear Me into Voice, *Tommy's interests include playing with toy cars, Lego, blocks, and bouncy balls. He also enjoys playing outside on the playground swing set. Parent and teacher both report that Tommy desires to be social and playful. The evaluating speech-language pathologist observed Tommy in the classroom on 2/3/19. During morning circle, he greeted every student in the class by pointing to them and verbally saying 'hi.' It was observed that Tommy thrives on positive reinforcement from his teacher and peers. His teacher stated that for every period of the day that he exhibits 'superstar' behavior, he earns a toy to keep with him throughout the day to play with during free time and recess. Tommy was observed handing a toy he earned to a peer next to him and flipping through his communication book. He pulled out the 'want' and 'play' icons and placed them on a Velcro® strip on the front cover of the book. The teacher read what Tommy had selected aloud and explained that Tommy was asking if the peer wanted to play with him. The peer agreed and they started to play. Tommy started flipping through his communication book again when the peer got up and walked away to*

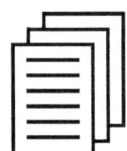

play with something else. Tommy became upset and started throwing toys, communication notebook and other items around him. After approximately ten minutes Tommy was better regulated. His teacher reminded him of his 'superstar' behavior and modeled how to ask another friend to play.

Oral mechanism: Note tone, mobility, and range of motion for the purpose of communication and swallowing.

Example: *The structure and function of the oral mechanism were informally assessed to determine adequacy for speech production. No concerns regarding chewing and swallowing were reported or observed during the assessment. Visual inspection of Tommy's dentition, palate, tongue, buccal cavity and other oral structures appear to be within normal limits. He demonstrated difficulty with oral functions such as imitation of consonant-vowel productions and imitating oral motor movements.*

V Assessment findings in the area of language

Note: Report formal and informal language test results, observations, and samples in this section. Provide examples of the child's receptive and expressive language by domain (i.e. phonology, morphology, syntax, semantics, pragmatics) as applicable. You may also choose to write a summary of findings by each assessment tool noting strengths and needs with examples. For children with a limited phonetic inventory consider providing a list of sound productions rather than a chart of sounds by position in which most of the chart would reflect deficits rather than ability.

VI Academic communication

Note: The results from the *Wisconsin Assistive Technology Initiative* (WATI; www.wati.org/), a free tool, are very helpful to inform this section. Indicate the child's present status and a statement on the use of assistive technology (AT), what AT has been tried with what success level and what AT needs to be considered. You may opt to include recommendations at the end of the report in the recommendations section.

- Math: Indicate the child's level in math, examples of problems, use of manipulatives, child's ability to line up written numbers on a page for effective calculations on a page, legibility, teaching strategies to support math, technology presently used, technology that would benefit the child.
- Reading: Indicate the child's reading level, technology and strategies presently used or should be tried including computer availability.
- Writing: Indicate the child's writing level and use of utensils and keyboard skills. What access can AT provide in the area of writing?
- Organization of self, time, materials, and information: What AT would benefit the child?

◉ Recreation and Leisure: Indicate how the client's current comprehension and production of language influence participation. What tools and devices support communication, participation, and access?

VII Seating and positioning

Note: In addition to your expertise, work with occupational and physical therapists to inform this section. Address the following bullet points on seating and positioning as applicable.

◉ State all seating and positions supports the child uses across environments (e.g. wheelchair, stander, elbow support in a chair, bouncy chair, cubby chair, couch, lying down, other)
◉ Postural considerations that support optimal respiration
◉ Postural considerations that optimize attention
◉ Lengths of time to be spent in different postural positions or require a change in position
◉ Postural considerations to comfortably access communication
◉ Attend to the relationship between the following:
  ◉ Head, neck, and trunk
  ◉ Arms and shoulders
  ◉ Pelvis, knee(s), and ankle(s)

◉ Note other positioning and seating recommendations or restrictions

VIII Nonverbal communication: how I use my head and body

Note: You may elect to write this section in a narrative format rather than completing the charts. Decide which format best represents the details you need to convey for the child. Consider a narrative in cases where many of the boxes in the chart are blank because they are not applicable.

Sample Narrative: *Tommy currently uses facial expressions, head nods, and oral sounds as a means of nonverbal communication. He uses facial expressions to communicate pleasure, discomfort, and other emotions at home and school. He has been observed to smile for social greetings, scrunch his eyebrows to show when he is upset/angry, and raises his eyebrows while smiling when excited. Tommy demonstrates use of head nods to indicate yes or no when asked questions or given choices. Vocalizations (e.g. crying, grunting) and word approximations (e.g. 'ju' for juice, 'ba' for ball, 'I wa' for I want) are used to request or protest.*

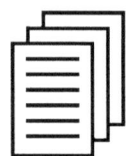

○ How I use my head for nonverbal communication

Head	Tried Indicate Yes, No, Not Viable	Presently Used With Examples by Environment	Recommend Trial, Train Team Members, Environments
Eyes	Yes: Home, school, library program, adaptive baseball	Eye gaze, eye blinks, uses peripheral vision, has left eye dominance at home and school	Need to try eye gaze with unfamiliar people in the community
Eyebrows	No	No	Trial in speech and language therapy
Forehead	No	No	Trial in speech and language therapy
Cheeks	Tried but was not viable	No	No
Lips/mouth	Yes, but the team is not sure if the smile is purposeful for choices	May be an emerging skill	Trial across settings to use a smile as a form of confirmation
Jaw position	Tried degrees of opening and closing – not viable	No	No
Head position	Yes	Turns away, towards, and tilt	Train school-based team members
Facial expression	Yes	Smile for social greeting	Trial using a smile to confirm a choice in speech and language therapy
Head movement for Yes and No	Yes	Indicate yes, no, or to give a direction	Not Required
Oral production • Vocalizations • Word approximations • Verbalizations	Yes	Vocal sigh, cry, vocal exhalation; Approximation: hung for hungry	Trial existing phonetic repertoire with other word approximations

○ How I use my body for nonverbal communication

Body	Tried Indicate Yes, No, Not Viable	Presently Used With Examples by Environment	Recommended Trial, Train Team Members, Environments
Gestures • Fingers/thumb • Hands • Feet • Arms • Shoulder	Yes Hands, fingers, and arm movements are viable; use of feet are not a viable option	Tommy moves his hands when excited; fine motor skills are better with the left hand; gross motor with the right arm	Team is presently trained. Monitor use of feet for future communicative benefit.
Sign language • Form (e.g. finger, cued) • Idiosyncratic	Not Viable	No	No
Body positioning • Makes a choice • States an opinion • States a direction	Yes	Optimal positioning is constantly monitored to maximize communication comprehension and expression.	Team members know to consult with the nurse, OT, and PT regarding current optimal body positioning.

IX Assistive technology for communication tools, devices, and access methods

Note: See *Section VI Technology II. Communication Using Aided Low to High Technology* to inform the content. You may elect to write this section in a narrative format rather than completing the charts. Decide which format best represents the details you need to convey for the child. Consider a narrative in cases where many of the communication tools and devices are not a viable option for the child.

○ Assistive technology for communication by tools and devices

Communication Tools and Devices	*Previously Tried* *Note Environments & Outcome*	*Presently Used* *Note Environments and Level of Success*	*Recommended* *Trial, Train Team Members, Environments*
Paper, dry erase boards, and writing utensils	Yes: dry erase boards	Used at school and home with 60 percent success	Use in school to offer quick choices
Boards, book, wallet, rings	Yes: communication board	Used for wants and needs	Add quick phrase commenting to communication boards; Make and trial a communication wallet
Static single message speech generating device	Yes: available to all students	Used at the art center and snack time at school	No
Static multiple message speech generating device	No	No	Yes: needed for verbalizing choices
Static sequenced message speech generating device	No	No	No: student would benefit from making novel utterances
Dynamic speech generating device	No	No	Yes: student requires voice output for quick messages and to formulate novel utterances across the purposes of communication
Visual scenes	No	Yes: photographs showing verbs in action support concept development	Consider expansion of visual scenes in a dynamic display speech generating device
Tablet applications • Static • Dynamic	Yes: static display communication apps at home and school	Yes: static display communication apps at home and school	Parent will consider trialing in the community over the next year
Text to speech tools	No	No	Introduce over the next school year
Other			

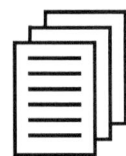

○ Communication access methods

Access Method	Previously Tried	Presently Used	Recommended
	Note Environments and Outcomes	Notes Environments and Level of Success	Trial, Train Team Members, Environments
Switches (e.g. plate, button, pillow, grasp, string, puffer, ribbon pneumatic)	Yes: plate access 70 percent success	Yes: used at school to activate electronic music players for books on CD	Consultation with vendors of switch access technology to determine other viable options
Key guard	No	No	No
Stylus	Yes: not viable, difficult to stabilize	No	No
Writing utensils	Yes	Yes: requires full motor support	No
Head or mouse pointer	No	No	No
Joystick	No	No	No
Mouse	No	No	No
Trackball	No	No	No
Eye gaze technology	No	No	Team requests an extended trial of eye gaze technology
Scanning • Visual • Auditory • Types: zoom, row/column, linear, group, step inverse, auto	No	No	Consider the best scanning options during dynamic display speech generating device trial
Mounts on chair/table	Yes: effective with prior AAC device; mount wore out	No	Team may require training for a floor mount with articulating arms to be used with a dynamic display speech generating device

Note: The following chart has more options with 'No' as the indicator. The information in this chart may be better written in a narrative format. See the following table for an example of the same content in a narrative format.

○ Sample narrative format for communication access methods

Tommy is presently successfully accessing electronic equipment to play music and read books on CD with his hands. A stylus was trialed to access tablet technology but less successful than anticipated. He prefers touch access. The team trialed eye gaze technology as a part of a dynamic display speech generating device trial to improve speed of production. He produced messages 20 percent faster than using touch with his finger.

X Modes of communication and topic choice by partner type

Note: The findings from *Social Networks* (Blackstone & Hunt-Berg, 2003) and *Hear Me into Voice* will inform this section. State the communication partners by type by familiar, less familiar, and unfamiliar communication partners. Indicate the modes of communication used with each person and the degree of effectiveness.

○ Modes of communication and topic choice by partner type

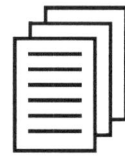

Partner	Type* (F, LF, UCP)	Modes of Communication	Topics and Comments
Parent, relative	Familiar	Eyes, smile, words, gesture	Tommy uses eye gaze to indicate to stay at the concert hall to listen to music.
Friend	Familiar	Laughing, smiling, eye contact	Tommy laughs to indicate comprehension that a horse in the living room is not where he should be.
Teacher	Familiar	Eye contact, pointing, SGD**	Tommy makes word choices to complete a journal entry given a word bank.
Coach	Less familiar	SGD single switch, eye contact, body posture	Tommy uses an AAC switch to say *Go* given the sequence *Ready, Set, Go!*
Clerk	Unknown communication partner	Eyes using a picture board, gestures, pointing	Tommy uses a picture menu to point to choices or uses eye gaze to make a selection

*Type: Familiar = F, Less Familiar = LF, Unfamiliar Communication Partner = UCP

**SGD = speech generating device

XI Symbolic communication representation

Note: State the what symbols the child comprehends and uses for expressive language. Indicate yes or no under the column titled, *Presently Used*. Offer examples under *Language Comprehension* and *Expressive Language*. The priority in selecting symbols is how salient the objects, images, or text is to the child.

○ Ways communication symbols are represented

Symbolic Method	Presently Used Yes or No	Language Comprehension and Expression
Tactile-texture	No	A tactile-texture based symbols are commonly used with children with a visually impairment.
		Example: Tommy does not use tactile-texture based symbols for communication.
Object-based	No	Objects may be used to support comprehension and expression in the initial stages of learning and using language and then photographs or line drawn images are implemented
		Example: Interventionists supported Tommy's development of photographs and line drawn symbols with object association. He no longer requires objects as a primary symbol for communication.
Photographs	Yes	Core and fringe vocabulary words may be represented in photographs.
		Example: Tommy effectively uses photographs to express core vocabulary words displayed around his classroom and located on low tech communication tools.

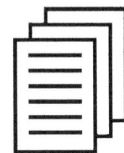

Line drawings	No	Core and fringe vocabulary words may be represented in photographs.
		Example: Tommy is emerging with his ability to recognizing objects in 10 trials with 60 percent accuracy.
Symbol sets	Yes	Companies develop complete sets of vocabulary for use in AAC tools and devices. See Symbol Set Comparison at www.spectronics.com.au/article/symbol-set-comparison.
		Example: Tommy's book contains colored symbol icons representing core and fringe vocabulary. He is able to receptively identify icons and point or hand them to a communication partner to express himself.
Writing	Yes	Written words or quick phrases are on each icon
		Example: Written words and quick phrases are on each icon to support Tommy's emerging reading and supports communication partners understanding of his intent.

XII Strategies used by communication partners to support expression

Note: Observe strategies that communication partners use to support the child's success with expressive communication. Ask yourself, *What strategies do communication partners and facilitators use to support the child's expressive communication?* The following represent a list of areas to consider and an example of how the strategy is used.

Gestures	Communication partners encourage the child to point and say *look* using the speech generating device
Request repetition	Note the range of repetitions a facilitator or communication partner may expect to use with the child. Integrate the reduction of repetitions in the goals
Aided language stimulation	Model of how to construct a message
Pacing tool	Use of a board or technique such as tapping that allows the child to improve intelligibility
Prompt	Visual, verbal, physical, use of time, or a number of prompts to indicate to the child to begin, repair, or use a word to generate a message with a communication board or device
Strategic support	Monitoring that AAC tools and devices are available, on, functioning; supporting communication partners
Co-constructing messages	Supporting the child with message development

XIII Strategies used by communication partners to support comprehension

Note: Observe strategies that communication partners use to support the child's success with comprehension. Ask yourself, *What strategies do communication partners and facilitators use to support the child's comprehension?* The following represent a list of areas to consider.

Unaided language supports

- Gestures: Communication partners gesture action verbs or point to icons to bridge understanding
- Repetition of a message

- Reducing the speaking rate to the AAC user
- Chunk the message into parts
- Reduce the complexity of messages
- Reduce the length of the message
- Increase or decrease speaker's voice volume

Aided language supports

- Modeling productions
- Co-constructing messages
- Calendars
- Maps or diagrams
- Pictured sequence
- Social stories
- Memory or remnant books, *All About Me* book
- Other novel strategies reported or observed by interventionists and communication partners

XIV Summary

Note: The following options A–H may be included in the summary section. Adjust wording as appropriate for the child especially within the parentheses. Remove the lettering. Generate a narrative. Each letter does not have to be its own paragraph but may be depending on the amount of content included.

A CHILD presents with a (note level: mild, moderate, severe) communication disorder secondary to the diagnosis of (e.g. autism). a) Formal testing (name of test) yielded a standard score of (X) and a percentile rank of (X). b) Dynamic/authentic/other(s) and informal measures addressed the child's communication in the areas of . . . c) A combination of standardized and dynamic assessment in the area of . . . Areas of strength demonstrated by (CHILD) include . . . (with examples). Ares of need include . . . (with examples).

B Type of Communicator
Note: Indicate the type of communicator the child's profile best represents. According to Beukelman and Mirenda (2013), AAC communicators function with varying degrees of facilitator and technology support. Based off of the AAC assessment, what type of communicator does the child represent at this point in time?

- Emerging communicator – limited to no reliable method of symbolic communication; may have non-symbolic modes of communication
- Context-dependent communicator – has symbolic and non-symbolic modes of communication with varying degrees of success by context, partner, or activity, broad range of skills, skill may be dependent upon degree of partner understanding of the person's communication
- Independent communicator – interacts with both familiar and unfamiliar partners in any context with any content, communicate novel messages

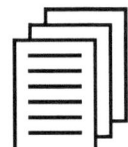

C AAC Purposes

Note: Light and McNaughton (2014) identified four purposes of AAC communication. Research by Rogers (1999) stated that the purposes of communication allow children to express their unique identity. Therefore, write a narrative and complete the purposes of communication chart summarizing the present and future communication plan. Completing the chart requires the assessor to think through how communication is impacted across modalities. A brief review of the purposes is included here.

○ Purposes of communication

1 Social etiquette: Politeness, greetings, closures, social regulation, offer recommendations.
2 Sharing information: Conveying thoughts and ideas, offer recommendations based on preferred activities and interests
3 Social closeness: Establishing, developing, maintaining relationships; jokes; emotions and feelings – love, anger, pain, joy, relief, offer recommendations
4 Wants and needs: How are the child's wants and needs presently being expressed to others? How do you plan on improving access to wants and needs?

Step 1. State the child's present communication status across each purpose in the chart. See the following table as an example.

Present and Recommended Communication Modalities across the Purposes of Communication

	Nonverbal	Vocal	Low Tech	High Tech
Social etiquette	Presently smiles to say hello and goodbye	Occasionally says the word approximation *hu* for hi	Recommend a communication wallet to use in the community	Vocabulary for social etiquette is programmed in high tech SGDs
Share information	Uses eye gaze and body posture	Understands but cannot vocally express an intent	Successfully trialed at private therapists single and multimessage SGD. Needed in school, home, and community	Required to share complex thoughts. Child is able to attend to conversations with no method of expressing ideas
Social closeness	Sustained eye gaze and physically moves closer	May sigh or may just be quiet	Vocabulary needs to be included on communication boards	Needs expanded vocabulary to express feelings and emotions
Wants and needs	Points or uses eye gaze	May cry or use vocal sounds	Presently uses communication boards for item choices. Needs expansion for self-regulation	Program fringe vocabulary to support core vocabulary that comes standard on a device

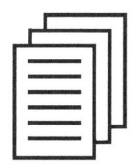

Step 2. Write a narrative of the rational or the plan to bridge the child's present communication status with the next steps to meet future goals. Funding agencies will expect trials across a number of speech generating devices along with data that proves benefit for activities of daily living including communication for medical necessity. Documentation may include data across a number of therapists. Include a video of the child's success. A well-designed progress monitoring collection tool will aid the team in documenting data and maintaining a collective focus on the priorities of the assessment across team members and environments.

Sample: To bridge Tommy's current communication status to that in the future plan, a high tech, tablet-based application was trialed with a set up display of 15 buttons (3x5 grid, 1"x1.5" cells) at a time. Tommy was initially shown how to make requests for preferred items (e.g. toy cars, Lego, bouncy balls) and then for self-help by building a 2-button message and tapping the message bar to play the entire message. The following table shows examples of Tommy's language generated after initial modeling of up two and three buttons (noun verb + object):

	1-Button Message *(object)*	*2-Button Message* *(noun verb + object)* *(more + object or action)*	*3-Button Message* *(noun verb + adjective + object)* *(noun or noun verb + more + object)*
Independently formed	*Lego, cars, ball, stuffed animal, goldfish cracker, book*	*I want + Lego;* *I want + ball;* *more + goldfish cracker;* *I need + break;* *more + help*	*I want + red + Lego;* *I want + blue + Lego;* *I want + more + Lego;* *Look + big + cars;* *I + go + car*

During the initial trial, Tommy showed interest in the device by holding it independently and trying to navigate through the folders to see the other vocabulary words. Tommy demonstrated understanding and intention with his requests as evidenced by pushing away an item when it was not the one he requested (e.g. if he requested Lego but was given a toy car, he would push away the car and re-request the Lego with an indirect gestural prompt back to the device). Additional data shows that Tommy used the message bar to communicate his message 10 times during this activity and independently cleared the screen if he selected the incorrect icon or accidently selected the icon twice (duplication) 3 times. He occasionally tried to verbally imitate the voice output of the speech generating device (e.g. said 'I wa ca' after the device said 'I want cars'). One, two, and three button messages were generated independently and functionally with dynamic display speech generating device communication.

D   AAC competencies

Note: Light (1989) identified four AAC communication competencies. A summary of the competencies is included here.

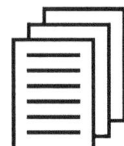

1 Linguistic: Summarize how the child comprehends and expresses language.
2 Operational: Summarize how the child physically signs or physically works with communication technology.
3 Social: Summarize how the child uses communication to interact with others.
4 Strategic: Summarize how the child uses communication to request help to access their communication devices or to clarify communication (e.g. Show a communication partner a card that says, *I need three choices to answer your question*).

Write a summary of the child's status with each of the four AAC competencies. Then use the AAC competencies to drive the goals and objectives. It is usually helpful to write an operational goal and language goals that incorporate the purposes of communication that foster a social connection. Goals may or may not be included in a report depending on organizational or administrative policy.

E   Summarize key communication facilitators and partners, topics, technology, and access methods.

F   Summarize an action plan for today (Beukelman & Mirenda, 2013): As appropriate note current abilities, immediate opportunities to increase communication, multimodal AAC technology for communication, assistive technology for access to home, school, and the environment. The greatest areas of need are developed into goals. A possible narrative template follows:

Tommy's communication strengths are . . . Tommy's communication needs are in the areas of . . . Immediate opportunities to increase communication are . . . A multimodal communication plan will support communication across environments at home, school, and the community (Add specific details pertinent to the child). Based on Tommy's need the goals will target . . .

G   Recommendations: Summarize a plan for tomorrow (Beukelman & Mirenda, 2013). Does the team anticipate natural abilities will change? What are the long-term communication needs of the child given the diagnosis (e.g. expected to improve in areas such as motor; expected to regress). Do you anticipate changes in access or opportunity barriers due to a change in residence, community experience, or school setting?

Include facilitator training that may be required for an effective AAC intervention program to be implemented. Include verbiage to justify direct and indirect speech-language pathologist services, funding, materials, and team member duties and responsibilities.

Bullet point a list of technology or materials required.

Bullet point a list of recommendations for the team to support intervention.

H   Prognosis and follow up: Generate a statement on quality of life or expected outcomes based on the findings from the assessment with a plan for follow up.

Sample: *Based on the findings from this assessment, Tommy's desire to communicate, and IEP team member support, Tommy's prognosis is favorable. An AAC assessment is not meant to be a one-time recommendation,*

but rather a part of a continuum of service that evolves as the child and communication partner's needs change. Therefore, a follow-up consultation with team members and Tommy is recommended every three months.

Closing statement to the family or referral source:

Sample: *It was a pleasure working with Tommy, his family, and the IEP team at the Hughes Academy. If there are any questions regarding the assessment or the information contained within the report, please contact me at (123)456–7890.*

_____

Name with credentials

Organizational structure name

Intervention planning: a way to structure an AAC session

The Augmentative & Assistive Communication (AAC) Intervention Session Planning Guide offers a way, but certainly not the only way, to design an AAC therapy session. Focus on planning AAC sessions to meet the language goals and objectives that specifically address communication to promote participation. The concepts introduced in this structure are addressed throughout the activities in each chapter from *Getting Started* through *Maximizing Participation*. The session structure in the following table starts with social greetings, offers an opportunity to share information like most typical interactions, an opportunity to practice ways to operate the body and technology for communication, a language focus, and finally a social closure or way to say goodbye. Remember to explicitly state the goals of the session. For example, *Our goal today is to express two ways to say hello, combine two words for a novel message, and generate one quick phrase, 'Go get 'em!' to a communication partner.* Look to the narrative after the table for further explanation of each column.

○ AAC intervention session structure

Activity #1: Practice social greetings

Forms of social etiquette help establish and maintain relationships. Engage in social greetings for the purpose of saying hello, and for the child to practice multiple ways of saying hello, so the child has choices or when the child needs options to say hello when the primary modality is not accessible or not appropriate to a situation. Be familiar with and apply the social customs of a child's culture to establish belonging and inclusion.

Priority #1: Communicative intent: The first priority in social greetings is to engage with the child by facilitating the initiation or response to a

Activity #1 Social Greeting	Activity #2 Share Information	Activity #3 Operational Practice	Activity #4 Language Intervention	Activity #5 Social Closure
Social greetings for communicative intent Social greetings as a therapeutic intervention Summary and status of communication between sessions with the child and facilitators Time: 1–5 min.	Determine optimal low-high tech tools Optimal seating and positioning Session topics Quick phrases to speak with communication partners Time: 1–5 min. or a session focal point	Body for communication Body as an access method Speech generating device functions Time: 5+ min. or a session focal point	Social interaction Communication activities Facilitator strategies Literacy Vocabulary AAC tools and access Time: Bulk of the session	Summary of the session Plan for the next session Social closure as a therapeutic intervention Social closure for communicative intent Time: 1–3 min.

Note: The time allotted to each activity will depend on the length of the session.

communication partner with a social greeting. The purpose is to generate a natural social greeting that includes the child and the communication partner. The extent of the greeting may include a simple '*hello*' or include social greeting schema (e.g. *Hello. How are you? I'm fine thank you. How are you?*). Modality options include nonverbal (e.g. wave, eye contact, hand or other body movement), verbal oral production, word or phrase approximation, vocalization, or assistive technology for social greeting messages.

Priority #2: Therapeutic intervention: The second priority in social greetings is generating the opportunity for the child to practice multiple ways of initiating or responding to a social greeting. For example: *Great job telling me 'hello' with your smile. Now tell me two ways. Use your hand, your voice, your single message speech generating device, or your high-tech speech generating device. Nice, now tell me three ways. Wonderful, we practice three or more ways, so you know you have options by choice or by need for saying, 'hi.'*

Summary and status of communication between sessions: Talk with team members about their summary impressions of the child's communication between sessions. Discuss factors that may influence communication such as diet, sleep patterns, medical updates, feelings and emotions, and fun things like trips to the library, park, or special events. True, knowledge is power. Knowledge is also fuel for communication topics and understanding for how and why a child is reacting and responding to communication partners.

Activity #2: Opportunity to share information

Before proceeding with the session check in with the child to be sure seating and positioning is optimal for comfort, access, and engagement with communication. Provide the opportunity for the child to discuss feelings and emotions, share topics or special interests, tell jokes, and ask communication partners to share information. Aim high! Spark thinking and interaction. Use a communication book, tip card, or speech generating device pages of topics about the child's favorite things to do, places to go, items, activities, and more. Use videos, bring in art, listen to different genres of music, explore science and sports. Remember to include quick phrases on pages for the child to ask the communication partner to share information (e.g. *What do you like to do? Where do you like to go? Tell me about your favorites. Know a funny joke!*).

Activity #3: Operational or strategic competency

Target goals to build the child's operational ability to use the body (e.g. finger or hand positions for pointing, activating access methods or direct select for a speech generating device) or assistive technology for communication (e.g. volume control, page and folder navigation, programming). The child may benefit from goals that support the child in learning to seek support, called strategic competency, to bridge a divide in communication such using body positioning or eye gaze to seek support for access to technology.

Building operational and strategic competency increase the AAC user's independence.

Activity #4: Language intervention plan

Social interaction: think 'language'

What purposes of communication are the focus for the session (i.e. social greeting, sharing information, social etiquette, wants and needs (Light, 1988)? What domains of language are being targeted such as morphosyntax, semantics, and pragmatics? Is the objective to generate a quick phrase message, a one-word request, combining words for a novel utterance? For example: AAC will verbalize a two-word message descriptive phrase using a speech generating device given picture or object stimulus in 2/3 trials with one verbal navigational cue in a structured setting across two consecutive sessions.

Facilitator strategies: communication partners need help too!

Decide what communication partners need to be successful to communicate with the child given the social interaction task or objective. Given the earlier task, make sure the parent knows how to use books or objects in the home to talk with the child and how long to focus on a task. Talk about how to see joint attention in the child. Model the communication exchange that includes aided language stimulation in both speaking the two-word description and generating the two-word production on the speech generating device (Goosens, 1989). Demonstrate how to promote participation by commenting more and asking fewer questions. Invite communication through turn-taking such as, *Let's talk about your picture. I will start and describe what I see then it will be your turn. Okay, my turn, I see the . . . Yellow-Sun. Now I am going to show you on your device where the icons are to say 'yellow-sun.' Now it is your turn. I know you are thinking of many things you can say. I can't wait to hear what you have to say about your picture.* Encourage communication partners to learn about the child's favorites, likes, and dislikes to drive communication and interaction.

Literacy: always!

Sprinkle, spoon in, or add a generous dollop of literacy into each session. Given the two-word production goal use a keyboard to spell out the words and read, use a dry erase board, markers, pencils, waxed string or any writing utensil that inspires the child and you to write and shape letters into words. Need more help with where to start and how to proceed with literacy? Read each chapter's sections on literacy and explore the materials and links to websites and documents that guide you through priorities in literacy for AAC users.

Vocabulary: think 'participation FIRST'

What words make sense for your child to participate in the social interaction and meet the targeted purpose of communication? There are lists of core words, high frequency words, words commonly used by children by age, and more. Simplify things. What words make sense to talk with communication partners about the task? Use yourself or the child's peers as models. What vocabulary, or words, are used when kids play games, draw, play music, and more? Don't forget fun words and phrases and vocabulary that allow a child to self-advocate (e.g. *Hey, it's my turn!*)

AAC tools and access: think multimodal

AAC tools and access methods are the child's voice when oral speech is limited or not an option either temporarily or permanently. Consider the variety of tools and ways the child can express language using nonverbal and the variety of verbal tools that include degrees of the human voice for words, word-approximations, vocalizations with communicative intent, and speech generating devices.

Activity #5: Session social closure

Therapeutic intervention

As the session comes to a close review the communicative success and activities completed. Ask what activities the child would like to do again? Discuss the plan for the next meeting including ways to incorporate communication for the child and communication partners throughout the daily schedule. As you end an intervention session with the child work on multiple ways to initiate or respond to a social closure. For example: *Now we are ready to say goodbye for today. Remember how we started our session? Yes, we practiced three ways to say 'hello.' Now let's practice three ways to say goodbye. Great job telling me 'see you later' with your eyes. Now tell me two ways, use your hand splay, your voice, your single message speech generating device, on your high-tech speech generating device. Well done. You told me three ways you can say 'goodbye.' You know you have options if one way is better for you on any day, time, person, situation, or environment.*

Communicative intent for participation

End the session focusing on the communicative intent of saying goodbye. The child may initiate or respond to a communication partner. Modalities may include nonverbal (e.g. wave, eye contact, hand or other body movement), verbal oral production, word or phrase approximation (e.g. Bye, See you later!), vocalization, or assistive technology for social greeting messages.

References

Beukelman, D. R. & Mirenda, P. (2013). *Augmentative and alternative communication: Supporting children and adults with complex communication needs* (4th ed.). Baltimore, MD: Paul H. Brookes Publishing.

Blackstone, S. & Hunt-Berg, M. (2003). *Social networks introductory package*. Verona, WI: Attainment Company, Inc.

Boavida, T., Aguiar, C. & McWilliam, R. A. (2014). A training program to improve IFSP-IEP goals and objectives through the routines-based interview. *Topics in Early Childhood Special Education*, *33*(4), 200–211.

Bronfenbrenner, U. (1986). The ecology of the family as a context or human development: Research perspectives. *Developmental Psychology*, *22*(6), 723–742.

Bruner, J. (1990). *Acts of meaning*. Cambridge, MA: Harvard University Press.

CAST. (2018). Universal design for learning guidelines version 2.2. Retrieved from http://udlguidelines.cast.org

Cress, C. J. & Marvin, C. A. (2003). Common questions about AAC services in early intervention. *Augmentative and Alternative Communication*, *19*(4), 254–272.

Damico, J. S. & Ball, M. J. (2010). Prolegomenon: Addressing the tyranny of old ideas. *Journal of International Research in Communication Disorders*, *1*(1), 1–29.

Delpit, L. (1995). *Other people's children: Cultural conflict in the classroom*. New York, NY: The New Press.

Duchan, J. (2004). *Framework in language and literacy: How theory informs practice*. New York, NY: Guilford Press.

Fried-Oken, M. & Granlund, M. (2012). AAC and the ICF: A good fit to emphasize outcomes. *Augmentative and Alternative Communication*, *28*(1), 1–2.

Gardner, H. (1993). *Frames of mind: The theory of multiple intelligences* (10th ed.). New York, NY: Basic Books.

Ginsburg, H. & Opper, S. (1988). *Piaget's theory of intellectual development* (3rd ed.). Englewood Cliffs, NJ: Prentice Hall.

Goosens, C. (1989). Aided communication intervention before assessment: A case study of a child with cerebral palsy. *Augmentative and Alternative Communication*, *5*, 14–26.

Granlund, M., Björck-Åkesson, E., Wilder, J. & Ylven, R. (2008). AAC interventions for children in a family environment: Implementing evidence in practice. *Augmentative and Alternative Communication*, *24*(3), 207–219.

Hammer, C. S. (2011). Expanding our knowledge base through qualitative research methods. *American Journal of Speech-Language Pathology*, *20*(3), 161–162.

Heath, S. (1983). *Way with words: Language, life and work in communities and classrooms*. Cambridge: Cambridge University Press.

Holland, A. (2007). *Counseling in communication disorders: A wellness perspective*. San Diego, CA: Plural Publishing, Inc.

Keller, H. (1903). *Optimism*. Boston, MA: The Merrymount Press.

Kleiman, L. I. (2003). *Functional communication profile-revised*. Austin, TX: PRO-ED, Inc.

Lash, J. (1974). *Helen and teacher: The story of Helen Keller and Annie Sullivan Macy*. New York, NY: Delacorte Press/Seymour Lawrence.

Light, J. (1988). Interaction involving individuals using augmentative and alternative communication systems: State of the art and future directions. *Augmentative and Alternative Communication*, *4*(2), 66–82.

Light, J. (1989). Toward a definition of communicative competence for individuals using augmentative and alternative communication systems. *Augmentative and Alternative Communication*, *5*(2), 137–144.

Light, J. & McNaughton, D. (2009). *Accessible literacy learning: Evidence-based reading instruction for individuals with autism, cerebral palsy, Down syndrome, and other disabilities*. San Diego, CA: Mayer Johnson.

Light, J. & McNaughton, D. (2014). Communicative competence for individuals who require augmentative and alternative communication: A new definition for a new era of communication? *Augmentative and Alternative Communication*, *30*(1), 1–18.

Light, J., McNaughton, D. & Caron, J. (2019). New and emerging AAC technology supports for children with complex communication needs and their communication partners: State of the science and future research directions. *Augmentative and Alternative Communication*, *35*(1), 26–41.

Mandak, K. & Light, J. (2018). Family-centered services for children with ASD and limited speech: The experiences of parents and speech-language pathologists. *Journal of Autism and Developmental Disorders*, *48*(4), 1311–1324.

McLeod, S. (2018). Communication rights: Fundamental human rights for all. *International Journal of Speech-Language Pathology*, *20*(1), 3–11.

McNaughton, D., Light, J., Beukelman, D., Klein, C., Nieder, D. & Nazareth, G. (2019). Building capacity in AAC: A person centred approach to supporting participation by people with complex communication needs. *Augmentative and Alternative Communication*, *35*(1), 56–68.

Millar, D. C., Light, J. C. & Schlosser, R. (2006). The impact of augmentative and alternative communication intervention on the speech production of individuals with developmental disabilities: A research review. *Journal of Speech Language Hearing Research*, *49*(2), 248–264.

Moll, L. C. (1990). Introduction. In L. C. Moll (Ed.), *Vygotsky and education: Instructional implications and applications of sociohistorical psychology* (pp. 1–30). Cambridge: Cambridge University Press.

Na, J., Wilkinson, K., Karny, M., Blackstone, S. & Stifter, C. (2016). A synthesis of relevant literature of the development of emotional competences: Implications for design of augmentative and alternative communication systems. *American Journal of Speech-Language Pathology*, *25*(3), 441–452.

Owens, R. (2014). *Language disorders: A functional approach to assessment and intervention* (6th ed.). New York, NY: Pearson Publishing.

Poplin, M. (1988a). The reductionistic fallacy in learning disabilities: Replicating the past by reducing the present. *Journal of Learning Disabilities*, *21*(7), 389–400.

Poplin, M. (1988b). Holistic/constructivist principles of teaching/learning: Implications for the field of learning disabilities. *Journal of Learning Disabilities*, *21*(7), 401–416.

Prizant, B. & Fields-Meyer, T. (2015). *Uniquely human: A different way of seeing autism*. New York, NY: Simon & Schuster.

Rogers, S. (1999). *Hearing them into voice: The hermeneutics of listening to children who cannot speak: A dynamic approach to assessing and teaching communication* (Unpublished doctoral dissertation). Claremont Graduate University, CA.

Romski, M., Sevcik, R., Adamson, L. B., Cheslock, M., Smith, A., Barker, R. M. & Batemen, R. (2010). Randomized comparison of augmented and nonaugmented language intervention for toddlers with developmental delays and their parents. *Journal of Speech Language Hearing Research*, *53*(2), 350–364.

Rose, D. H. & Meyer, A. (2002). *Teaching every student in the digital age: Universal design for learning*. Alexandria, VA: Association for Supervision and Curriculum Development.

Schlosser, R. & Wendt, O. (2008). Effects of augmentative and alternative communication on speech production in children with autism: A systematic review. *American Journal of Speech Language Pathology*, *17*(3), 212–230.

Snow, C. E., Burns, S. & Griffin, P. (Eds.). (1998). *Preventing reading difficulties in young children*. Washington, DC: National Academy Press.

Spectronics. (2019). Symbol set comparison. Retrieved from www.spectronics.com.au/article/symbol-set-comparison

Stone, C. A., Silliman, E., Ehren, B. & Apel, K. (Eds). (2004). *Handbook of language and literacy: Development and disorders*. New York, NY: Guilford Press.

Strobel-Sabatino, T. (2019). *AAC assessment report project* (Unpublished). Riverside, CA.

Thomas, S. & Oldfather, P. (1997). Intrinsic motivation, literacy, and assessment practices: "That's my grade. That's me". *Educational Psychologist*, *32*(2), 107–123.

Travis, T. & Worrall, L. (2004). Classifying communication disability using the ICF. *Advances in speech-language pathology*, *6*(1), 53–62.

UN General Assembly, Convention on the rights of persons with disabilities: resolution/adopted by the General Assembly, 24 January 2007, Article 30: Participation in cultural life, recreation, leisure and sport. A/RES/61/106. Retrieved from www.refworld.org/docid/45f973632.html

Vygotsky, L. (1986). *Thought and language* (A. Kozulin, Ed.). Cambridge, MA: MIT Press.

Wallach, G. (2018, Spring). Language is literacy and literacy is language: The challenge for speech language pathologists. *California Speech Language Hearing Association Magazine*, 21–27.

Westby, C. (2019, February 22). Play and language: The roots of literacy [Live Webinar]. Retrieved from https://catalog.pesi.com/item/play-language-roots-literacy-35343#tabDescription

Wisconsin Assistive Technology Initiative. (2018). Student information processing guides.Retrieved from www.wati.org/free-publications/wati-student-information-guide-process-forms/

World Health Organization. (2007). *ICF-CY. International classification of functioning, disability and health: Children and youth version*. Geneva: Author.

Yoder, D. (2001). Having my say. *Augmentative and Alternative Communication*, *17*(1), 2–10.

PART II

AAC intervention plan with case studies

Getting Started with social interaction

Building intentional communication

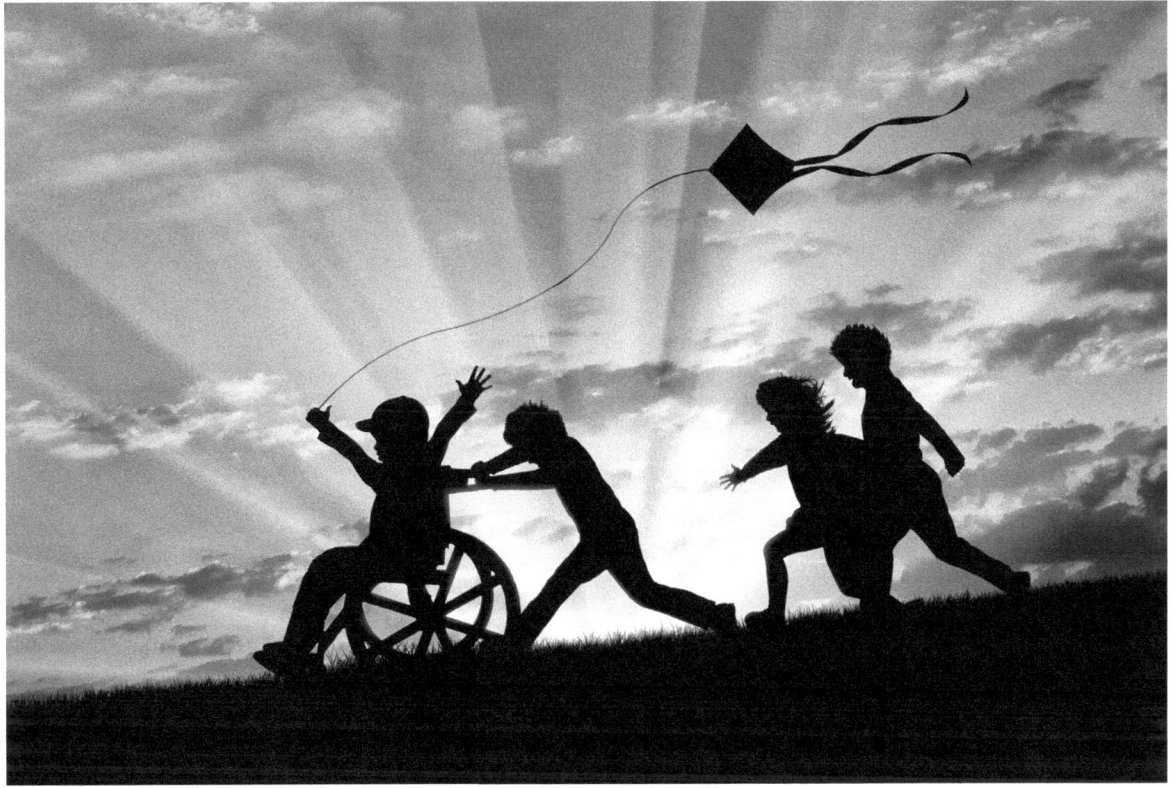

Our children . . . teach us the wonder of life and joy of achievement. They teach us unending patience and perseverance. They do not give up, and neither can we.

–Parent (Rogers, 1999)

Here we are at the very beginning. Congratulations! Let's get started. You are probably asking yourself many questions. *Where do I begin in building intentional communication for my child, student, or client with a complex communication profile? What does intentional communication mean for my child and all communication partners?* Snell et al. (2010) state that is important to address the intentional functionality in service delivery from assessment to intervention. Step one with *Getting Started* is simple and powerful: Complete the protocol *Hear Me into Voice* to collect an inventory of what and how your child is communicating. Next, identify the successes you and your child experience given the tips and strategies in *My Tool Box* and *My Child's Tool Box*. Finally, read Diego's Story as an example of *Getting Started* with the six sections of developing participation for a beginning communicator with social interaction, communication activities, facilitator strategies, literacy, vocabulary, and tools and access.

Intentionality starts with joint attention

What is joint attention? *Getting Started* with communication involves joint attention between the child and communication partners who share a visual focus on an object, an action, or objects in action! What a great way to start communication. Joint attention is one of the first intentional communication acts that emerge from human experience making it a very important skill for both a child to demonstrate and the adults to respond and shape successful communication. A child or adult may initiate joint attention through eye gaze, giving, pointing, and showing. According to Kaderavek (2015), joint visual attention demonstrates the ability for your child to initiate and respond to eye gaze. This means that the child and the communication partner are focused on the same object or idea at the same time. For a child with a vision impairment, look for a head-turn and body posture pause that tells you your child is attending to what he is hearing. People may engage in joint attention using any or all of the senses including vision, hearing, taste, smell, and touch. You may ask yourself, *How will I know if a behavior is an intentional communication behavior or not an intentional communication behavior?* Sometimes a behavior can be an intentional communication behavior and sometimes the same behavior can be non-intentional. For example, a smile may intentionally express *hello* or it may be a reflexive in response to gastro-intestinal issues or a seizure. A smile may also be an expression of an internal state of happiness such as thinking of a memory that communicates your child's emotional state but not a message. Look at your child's behavior as a discoverable opportunity. Make the *least dangerous assumption* that your child's behavior carries meaning, and if you are not sure, recognize the opportunity that a behavior you see in your child may become meaningful. Do not get discouraged if a behavior you observe is not intentional. A behavior that is not intentional today may be intentional tomorrow.

○ My intentional communication tool box

Begin recognizing joint attention! *What am I doing to build and sustain joint attention?* Look at *My Tool Box* for a list of tips and strategies to elicit a skill such as joint attention. Reflect on the list of tips and strategies and use the following page to write them down. Why? This is your *Getting Started*, list of communication behaviors that you see in your child, and successful communication you use with your child, that can be shared with other communication partners.

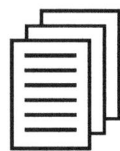

○ **What am I doing? I am going to use my tool box!**

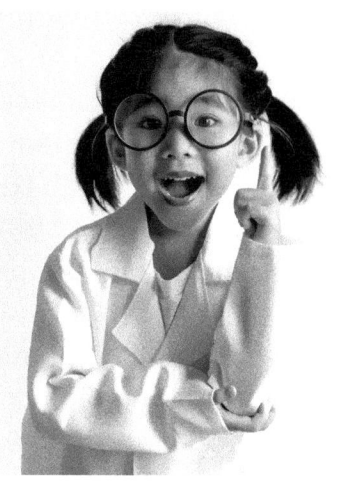

◉ **My Tool Box!**

◉ I gain eye contact with my child

◉ I smile at my child

◉ I say my child's name and watch for a response

◉ I point out how people of all ages are engaged in communication and the environment at home, at school, and in community

◉ I demonstrate affection with my child by using eyes, smiles, body postures, hugs, closeness, and body positioning

○ **What is my child doing? I will define my child's tool box!**

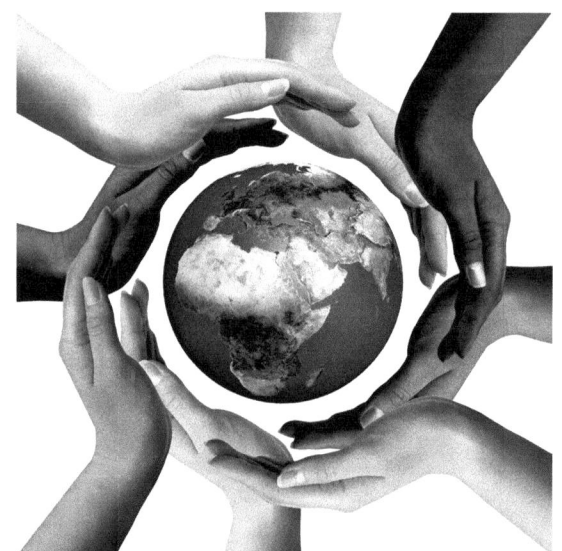

⊙ My Child's Tool Box

- ◎ My child looks at and watches me or the communication partner's eyes and face

- ◎ My child smiles at a communication partner

- ◎ My child responds to music by humming, moving or tapping to the rhythm, smiling, singing along with words or word approximations

- ◎ My child observes interactions of people of all ages at home, school, and in the community

- ◎ My child demonstrates affection using eyes, smiles, body posture, hugs, closeness, and body positioning

- ◎ My child gains attention by laughing, cooing, vocalizing, crying

- ◎ My child listens attentively to conversations, TV, music, others

- ◎ My child makes requests such as being held or asking for more using vocalizations, nonverbal gestures, communication tools and devices

○ Using my tool box: joint interaction success

Establishing joint attention: Indicate what success looks like for your child. Use Use the chart titled *Joint interaction success* on page 72 by writing in the date and/or number of times an item is demonstrated. In the comments section write notes to share with team members about the child's communication. Consider writing notes about behaviors that you work on at home, school, and in the community.

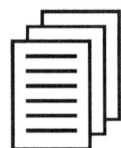

Joint interaction success

Communication	Success	Success	Success	Success	Success
My child looks at and watches communication partners' eyes and face					
My child smiles at a communication partner					
My child responds to music by humming; moving or tapping to the rhythm; singing along with words or word approximations					
My child observes interactions of people of all ages at home school, and in the community					
My child demonstrates affection by using my eyes, smiles, body posture, hugs, closeness, and body positioning					
My child gains attention by laughing, cooing, vocalizing					
My child listens to conversations, TV, music, others					
My child makes requests such as being held or asking for more using vocalizations, non-verbal gestures, communication tools and devices, other					

Comments and Notes:

_____

_____

_____

_____

_____

_____

_____

_____

_____

_____

_____

_____

Joint Attention

A case study in *Getting Started*: meet Diego

Meet Diego, a son, a brother, and a friend who is *Getting Started* with communication. We follow Diego, bilingual in Spanish and English, from age three through age 10. You may be thinking, how is a 10-year-old child just Getting Started with communication? Maybe the answer is we are all *Getting Started* with communication each time we meet someone new or tackle a complicated interaction. *Getting Started* with AAC begins at any age when communication needs to be augmented or assisted for any purpose. Diego was a vibrant communicator every day as an infant and toddler. Diego experienced a traumatic brain injury as a result of a near drowning accident at age three when he experienced hypoxia, a lack of oxygen to the brain halting his verbal communication. Learn more about Diego.

Infancy: Diego is welcomed into his family, his loving parents, and his two delightful sisters, one older and one younger. He learns to take his first steps, explore the house and outdoors, name his favorite person, and follow his older sister. He enjoys his family and they enjoy him.

Life changing moment: On a warm summer evening with tangerine skies, a neighborhood block party commences. Families opened their homes and yards to each other as they gathered in the street for a meal and to share summer stories. Diego, a curious three-year old boy, wanders in and out of neighbors' yards as so many children do that evening. He scampers into the home next door where he sees an inviting pool. Moments later, a quiet stillness and devastating panic sweeps over his parents. *Diego!* Family and friends call and search for Diego. What takes place only minutes later is a flurry of chaos, emergency personnel, hospitals, a six-week coma, and the lifelong impact of a near drowning.

Recovery: Diego, once an active boy, is now a patient in a hospital with a traumatic brain injury. His body does not respond to sounds or sights despite the best care possible. His family is vigilant in keeping watch for months. The seemingly one-sided interaction by his family is centered on watching for any changes in Diego's breathing or movement. The hospital staff releases Diego when he finally opens his eyes. As he recovers at home, his family listens for the deeper breaths he takes and the sounds he makes with his voice. They interpret his quietness as his time to process. He is happy to be home.

Adapting to change: His family recognizes that his eyes and smiles express subtle communication. They know they are his sensitive interpreters. When they succeed Diego gives them definite nonverbal responses. Diego is a communicator and a participant again in his environment and activities of each day. He participates in the same activities as before the accident but now he participates differently.

As Diego and his family learn to establish joint attention, close family and experienced caregivers begin to recognize and reinforce his unique modes of communication. Sometimes he uses his voice to express concern for his sister. Other times he is silent yet listening. The recovery from the accident changed his communication and physical movement. What did not change is that Diego continues to enrich his communication partners' understanding that he has a powerful nonverbal message of love and understanding to share. His family and team continue to ask the right questions. *What does Diego understand? How can Diego get started expressing verbal and nonverbal communication? How do we find a way to continue to help Diego participate and aid others in understanding what he has to say? Getting Started* is a time to discover a person's communication in all of its forms and connect intentional communication with communication partners, participation in activities, and events across environments. As you read more about Diego consider the guiding questions directed at how discovering and recognizing language, both his comprehension and expression, impact his participation with others through AAC.

○ Section 1 Social interaction: How does Diego demonstrate his communication strengths and motivations in interacting with others?

Diego makes connections with each of his family members. He opens his eyes to listen attentively to the conversations of his parents and sisters. He smiles when he hears a particular sound like a door closing that signals his sister may be home. His eyes sometimes open wide in surprise when she comes to his room. Caregivers learn to be sensitive to Diego's best communication nonverbally and to rely on his mother's interpretations of his subtle movements. His mother offers him breakfast choices of eggs or cereal. While his mother feeds him, she speaks to him about the day's schedule, sometimes fluently switching between Spanish, her native language, and English, the language spoken with his two siblings. Diego enters into the conversation by listening as he sits silently in his wheelchair.

Communicating with less familiar communication partners is where Diego and his family need the most help in *Getting Started* to transfer successes into school and the community. Completing the protocol, *Hear Me into Voice*, detailed Diego's eight best ways to comprehend and express himself. He lets others know he enjoys listening to the sound of their voices as he turns his head toward the conversation and uses engaging smiles. Many less familiar communication partners are at a loss in interpreting Diego's voice, body posture, and glances. Diego's silence is often misunderstood as a lack of motivation, interest, or comprehension. His voice inflections express approval or rejection. His vocalizations fluctuate to share experiences with his family and show feelings of satisfaction and dismay. By turning his head toward sound, he lets others know he is aware of other people, things in his environment, and to make choices. His silence or smiles means *yes* and *Nnn* means, *No, that is not a good idea.* These help his parents and communication partners make choices for types of exercises, selecting clothes, and foods to enjoy.

Diego is an active member of the family as they talk together at dinner about the day's activities. His dad, a construction supervisor, has more vocal exchanges with Diego than any other person. On the way to see the new movie release of *Godzilla* Diego saw his father's truck and protested with vocalizations as if to be exclaiming, *Get me out of this car. I want to see my dad!* His mother thought quickly, *I know you want to see Dad. He has to work now. You will get to see him tonight. Wouldn't your friends be jealous to hear that you saw the movie first?* Diego responded with a deeply triumphant smile of satisfaction. The next day was Sunday and they would sit together to watch the games. His family recognizes the uniqueness and lovingness Diego brings to the family. Diego is quite attentive to his sister when she tells him about her friends and struggles at school. She feels his compassion toward her as she sits beside Diego and talks with him each day. She wrote a senior essay about, *Her silent guardian who gives her strength.* He expresses his concern with his voice when his mother speaks to him about his sister taking the SAT test and moving away to go to college. His mother notes, *We assume that he understands more than anyone gives him credit for. He is dear to us even if we do not always understand, because he teaches us the wonder of life and joy of achievement.*

His mother only hires caregivers who believe in Diego's potential and also take responsibility for his day-to-day participation in activities. His mother conducts interviews asking each potential caregiver a simple question, *What does an ideal day with Diego look like?* The caregivers' response shows Diego's mother how creatively and imaginatively they will match both as people and interests and talents to daily activities. *There is always a match*, says his mother. How did the potential caregiver, as a communication partner and potential facilitator, respond to his smiles, eye gazes, and facial expressions? How would the person offer choices to Diego? Did this person enter into a conversation with expectations, enthusiasm, and patience in waiting for his communication in whatever form? At school, educators and therapists including physical, occupational, and speech-language pathologists who work with Diego, *believe that his comprehension is much greater than his motor system allows him to express. That was the place to begin*, his mother insisted. His intervention team agreed.

⊙ Questions for Reflection

Section 1 Social Interaction: What were Diego's communication strengths and motivations?

1   Match the ways Diego communicated with the importance of his intent of the message.

a	Smiles	1	_____ Often misunderstood by unfamiliar communication partners as not comprehending; A way to nonverbally emphasize or express understanding and attention
b	Vocalizations	2	_____ Nonverbal facial agreement, expression of joy and humor

	c	Head turning	3	_____ Used to make choices between two objects
	d	Eye gaze	4	_____ Nnn = no
	e	Silence	5	_____ A way to participate and share experiences in the moment through sound showing satisfaction or dismay
	f	Word approximation	6	_____ Body posture used to support attention to the environment or people, rejection

2 What are three ways interventionists support Diego's motivation?
   a He makes choices about therapy exercises performed
   b Participation is restricted to family members to reduce disappointments with unfamiliar communication partners
   c He makes choices about clothes to wear and food to eat
   d Interventionists believe in Diego and creatively and imaginatively interact with him

Answers

1 1=e   2=a   3=d   4=f   5=b   6=c
   Diego has many communication strengths and motivations from listening intently with his sister, the intensity of his face to indicate engagement, along with his eyes, smiles, silence, and vocalizations. By turning his head or his eyes toward sound he let others know he is aware of other people and wants to make choices in his environment.

2 Letters a., c., and d. are the correct answers. Each interventionist providing services to Diego takes an active role making sure that he is not a passive recipient of care. These services were most successful when they built on Diego's communication strengths in the context of what is most important to him. Letter b. is an incorrect choice as the family nor Diego need not be isolated because of this life changing moment.

O Section 2 Communication Activities: How was Diego's participation in activities reciprocal with his successful communication?

Diego relishes participation and his mother appreciates Diego's thoughts, his unique ways of expressing himself, and his delight in being with his family. His mother offers, *Do you want the shirt that Silvia bought you for your birthday or the red one?* Often, she repeats the choices before he responds. She expects responses and he learns that his responses matter. His younger sister, fond of poetry, includes him in her writing experiences. She bounces ideas off of Diego reading his gilded smiles as enjoyment of her work and approval of her words. His silence is read as either complete captivation with the imagery she created or . . . *maybe sister you should try that again because I have no idea what you are saying.* His communication makes a difference. His communication is valued.

Diego's eyes brighten when he hears music on the radio or television. His caregiver offers Diego an activity of listening to music. Then she asks, *Which station would you like to hear, Latin music or classical?* Diego turns his head when she says Latin music, so she turns the radio to the Spanish speaking station they prefer. They often sing together as they listen.

Eating away from home in the community is a fun event. They name three to four restaurants that he chooses from. Diego smiles when his favorite is named. *Mijares, yes!* Diego has distinct preferences for menu options, often selecting the spiciest Mexican foods possible. He also flirts to no end with the wait staff making outings embarrassingly entertaining for all.

Diego likes to travel, as indicated by his smiles in the car when the family talks together during the ride. His mother notices his contentment during the ride now that he is tall enough to look out the window from his car seat. Diego hears a plane flying over his head and looks at his mother. *He likes planes*, his mother says, recalling the smiles and alertness Diego showed during the flight to visit his father's parents in Ukraine. Diego thrives on the rush movement brings to him, the places he can see in the environment and the participation in the world that is unique from his daily experiences at home and school.

Diego's at-home caregiver gradually learns to notice how Diego looks up and smiles when she volunteers to turn the television on to watch an action movie. Diego quiets with anticipation of the film starting when the TV announcer counts down *5-4-3-2-1*. She watches the way he turns his head and or uses his eyes to express pleasure, concern, or protest.

Diego likes to go with his family to watch movies in the theater too. Diego watches the big screen and pays attention to every scene of the feature length film. His mother recalled, only once did Diego become very upset when they were watching the dramatic film *Titanic*, Diego cried out so loudly that they took him to the theater lobby to calm his frantic cries. She asked why he was so upset by that scene. *Was it that the ship was sinking or that the passengers were struggling to swim to safety?* she asked. Finally, she thought to understand his feelings of overwhelming sadness by framing another question. She asked, *Were you sad because the water was coming over them?* Only then did Diego's crying stop. He communicated with his crying and silence that he understood and empathized with the characters. She recognized, *He senses others' pain.* Perhaps the fear of water from his past experience rushed back to him.

Diego has his favorite therapists and educators. He uses his smiles and vocalizations to continue conversations with them. He smiles at Rodriguez, his educational aid, when he tickles his arm with a feather to alert him to a new activity. His smile continues as Rodriguez makes sure he participates with peers during physical education whether catching a ball or moving on the field with the soccer team. Diego activates a switch that counts down for the children to play their recorders during music class.

⊙ Questions for Reflection

Section 2 Communication activities: What activities did Diego enjoy participating in? How are participation and communication reciprocal?

1 Circle the activities that Diego preferred:

- ⊙ Action movies
- ⊙ Counting down
- ⊙ Latin and classical music

- ⊙ Making food choices
- ⊙ Staying home to eat
- ⊙ Art work

- ⊙ Being with peers
- ⊙ Going to restaurants
- ⊙ Movement and travel

2 Match these social interactions with the family members and caregivers

Communication Partners	Communication Activities
1 _____ Dad	a Wrote poetry with Diego; Talked about good and challenging things in her life with him and considered Diego her silent guardian angel
2 _____ Mom	b Played Latin and classical music for Diego; Watched action movies together; Focused on his abilities
3 _____ Sisters	c Loved watching sports with Diego; Going out to dinner; Traveling around in the community and car
4 _____ Caregiver	d Expected communication from Diego; Offered choices for food, fun, clothes; Adamant to find people who fostered Diego's strengths

Answers

1 Diego's preferred activities are all of the options *less* staying at home to eat. Look at the question again and notice that Diego enjoys the same activities as most children.

2 1=c 2=d. 3=a. 4=b.
Diego's family and interventionists validate his communication and believe in him. His sisters made him a part of their world through poetry and conversations about rich and meaningful topics in their lives.
Silence was not absence of thought or meaning. Silence was empowerment as others read the meaning in his eyes and from his body.

○ Section 3 Facilitator strategies: What strategies were used to support Diego's communication at home and school?

At home, Diego's mother uses many strategies to support his communication. She uses a counting down system to give him time to organize himself and respond while still holding on to the expectation that he follows her directions. If his mother does not sense a clear response, she rubs *his upper lip which brings back energy and helps him concentrate.* Then she rephrases her request. Sometimes teasing and being silly are familiar routines at home. Diego brightens up when others talk with him like they would with any other 10-year-old boy. He shuts down when people talk over him like he is not there.

At school, Diego's education team and peers are his communication partners. They motivate his thinking with language through exposure to extensive vocabulary and grammar in Spanish and English, tools for creating stories, communication modalities for sharing information, and foster their relationships through fun and schoolwork. When it is time for Diego to start 4th grade the team seeks a change to find a full inclusion classroom. Mr. Cortines teaches a bilingual class of mostly 10-year-olds, which is perfect. This is when Rodriguez is hired as Diego's educational aide. The speech-language pathologist coaches Mr. Cortines and Rodriguez to observe Diego's responses to interpret meaning. Diego learns to squeeze Rodriguez's finger or smile to indicate his *yes* in making choices from the auditory options he was given. Mr. Cortines and Rodriguez learned to follow through with Diego's choices using his body, using communication boards, and single message speech generating devices. His mother makes the thoughtful step of talking to the kids and any adults about what to expect of Diego. Diego's mother tells them about his strengths and explains that the near drowning accident caused his present motor difficulties so his participation and communication would be different. The students learn that they simply had to wait and watch for the smile, even when his responses came slowly. She offered they try counting down in their mind to keep them from talking too soon and to give Diego more time to respond. She introduces Rodriguez and explains his duties with Diego that target increasing participation with peers and schoolwork such as using headphones to listen to text, interpreting concepts, eating, and restroom needs. Finally, Diego's mother tells them how excited Diego is to be with them in this bilingual class. Not only was Diego *Getting Started* with communication and participation but so were his classmates and educators. Finally!

The principal encourages the educator, Mr. Cortines, to plan for peers to be included with Diego using a software program that translates movement on a pressure sensitive keyboard to create music together. Peers love trying out

Diego's new adaptive technologies. One of Diego's classmates moves Diego's right hand in rotating motions on the keyboard to create a new melody. Both smiled. Diego flourishes. From day to day, Diego's smiles catch the other students' attention and so begins a new friendship. Being with other active students brings out his interest and participation each day. One day as they were assigning instruments in music class, a peer volunteered to be Diego's partner and made sure Diego had a maraca in his hand. He brought his own instrument beside Diego so they could play the music together.

His mother agrees with the teacher who comments on the first quarter's report card that, *Diego clearly responds to social interaction.* He was far from being bored and was one of the gang with the other students, the teacher, and of course Rodriguez. In fact, one student described how special he felt to have Diego in his class. The staff note, *He lights up for these kids at school and they light up for him.* Diego's mother noted, the students became very comfortable playing with each other. *It was a real nice bonding experience for all these kids.* Diego has new communication partners in the educator, Rodriguez, and in his classmates that lead to friendship, knowledge, and participation for Diego.

⊙ Questions for Reflection

Section 3 Facilitator Strategies: What strategies were used to support Diego's communication at home and school?

1   Circle the important strategies that his family used to encourage his participation.

- ⊙ Recognized Diego's effort needed to respond
- ⊙ Rephrased their requests
- ⊙ Counted down to give him time to respond
- ⊙ Rubbed his upper lip
- ⊙ Teased and joked with him
- ⊙ Modeled verbal language

2   What strategies did Diego's peers use to support Diego's communication? Indicate T=True or F=False.
   a   _____ Talked to him in both Spanish and English
   b   _____ Not treated as 'one of the gang'
   c   _____ Talked about upcoming events
   d   _____ Hand him a musical instrument during music class
   e   _____ Felt that they were special because of Diego was assigned to their class

○ **Section 4 Literacy: How was Diego's team equipped with strategies and ideology to support his strengths in accessing literacy?**

Diego's educational team know that he understands words and sentences in Spanish and English though they cannot always quantifiably measure it. Others falsely assume that due to his visual and physical limitations, Diego will not be able to read or write. Researcher, Yoder (2001) of the Center for Literacy and Disability Studies, states *No child is too anything to be able to read and write*. A major portion of a 4th grader's instructional day is dedicated to literacy. In Diego's class, students write a response on the topic of the day. Diego engages in the same task with Rodriguez through guided support of his hand, a felt tip pen, and a large sheet of paper attached to his wheelchair tray. He draws his reflection of his personal experience of the topic. Diego works with two to three classmates on writing a story about his dog jumping on his bed with wet feet. They take turns choosing a character, an action, or a setting to add to the story. A computer-generated publication of their story creation is complete with a title and a subtitle. The story development of the characters in some ways mimics the movies he watches intently at home and on the big screen in theaters. The threading of personal experience with new experiences connects Diego to his motivations, experiences, and success in school. The whole class loves to listen to and read the story they created. Diego's friends enjoy listening to and creating these stories with Diego. They covet, in fact fight over, being chosen to read with Diego.

The afterschool program incorporates many Mexican folk tales, which the students read in class and act out. Diego listens to the dance director give instructions. He feels the stories come to life in physical and emotional dimensions as the class rehearses them and the musicians accompany their actions. A peer volunteer guides Diego in the wheelchair around the stage as they move like eagles, coyotes, or deer. They become animals that find water to drink, chase other animals, and leap into the air. One student takes delight in Diego's smile when he helps Diego lift his arms and legs in imitation of a leaping deer. For Diego and his peers, the predictable language and voices spoken and heard strengthens their learning of a second language. They are motivated knowing their parents will watch the final performance. Literacy tasks built upon Diego's existing knowledge. He is engaged through interactions with peers, fostered through story development, and purposefully embedded into his daily schedule. *Getting Started* with literacy had begun.

⊙ Questions for reflection

Section 4 Literacy questions: How was Diego's team equipped with strategies and ideology to support his strengths in accessing literacy?

1   Through which reading and writing activities did Diego access literacy? Circle 3 activities.
    a   Listening to stories in Spanish and English
    b   Watching the dog jump onto his bed
    c   Generating drawings with Rodriquez based on a writing prompt
    d   Making choices of peers to work with in class
    e   Acting out stories

2   What activities further promoted Diego's language and literacy? Indicate T=True or F=False
    a   _____ Learning about and seeing his name written
    b   _____ Making choices of characters, modes of transportation
    c   _____ Seeing and hearing the story he created with his peers

Answers

1   Letters a., c., and e. are the best answers. Diego was quite attentive listening to stories in Spanish and English. He participates in literacy tasks. Acting out stories is a way to bridge knowledge he hears. Answers b. watching the dog jump onto his bed and d. making choices for peers to work with are fun events he can anticipate in as a part of his routine, but they did not directly contribute to his literacy development.
2   Letters a., b., and c. are all True. Seeing his name and learning about his family attached emotional meaning to letters on the page. Making choices of characters involve him in making a story. Of course, seeing and hearing the text of the story with his peers was motivating.

○ Section 5 Vocabulary: What vocabulary does Diego need for participation?

Diego's team considers what vocabulary he will need access to as they develop his augmentative and assistive communication plan. As a start, Diego needs quick phrases with messages to interact with peers that say, *Could we keep on talking?* Diego needs to construct his reason for rejecting a movie such as, *Not enough action*, or *I have seen that before.* Simply being able to say, *Stop* was necessary as he participates in certain physical exercises his therapist wants him to try. How much better would it be for him to communicate what part of his body was physically uncomfortable or why he did not want to try a new activity? *Help, please. I have been standing long enough!* Quick phrases and words will give Diego a way to control his environment.

Based on the findings from *Hear Me into Voice*, Diego's education team consider his current mastery of words including, *mom, dad, bye, come*, and *no*, and the quick phrase, *see you later.* They decided he needs access to the basic conversation vocabulary of his peers Emily and Patrick and family such as *my turn, forget it, come be with me, okay.* From basic social greetings and social etiquette of *hi* and *bye*, to expressing his wants and needs, *Please make my eggs hotter*, to voicing his feelings *I am afraid*, to sharing information from the story he created, *I know that horses can't throw boomerangs*, and offering his own unique identity, *My name is the same as my Dad's. My grandparents lived in the Ukraine and Mexico*. In *Getting Started* with vocabulary Diego's world of vocabulary had begun across many purposes of communication.

Diego's understanding of words that he hears include the vocabulary he embraces as he participates with everyday **core words** such as, *put, get*, and *want*, pronouns such as *mine, he*, and *she*, and words like as *this, that, here*, and *there*. He also needs access to **fringe words** or words specific to people, places, and things such as classmates and family names, favorite restaurants, book names, and places he travels. Having access to quick phrases is a great resource and supply for vocabulary in *Getting Started* with vocabulary.

While many facial expressions and vocalizations express emotions, Diego, as any child, needs a way to describe his unique identity whether it be his everyday feelings, his wanting to tease or make jokes, and switching from English to Spanish for his classmates and teachers. For example, he shares the delight in simply belonging with his classmates saying, *Thanks for talking with me.* He can express, *I am awesome*, after achieving a goal. For enjoying turn taking in playing a game, Diego conveys more abstract words and concepts he needs to use negation and adjectives *Don't be silly. I am teasing you.*

Quick phrases to use as Diego watches sports need to be included such as, *He missed that shot, now what?* and *What's the score now?* Having access to saying *ready, set, go* will allow him to call the start of the miniature car races with his cousins. Quick phrases give Diego a way to participate easily and enthusiastically in everyday events and environments. The vocabulary is broad enough to serve the purposes of his social interaction and social etiquette, sharing information, wants and needs, and expressing his inner language as a unique person. Diego, like other children, increases his understanding of various meanings and usage of words that are simply a way to get started with communication and strengthened his and others' motivation.

⊙ Questions for reflection

Section 5 Vocabulary: What vocabulary did Diego need for participation?

1   Match the four purposes of communication with Diego's vocabulary words and quick messages?

Purposes of Communication	Getting Started Words and Phrases
a Social closeness	1 _____ He missed that shot, now what?
b Social etiquette	2 _____ Come be with me; I want to be alone
c Sharing information	3 _____ Spicy food, hip pain, movie choices, activity choices
d Wants and needs	4 _____ Hi; Goodbye; Thanks for talking with me.

2   Diego's motivation of selecting initial vocabulary would include all EXCEPT which one of the following:
   a   Accessing only the words the adults want him to say
   b   Expressing his likes and dislikes, feelings, and preferences
   c   Inviting others engage in greetings and sharing information about sports
   d   Knowing others will repeat vocabulary to confirm his intent

Answers

1   1=c Sharing information: He missed that shot, now what?
    2=a Social closeness: Come be with me; I want to be alone.
    3=d. Wants and needs: Spicy food, movie choices, activity choices
    4=b Social etiquette: Hi; Goodbye; Thanks for talking with me
2   Letter a. is the exception to Diego's motivation for vocabulary comes from interactions with adults and children. Letters b., c., and d. are motivating for him to be able to express his likes and dislikes, feelings, and preferences. He knows he can rely on others to support his vocabulary choices so he can share his intent.

○ Section 6 Tools and access: What assistive communication tools have helped Diego get started with participating at school?

The more the team listens, the more they see Diego's actions, and the more they find ways for him to respond. Diego is alert to participation. Diego is motivated by being with peers, however, his expressive language is limited to vocalizations. They rule out teaching Diego braille because of his limited physical dexterity and sensitivity to touch. The speech-language pathologist suggests the Ablenet BigMack© speech generating device that is easily programmable in the moment to match the communication need. It can have a line drawing or photo symbol icon along with the words or phrases on top or at the bottom of each icon. Rodriguez suggests his friend Riley record the greeting, *Hey, what's up?* to generate a more authentic experience. The next day Rodriguez mounts the device on his wheelchair tray and they start greeting many friends each day with Rodriguez supporting Diego at the elbow to get to the speech generating device. As Diego gets off the bus, Rodriguez reminds him of the greeting they will practice with a student. Rodriguez pushes Diego's wheelchair along the school corridor. He coaches Diego to raise his hand and presses the BigMack© when he hears another student go by. However, when Diego attempts to use the device independently the child had passed Diego by. So much for a motivating greeting this morning! Now what? One of the team members decides to look for a *light touch* switch that will allow Diego to respond more quickly. They find the Ablenet Microlight Switch© requires only .4 ounce of pressure, compared to the 5.5 ounces needed to activate the BigMack©. Success. Two students hurrying along to their classroom looked up. One stops, looks at Diego, and says, *hi.* Diego responds, *Hey, what's up?* Then his classmate says to his friend walking along beside him, *See, he knows me.*

Diego's inclusion specialist observed Diego thrive when he used a head switch to drive a toy car and decides to transfer that skill to music. She set up the radio with the switch attached between his headrest and the radio. The specialist recalls to her delight, *Within seconds he pressed the switch with his head. There is a whole lot of real control going on. And we were just floored!* When they asked Diego to play the music again, he sat quietly with not a single hint of movement. He did not smile. He did not turn his head to find the switch, nor did he even make a sound with his voice. After about 20 more minutes, the desperate but determined speech-language pathologist who had been watching with some degree of frustration, interrupted, and jokingly said, *Ok, Diego I will dance when you turn your head to play the music.* Diego's eyes brightened and within much less than a half of a second, Diego smiled, moved his head, hit the switch, and the music started playing. The speech-language pathologist begin her dance. The inclusion specialist, Rodriguez, the speech-language pathologist, and his favorite classmates see the big smile on Diego's face and they laugh out loud. He knows what to do. That is participation. That is fun.

Questions for Reflection

Section 6 Tools and Access: What assistive communication tools have helped Diego get started with participating at school?

1   Rank the questions 1–4 that the team answered to select the first AAC tool for Diego.
    a   _____ How will he access a speech generating device like the BigMack©?
    b   _____ How will adding an icon, line drawing or photo, and words or phrases on the icons make his communication more meaningful?
    c   _____ How much pressure will he need to get the switch to speak his message?
    d   _____ Based on Diego's interaction and participation with peers and adults, what messages and device will match his communicative situation?

2   Circle words within the parenthesis that best complete the sentences about Diego's AAC tools and devices.
    a   The child's lack of use (is/is not) a sign of rejecting/ignoring a message that has no meaning for him.
    b   Building upon the child's (strengths/weaknesses) (e.g. auditory, visual, tactile, kinesthetic, gustatory) leads to the greater communication.
    c   Deciding on approaches to assistive communication needed to be (fun/punishment) because communication is most satisfying as a (two-way street/dead end/one-way performance) with partners.

Answers

1   The rank order is d =1, a =2, c =3, b =4
    Diego's educational team makes careful decisions recognizing that each step is important starting with what messages Diego needs to express and then decides on the required tools and devices, access, and best way to represent language. What is really important is that the team keeps asking questions and seeking answers.

2   The words within the parenthesis that best complete the sentences about Diego's AAC tools and devices are the following.
    a   The child's lack of use is not a sign of rejecting or ignoring a message that has no meaning for him. Diego was not rejecting AAC, he was looking for motivation.
    b   Building upon the child's strengths (e.g. auditory, visual, tactile, kinesthetic, gustatory) leads to greater communication. Diego's family and education team build upon his sensory strengths in providing assistive communication.
    c   Deciding on approaches to assistive communication need to be motivating because communication is most satisfying as a two-way street with partners. Communication partners influencing the other based on a motivation that may not always be fun but is necessary, needed, or wanted.

Case Study Closing Thoughts

Getting Started with participation and communication for Diego includes his family and educational team who acknowledge his preferences and unique expressions after his traumatic brain injury due to a near drowning incident. His family and educators learn, watch, and listen to detail his social interaction skill. They nurture an extraordinary relationship with him in Spanish and English about movies and race cars, wet dogs on beds, spicy Mexican food and eggs, reading and drawing, hearing stories and acting them out. They identify opportunities to incorporate strategies to promote Diego's attention and interaction with peers and his academic program at school. Not limiting his verbal messages to greetings but finding a way to share information about hearing his favorite music and beginning reading and writing to construct his own messages allow others to experience his unique personality. The team learns to match AAC tools and devices to the situation to give him a voice along with reading his facial expressions and movement. This process of discovery became a delight, a novel experience where creativity and knowledge combined to see into who Diego is and support his development. His most successful communication partners recognize that participation is invigorating. They said about communication, *If we are having fun, Diego is having fun too. Look, his eyes are smiling too.* His mother and interventionists hold high expectations of Diego. His mother noted, *Our children who are dear to us, teach us the wonder of life and joy of achievement. They teach us unending patience and perseverance even as we feel and fill ourselves with self-doubt and puzzlement. They do not give up, and neither can we.*

Getting Started with communication activities

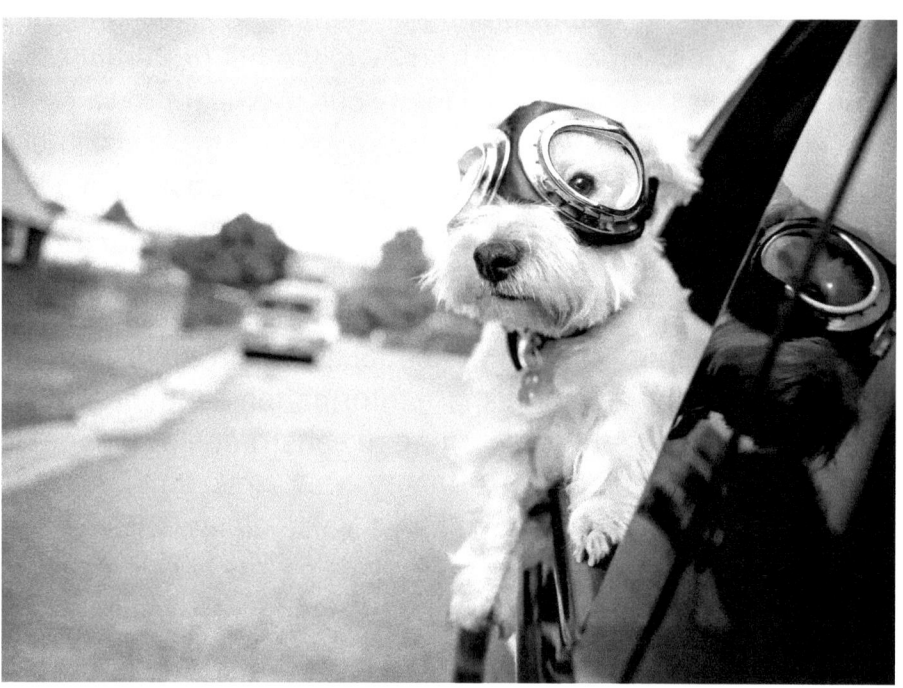

○ Motivation

Getting Started with communication activities is about awareness of communication in everyday events and routines and not about adding to your already busy schedule. Keep in mind that we will always want to monitor the status of joint attention in order to maximize communication opportunities and communication participation. Start playing; have fun! Start incorporating; teach routines. Use the communication activities to let interaction happen. Recognize and create communication opportunities.

The activity pages include vocabulary recommendations. Vocabulary represented as images and words for an AAC communication boards are symbols of language, often called icons, that are printed on paper and used to represent objects and ideas. Symbols on speech generating devices are programmed images and words, often called buttons. Your child may need to establish symbolic understanding. For a child learning symbol association for the first time, use an identical object for the child to reach or point to and then the child will receive the identical object. Transition the child from an exact copy of an object to a photo of the object to a generalized image of the object. For example, a line drawing with or without color, may represent an *orange*. It may be necessary to use a transitional object such as a part of an object or a mini object to help the child understand that one item represents the desired object. Think about the least cognitive demand that is put on your child to learn the symbolic understanding. Often times the best transition is from the exact object representing the exact desired object to a picture. In the case of a child with a vision impairment, the use of a miniature object serves as a tactile choice. As the child's symbolic understanding emerges, expose your child to two choices. To drive home understanding that the symbol represents an object include the preferred item and a non-preferred item. The non-preferred item will increase the child's attention to the symbols especially if your child receives a tissue instead of their favorite action figure. Use the vocabulary offered in each activity as a guide. Starting with one icon is fine! Build to two icons when your child can discriminate between two symbols to make an intentional choice. Build to the number of icons that works best for your child. Investigate Project Core from the Center for Literacy and Disability Studies at www.project-core.com free resources and educational guidance about universal core vocabulary for children *Getting Started* with communication. Explore the number of vocabulary apps and products as a marvelous way to guide decision making. The range of vocabulary readiness will vary for each child. Focus on successes, your child's communication, and participation. Enjoy.

Communication activities

1 Get into the Rhythm
2 Art Time Descriptors
3 Let's Get Moving
4 Ready, Set, Activate, Go!
5 Balls, Helicopters, Blocks, Bubbles, and More
6 Puzzle Time!
7 Flashlight Play
8 Walkabout

Activity: Get Into the Rhythm

A place to start

Music and rhyme: What a glorious place to start! Music is fun which means it engages the senses of our body, our brain. Music registers emotionally and physically. It calms and excites. Music can be an independent and a shared experience with the opportunity to experience the rhythm of melody with or without language. Nursery rhymes are the perfect *Getting Started* balance of literacy and song, fun and form, mind and body interaction with others. Poetry is a marvelous form of rhyme for older children! Download a poetry application or complete a quick internet search. Participation with music is implied through dancing, movement, and signing. Use music and rhyme as an opportunity for your child to participate with you, peers, and others.

- Sing to and with your child
- Read or listen to poetry
- Play recorded songs on a disc, tape, radio, internet, or other devices
- Use video as a visual support of eye contact and body movement with songs
- Point out music played in the background in the community in stores and other places

Communication partner: what I am doing with my child

Singing songs and reading rhyming poems or stories with your child engages your child's mind and body. Add physical movement to music by putting your or your child's arms down and up, out and in, over the head, and across the chest to open up the air way and encourage vocalizations and teach concepts. Use the same routine each time you sing a song to teach predictability. Notice how the child responds and give words to the child's feelings and emotions (e.g. excited, calm, irritated).

My Tool Box

- Phone, car radio, TV, tablet or other device, sounds in the environment, internet sources

- Make the nursery rhyme visual using media or a board book, print outs of the nursery rhyme including words, follow along in the pages of the rhyme in poetry

- Sing the song to the child and turn pages to the book pointing to each word of the story

- After reading the nursery rhyme, act out the nursery rhyme with actions

- Ask your child what they want to do again, reading or acting out the nursery rhyme

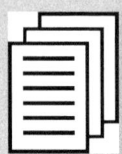

What my child is doing with me

My child is having fun with songs and rhyme, connecting sounds of language and rhythm with movement. The movements stimulate the mechanism we use to speak including *respiration* (breathing and control), *phonation* or making sound, *resonation* of sound through our body, and *articulation* of sounds all while singing songs. Use the vocabulary below to connect music and rhyme to communicative intent by giving, pointing, and showing icons. Create visual supports using pictures from stories that can be made into icons. Your child makes choices from icons to choose music or a rhyme, use eye gaze to see and follow each word on the page, point with the appropriate physical support at the shoulder, elbow, hand or finger.

Vocabulary targets for nursery rhymes

I pick	I go	You pick	Again	Sing	Read	Dance
Act it out	Yes	No	All done	Look	Break	Help

Nursery rhyme options: Where is Thumbkin?; Mary Had a Little Lamb; Itsy Bitsy Spider; Jack & Jill; Row, Row, Row Your Boat; Hey Diddle Diddle; Little Miss Muffet; Humpty Dumpty

Poetry options: Poems for Kids (2019) https://poets.org/poems-kids; Ken Nesbitt's Poetry 4 Kids www.poetry4kids.com/

Activity: Art Time!

A place to start

Blades of grass and fallen leaves can be shaped and taped or glued onto paper in the image of a house, a cat, or a car. Shred and reshape pages of magazines and fliers into objects. Creativity through art activities is fun. It is a safe place for success and many *oops* opportunities (e.g. oops too much glue, oops the wind blew our leaves away). It is a fun time to make choices, give commands, and follow commands for materials, and explore concepts such as color, texture, size, shapes, quantity ... and laugh when the wind blows your project awry.

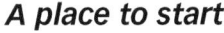 What sounds like fun to you will likely be fun for your child too! A great rule of thumb, *If I am having fun, then the child is having fun. – Dr. Mayne*

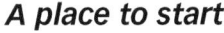 Use materials you have inside your home or available outside in the environment as tools

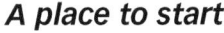 It is okay to start a project and finish it later

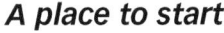 Find a way around any barrier to make communication, interaction, participation, and the craft fun. Or . . . have fun and you will find a way around any barrier

Communication partner: what I am doing with my child

A child with a complex communication profile may have physical limitations in accessing and using art supplies to make crafts independently but that will not stop you. Children love the creative process. Teach the child to use and expand on communication modalities such as using a smile to make a choice. Learn to differentiate between a smile that represents a choice, a response to an internal state (e.g. smile during or after a seizure), and joy. Encourage these communication options with your child including smiling, eye gaze, head placement or movement in a direction, pointing to the object (e.g. a pen, a brush) or an icon on a choice board, vocalizing, word imitation given sign language (e.g. want, stop, again), word imitation given a verbalization or speech generating device, word approximation, verbalizing through voice or a speech generating device.

My Tool Box

- Scissors, glue, tacky glue, hole punch, crayons, paint, markers, twisty ties
- Construction paper, paper, mail flyers, magazines
- Pom-poms, pipe cleaners, waxy string, googly eyes
- Fallen leaves, blades of grass, sticks, and pebbles

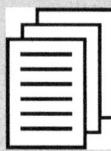

What my child is doing with me

- ◉ I can make a choice for what we will make today using a communication modality such as my eyes, a communication board, a single or multimessage speech generating device
- ◉ I can make a choice for materials to be used using a communication modality
- ◉ I can comment on how much fun I am having and when I am done

Vocabulary targets for art time

More	Keep going	That one	Yes	No	All Done
Stop	I want a different choice				

Activity: Ready! Set! Activate and Go!

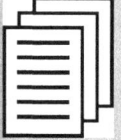

A place to start

Time for battery operated toys! Time for battery adapters! Time for a switch! When we are Getting Started with play, we want our children to have fun and recognize they caused an effect on others or the environment. For children with physical impairments and complex communication profiles, access to motion based toys is usually experienced by watching or hearing others play. Let's get the play into the control of the child! Using switch activated toys gives children an active part in participation and communication by moving battery operated toys such as toys that move and/or make animal sounds, setting cars off to head down a ramp, activating a spinner for musical toys, coloring and painting toys, and many others. Look into switch toys at *Ablenet, Adaptive Tech Solutions, Beyond Play, Enabling Devices, Enablemart, Flag House, Special Needs Toys*, and *Rehab Mart* to get you started.

Communication partner: what I am doing with my child

You are showing your child that he or she can cause an effect on something else and control the experience. You are helping the child put language to the emotional experience, promoting joint attention, building reciprocity through turn taking, and commenting on the experience. Consider having more than one switch accessible toy available for choice making. Expand the environments where you play with the child such as the park or backyard in addition to indoor play so the child learns to accommodate for different environmental sounds, lights, temperatures, and hopefully play partners.

⊙ My Tool Box

- ◉ Battery operated toys
- ◉ Battery adapter for AA/A and or C/D batteries
- ◉ Communication switch adapter, Bluetooth switch
- ◉ A communication board or speech generating device for commenting

What my child is doing with me

- ◉ I can request to play with a switch activated toy from a choice board of activities
- ◉ I can ask for a turn
- ◉ I can say about whose turn it is
- ◉ I can talk about how the toy is fun, silly, or scary
- ◉ I can make comments in exclamation such as *yeah* or *oh no* my toy fell over/stopped

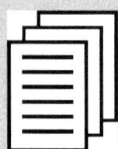

Vocabulary targets for Ready! Set! Activate and Go!

My turn	Yeah	Again	This is fun!
Your turn	Oh no	Stop	This toy is scary!

The following list represents selected companies that sell accessible toys.

- Ablenet www.ablenet.com
- Adaptive Tech Solutions www.adaptivetechsolutions.com
- Beyond Play www.beyondplay.com
- Enablemart www.enablemart.com
- Enabling Devices www.enablingdevices.com
- Flag House www.flaghouse.com
- Special Needs Toys www.specialneedstoys.com
- RehabMart www.rehabmart.com

Activity: Balls, Helicopters, Blocks, Bubbles, and More

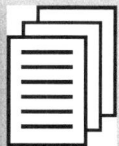

A place to start

Get to the basics of play. Engaging in play with balls is fun. Let's face it, some people make millions of dollars playing ball. Remember what Yoder (2001) says, *You are not too anything to acquire communicative competence.* You are also never too young to play with balls, helicopters, blocks, and more. Let's add toy cars, motorcycles, airplanes, bubbles, and whatever else suits you and your child's fancy.

Communication partner: what I am doing with my child?

Consider the participation and communication possibilities! It is okay to hold your child's arm to motor the child through pushing, catching, flying, building, or blowing bubbles. Promote joint attention using eye contact and pausing for the child to ask for more to continue communication using nonverbal skills such as eye gaze, smiles, or body positioning. Use pausing to create the impetus for the child to communicate. Offer a nonverbal eye gaze or smile, a word approximation, a physical gesture, pointing to or exchanging an icon, or a voice output utterance from a speech generating device to prompt communication. Consider enlisting a family member, peer, or interventionist to either support the child physically as needed or model the play while the other person serves as the turn taking partner during the play. Feel free to have a number of different types of toys around to keep the activity interesting. You can always take the play into different environments such as different rooms of the home or clinic, outside of the home, into the park, in the car (excluding the driver of course) and any location that is conducive for play. Build upon the number of meaningful communication cycles of exchange (My Turn + My Child's Turn = 1 Cycle). Have fun with play, participation, and communication. Reinforce communication using comments such as, *You told me with your eyes that you want me to blow the bubbles. Now tell me another way. You can use your smile, your communication button, your activity choice board, or point!*

My Tool Box

- Balls: big, small, light, textured (Ask yourself if the size, weight, color, and texture is appropriate for your child)
- Toy vehicles: miniature cars, fire trucks, helicopters, airplanes, motorcycles, sport trucks, utility trucks (Ask yourself if the size and weight is appropriate for the child)
- Variety of different bubble wands from big to small
- A choice board of activities
- A communication board for commenting

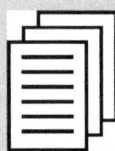

What my child is doing with me

- I can request a toy from a choice board of activities
- I can tell you to *go, fly*, or *push*
- I can tell you about whose turn it is
- I can ask for *more* or to *stop*
- I can request bubbles from a choice board of activities
- I can request the size of the bubbles I want to blow or want you to blow
- I can tell you about whose turn it is
- I can ask for you to blow bubbles again or to stop
- I can say I want the bubbles bigger or smaller

Vocabulary targets for Balls, Helicopters, Blocks, Bubbles, and More

| Push | My turn | Go | More | Open | Blow | Again | Bigger |
| Fly | Your turn | Stop | All done | Close | Pop | Oh no! | Smaller |

Vocabulary choice board-specific interests and activities

Offer your child a choice board for specific activities your child enjoys like balls, helicopters, cars, and books. Consider action figures, light up toys, musical toys, and sensory toys.

Activity: Flashlight Play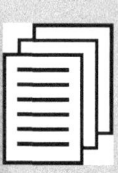

A place to start

Let's see what we can find! Collect a flashlight and create your own version of *I Spy*. Go into a room the child is familiar with and tell the child you will be using the flashlight to find objects, colors, sizes, and shapes. Comment on what they like or do not like. Turn the lights down or off or even keep them on if the child is scared of darkened rooms. Flashlight play is fun way to practice communication skills.

Communication partner: what I am doing with my child

Create a fun environment in which to play with language using light to create a contrast between objects. You can take turns with your child labeling and describing using a flashlight. You can model language expansion. If my child says, *Look!* You can respond with *Look, ball!* You may choose to use vocabulary words such as *look, that, go, stop*, core words that describe basic items in a room, or fringe words such as people's names seen in pictures, names of stuffed animals, or names of pets, and items that are important to your child.

⊙ My Tool Box

- ◎ Flashlight
- ◎ Environments to explore such as the child's room, play room, or outside
- ◎ Communication board for commenting with core board and fringe words

What my child is doing with me

- ◎ I can point the flashlight and my communication partner can tell me what I showed them. This will build my vocabulary and improve my joint attention
- ◎ I can use my communication board to ask a question
- ◎ I can use my communication board to make a comment

Vocabulary targets for Flashlight Play

What do you see?	My turn	Look	Again	No	Your turn	That	All done

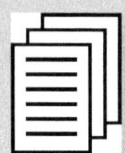

Activity: Puzzle Time!

A place to start

Puzzles are the perfect socio-relational and cognitive-linguistic task! Was that too much? Okay, let's try again. Puzzles are AWESOME! Puzzles are a time to show a social interest in others, building communication between people and engaging with objects (that is the socio-relational part). Build cognition, or thinking skills, addressing attention, memory, communication, and problem solving (that is the cognitive-linguistic part). Use inset puzzle boards, 2–4 item interlocking puzzle boards, or image puzzles that have the letters at the bottom such as a three-item puzzle of a whimsical cat with each letter of c-a-t on a different puzzle piece. My favorite way to play with puzzles, build pragmatic skills, and language is by playing *shopkeeper*. The communication partner keeps the pieces and the child can point, vocalize, hand an icon or use a switch to say for example, *That one!* The *shopkeeper* hands the child the piece and provides the appropriate amount of physical and/or verbal support. All that great learning wrapped up in a fun, usually colorful and interactive puzzle.

Communication partner: what I am doing with my child

I am building attention skills by pointing out each piece and using short sentences with words my child can or will come to understand. I can point out whole relationships using an inset puzzle highlighting the shape of the piece and its corresponding location on the board. I can point out part to whole relationships for example pointing out the shoe of the boy goes on the bottom and matching up the part of the shape to the shaped space on the board. Talk about shapes and colors and sizes and names of the parts and of the whole of the puzzle of your choice.

My Tool Box

- Inset puzzles have piece in which one piece fits into one space (e.g. the whole bird puzzle piece is set in the whole bird shape space, the cow shaped piece is placed in the whole cow shape space)

- Interlocking puzzles have pieces that fit together to make an image using 2-4-6-8 or more puzzle pieces. Puzzles with fewer piece are fine to start with. Fewer pieces may help establish success with construction, build language skills, and promote social skills such as turn taking and eye contact

- A communication board for commenting with core words and additional boards with descriptor words for colors, shapes, and sizes

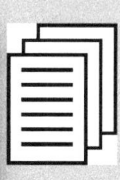

What my child is doing with me

- My child is connecting language while having fun with a puzzle and building cognitive problem-solving skills
- My child is learning to connect to a communication partner while selecting or placing puzzles pieces or giving directions to others for placing puzzle pieces
- I can say what I see on the image nonverbally by using my head, face, or body, vocally, a word approximation, or verbally using a word, or a speech generating device

Vocabulary targets for Puzzles

That one	My turn	Your Turn	Look	Yes	No
Put it there	Move it down	That	No	Move it up	

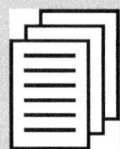

Activity: Walkabout!

A place to start

Let's take communication outside! Go on a walkabout. Okay you do not need to go to Australia, although if you can, that would be advisable! What you can do is take your opportunity for communication outside of your home, school, or clinic. Sometimes people think the idea of integrating language and communication can only be completed indoors at a tabletop but getting outside provides us with some fresh air and a way to practice communication skills. So where can you start? Head out the door of whatever building you are in and head down the path, road, or sidewalk.

Communication partner: what I am doing with my child

Head outside with communication and physical access for your child. Take or attach a communication board, a card ring, or a speech generating device using a mount so the child can comment on the environment. If the best physical access is a wheelchair or stroller, then great. Think about what the child can communicate. The child can talk about when you walk and when you stop. The leaves, grass, stones, tree trunks, and flowers provide your child a chance to explore and be surprised! Talk about textures such as *soft, bumpy, rough*, and *smooth*. Talk about size (e.g. big as your hand, little as your fingernail) and quantity. Consider collecting leaves and sticks. Bring tape and paper. Tape the sticks and leaves onto the paper making a rocket or house. Consider using a multi-message device to state messages such as, *Let's go. Wait. Touch.* Add vocabulary such as *leaf, grass, stone, tree, flower*.

My Tool box

- Stroller, wheelchair, or other forms of physical support
- Hat, sunglasses, sun lotion or jackets other forms of protection given the weather
- A communication board, a card ring
- Velcro® or straps to attach communication tools or devices
- Single or multi-message speech generating device
- Tape, glue, paper, construction paper
- A communication board for commenting
- A choice board for colors, shapes, and sizes

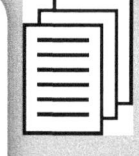

What my child is doing with me

Your child can give commands on the walk by saying, *Let's go!* or *Wait*. Your child can request to *touch* and talk about the textures. Provide commenting opportunities to state *that* or *look. I like that* (e.g. the rock, leaf, or blade of grass), or, *Put that down*. For fun, make a picture from the sticks, leaves, and blades of grass during the walkabout.

Vocabulary targets for a Walkabout!

Let's go	Touch	Feel	Look	I like that
Wait	More	That	Yuck	Put that down

Getting Started with facilitator strategies

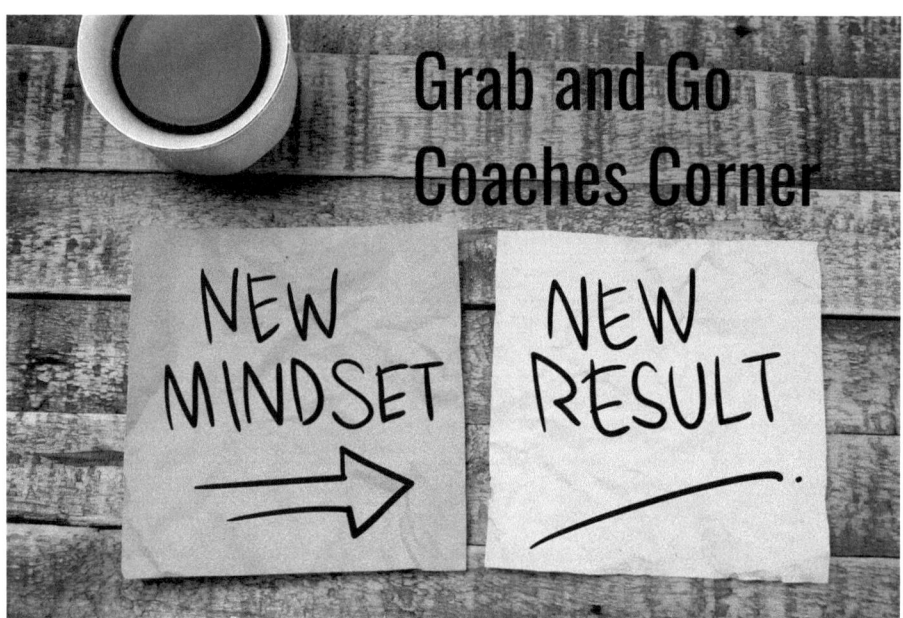

O Grab and Go Coaches' Corner

Getting Started with communication is a multi-person task. We learn language and participation by interacting with other adults and peers. Research shows the more responsiveness and reciprocity communication partners have with children the more children's language skills will increase (Brady, Thiemann-Bourque, Fleming & Matthews, 2013; Donaldson & Stahmer, 2014; Lund & Light, 2007; Woods, Wetherby, Kashinath & Holland, 2012). This starts with joint attention and leads straight into using attention to be aware of other people and their intentions and objects and their functions. Research also tells us that children with communication impairments are spoken to less than typically developing children and for fewer communication purposes such as making choices and sharing information (Johnston, Reichle & Evans, 2004; Lund & Light, 2007). Use the *Grab and Go Coaches' Corner Facilitator Tips* to expose and promote language skills for our children just Getting Started with communication.

Topics:

1 Getting Started with Routines
2 Working with the Theory of Natural Consequences
3 Understanding What My Child Needs to Know in Order to Say *Yes* or *No*
4 AAC Communication Tip Card
5 Tips for Modeling Language
   a   Modeling Expressive Language with AAC
   b   Modeling Receptive Language with AAC
6 Communication Temptations! Creating Opportunities for Communication

7   I Can Offer Choices!
8   Comment More, Question Less
9   How Many Turns Can We Take?

○ *Facilitator decision making tips and steps in* Getting Started *with communication*

1 *Getting everyone started with routines*

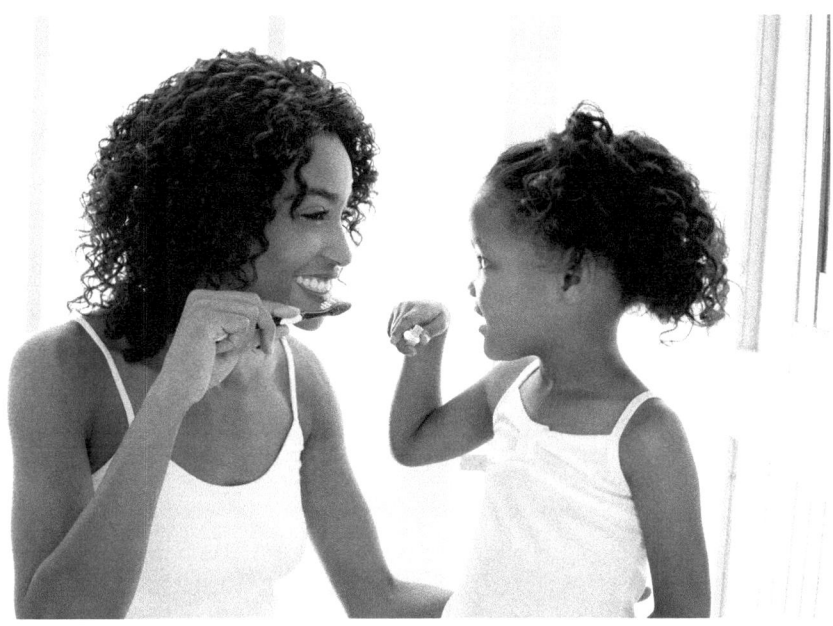

Identify opportunities for communication in daily routines such as dressing, cooking, cleaning, bath time, riding in the car, going to the store, playing in the park or yard, participating in art classes, joining sport teams, watching sports or events, or anything! Make routines visual with a low-tech picture schedule with braille for vision impairment or use technology that may include auditory messages. Start with one routine to establish success!

Do: Pick a routine that works for you, your schedule, and your child

Do: Pick a routine that you can incorporate a communication tool or device

Do: Pick one thing the child can comment on or request

Do: Check to make sure that you child is able to complete the steps or demands of the routine

Do: Check to make sure that your child is able and understands what he or she can and will communicate within the routine

Do: Be willing to ask yourself what may help make the interaction more successful. Enlist interventionists to talk through ways to adjust the words or situations

Don't: Add one more thing to an already busy moment that may deter your motivation to continue to help your child communicate. Remember to create an opportunity for success

Generate three picture sequences of daily routines such as a play activity using real pictures of your child and belongings or images your child understands. Then select a sequence for playing or regulating the length of play such as 1) I choose a toy, 2) I request *more*, 3) I state, *all done*. Monitor how many steps your child can attend to or can be directed through. Certainly, the play sequence can be expanded many ways. It is okay to start with a few pictures that provide discrete steps. Add more language to the cards as appropriate. For example, the *more* picture could say, *I want more*.

2 *Working with the theory of natural consequences*

The theory of natural consequences states that if a child makes a choice, the communication partner follows through in providing the child with the choice even if the communication partner thinks the child made a mistake. It is important that your child is aware of the choices, has an opinion about the choice, makes a choice, and knows that you the communication partner will follow through with the request even if it is to opposite of what you think it should be or is a mistake. The communication partner can provide the child with another opportunity to make a different choice. The following scenario and examples illustrate the point of the Theory of Natural Consequences.

Scenario: You can see our client Ella does not want ice cream today. Her communication partner Brooke knows Ella well including choices she is likely to make. Therefore, it would be natural for Brooke to give Ella what she knows she likes rather than what Ella actually requests using AAC such as pointing or reaching for the picture icons. Read the following poor example. Then read the good example and see how the theory of Natural Consequences supports a child in learning that communicative intent matters.

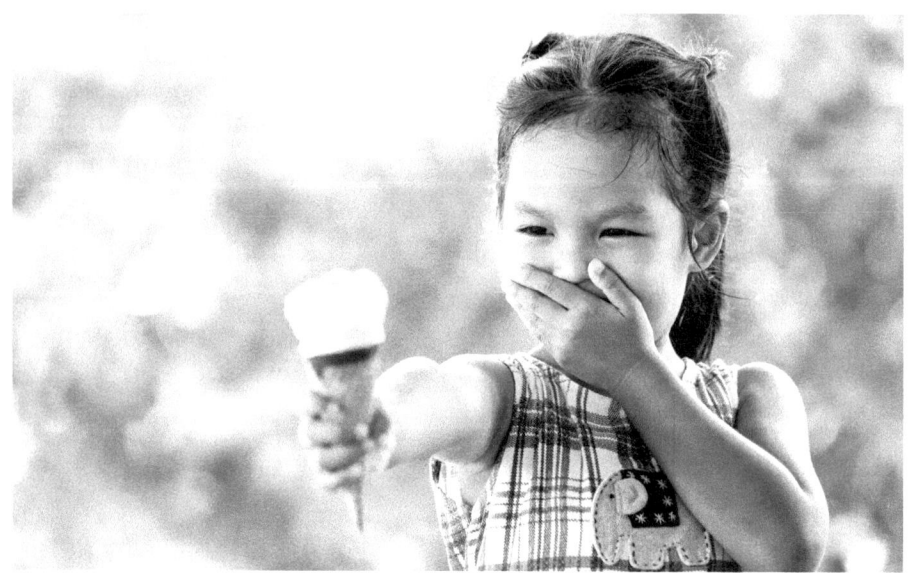

Brooke and child Ella:

Poor Example of Employing the Theory of Natural Consequences for Communication

- Brooke says, *Ella, do you want ice cream or a cookie?*
- Ella points to an icon of the cookie.
- Brooke thinks Ella wants the ice cream because she always picks ice cream. Brooke gives Ella ice cream and not the cookie.
- Ella gets a treat that she likes but does not learn that her choice matters.

Good Example of Employing the Theory of Natural Consequences for Communication

- Brooke says, *Do you want the ice cream or the cookie?*
- Ella looks at the cookie icon.
- Brooke says, *You want the cookie*.
- Brooke gives Ella the cookie.
- Note: If Ella protests, she is given another opportunity to make a choice. Maybe today Ella wants a cookie.

3 Understanding what my child needs to know in order to say yes or no

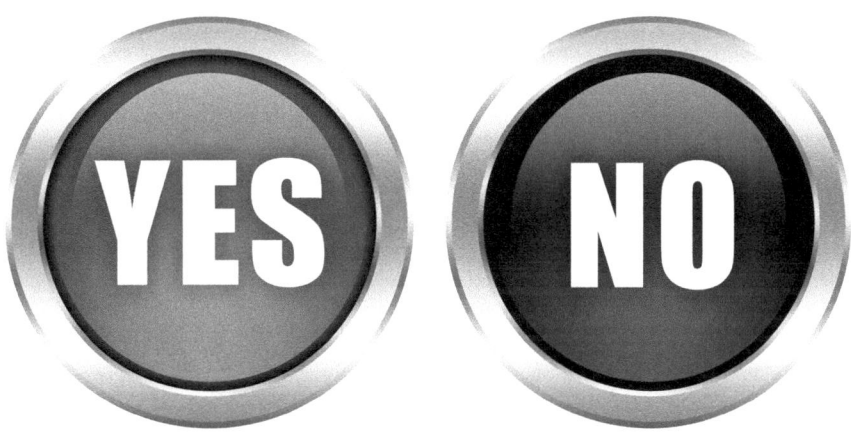

Saying *Yes* or *No* seems like a simple enough of a task, but wait a minute, take a look at all of the steps it takes to actually state *Yes* or *No.*

- The child needs to have the opportunity to say *yes* or *no*
- The child needs to have one or more ways to say *yes* or *no* (e.g. nonverbal, verbal, communication board, static or dynamic speech generating device)
- The child needs to know the difference between the options
- The child needs to have a preference
- The child needs to remember what choice was made
- The child must know the choice made will be acknowledged and acted upon using the Theory of Natural Consequences

4 AAC communication tip card

Talk with Me Tips!

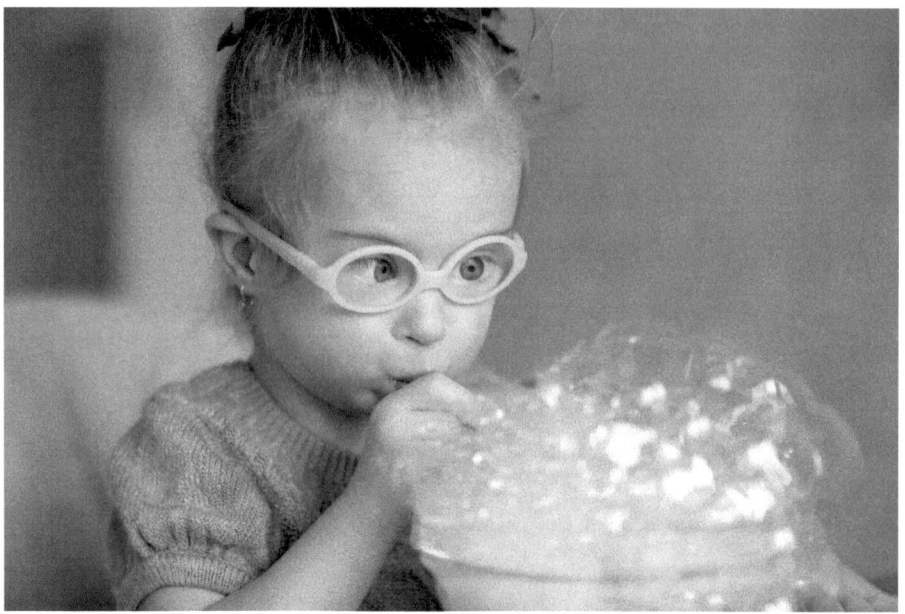

I show you I understand when I...

- Smile
- Squeeze your finger
- Look into your eyes
- Shake my head to say *no*
- Talk with my speech generating device

Create a 4x6 or 5x7 card with information about how your child communicates. Include information such as the following and as appropriate for your child.

- I am 10 years old, so please feel free to talk to me like you would any 10-year-old kid.
- I understand everything you say. *Or* I understand short sentences.
- Give me three choices to answer your question.
- I like to talk about photography, what people like to do, and movies.
- I would like to hear about what you like to do . . . what have you been up to lately?

Place a few pictures on the card. Consider placing a photo of the child on the card. Consider one or two images of the child engaging in fun with peers or a situation that would provide a good topic for starting a conversation with the child. Then, laminate the card or put it in a zip lock bag and hang it from string on a wheelchair, an AAC device, or anywhere a communication partner will be likely to see it.

5 Tips for modeling language

We can model language two ways, expressively and receptively. Ask yourself two questions. 1) Expressive language: What do I want my child to say? 2) Receptive language: How do I want my child to know and express comprehension of my message or messages from peers and other adults? Use the ideas offered next and adjust them to meet the communication goal for your child. This means you need to know what the goals are. Visit or revisit your child's intervention goals as needed. Everyone needs a refresher now and again. Ask for clarification if necessary.

- Determine the purpose of communication you want your child to express (i.e. social greeting, social etiquette, sharing information, a want or need) or understand (e.g. nouns, verbs, phrases, etc.).
- Provide your child with one or more communication modalities. Identify if a gesture or sign language would express the message. Employ a communication board, card ring, single message or multimessage speech generating device.
- Model the intended message so your child can hear your words, see the motor plan or steps, and feel the gestures or signs you used to generate the message. You may support your child with physical prompts to indicate the sequence and reduce the level of prompting to increase independence as skills are learned.
- Remember to model at least one modality, but ideally two or three modalities. Learning to express a message across modalities gives your child greater independence and options for expression under different circumstances. For example, your child can use a speech generating device to voice the message, *hello*, wave to say *hi* to a child across the yard, or point to an icon with an image with the word *hi* on a communication board or other tool.
  a   Modeling Expressive Language
      Talk about what the child is doing, smelling, seeing, touching, tasting, and experiencing with people and the situation. As the child comments, state what the child has communicated (e.g. *Hey I see your smile that told me you liked that picture, or you just told me with your eyes that you noticed that bird that just flew by*). Reinforcing the child's communication lets your child know the message resonated with you.

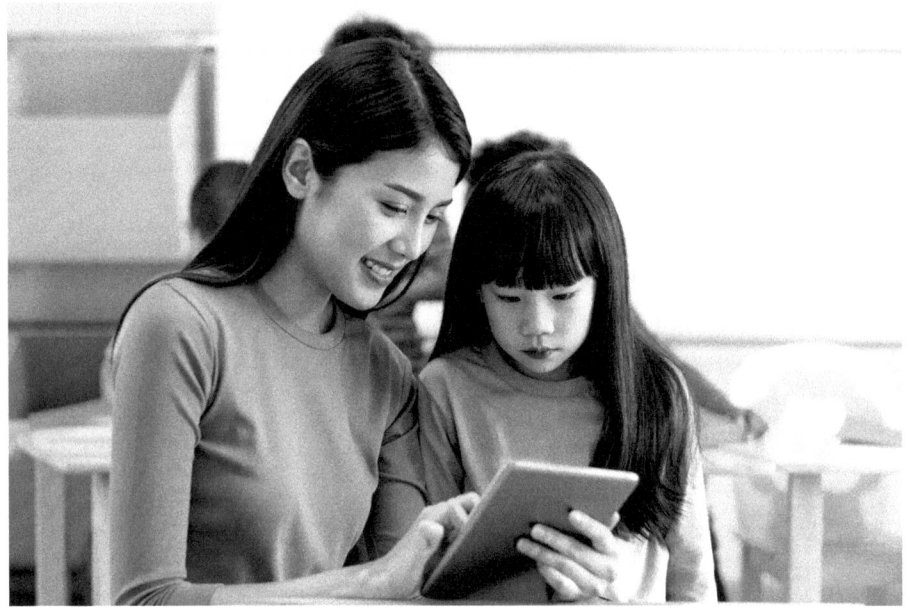

b Modeling the Use of Gestures, Sign Language, Communication Boards and Speech Generating Devices to Build Your Child's Receptive Language

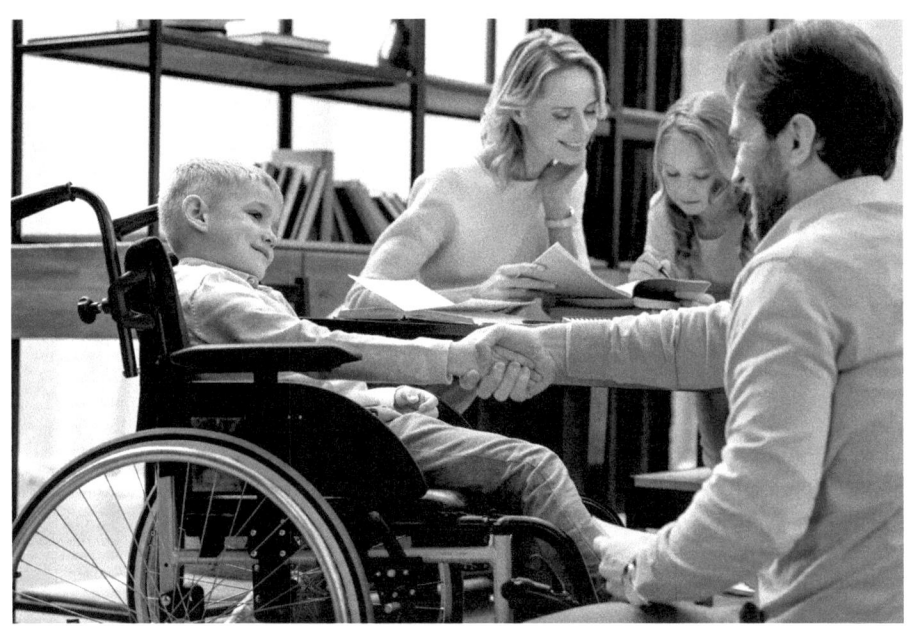

Here is your opportunity to talk to your child with the purpose of explicitly showing your child how to formulate language. Use complete sentences to talk about the bird you see *flying up to the trees* and the *big round ball that is bouncing across the grass*. Decide how much language would be appropriate for your child to be exposed to receptively understand your message. Explain a little more of what the child is seeing, feeling, hearing, experiencing. Monitor your language matching the receptive language level of the child (e.g. If you both saw and acknowledge the presence of a bird, you can model the word, *bird*, or *blue bird*, or *The bird is flying*. Feel free to expand your language to help your child's language grow but monitor your child's receptive language abilities. Comment on what you see as you walk around outside like the clouds in the sky. Comment on your actions and the actions of others. Comment on what you hear. Comment on emotions you see and feel with in others. As you comment, model language using your child's communication boards or speech generating devices.

6 Communication temptation! Creating opportunities for communication

Communication temptations and environmental sabotage are strategies designed to elicit a response from your child to continue or complete an activity. For example, you may 'forget' a step in a process in order to increase expectancy and elicit communication in the form of eye gaze or verbal expression. Try some of these communication temptation strategies. Praise the types of communication modalities the child uses (e.g. *You said, 'keep going' with your eyes! Here we go.*)

Communication temptation strategy

- Pausing: Insert wait time when normally there would be no wait time. For example, fly a toy airplane, stop, and wait for a request to continue. Work with crafts, pause, and wait for a message to *keep cutting, keep gluing, keep painting* programmed on a single message speech generating device.
- Withholding access: Retaining access to toys, food, or any desired object until a request has been made. For example, keep toys up on a shelf for child to request. Post icons of snack choices on the cupboard for your child to make a request.
- Feign confusion: Pretend you forgot a step or steps to complete next. For example, require the child cue you to take the cap off the bubble bottle. Forget how to turn on a blender.
- Expand descriptions: When a child gives a request, ask for further information/ probing. For example, *You want the ball*. Pretend you do not know which ball or which toy to choose from. *Do you want the blue ball or the red ball?*

7 Dive into making choices!

I can ask questions, offer two to three choices, and model answers about daily routines, stories, and play activities. Look at the sample questions, options for offering choices, and activities to get you started.

- Sample questions: *Do you want rice or bread? Do you want your shirt on first or your pants? Do you want a bath book or bath crayons? Do you want to go to the park or play in the back yard? Do you want a book or a book on CD?*
- Choice options: Food. Crafts. Clothing. Which article of clothing will go on first? Choose an activity for car rides, activities to play with when visiting friends, or art tools
- Activities: Meals, getting dressed, bath/shower, transportation, visiting friends or family, playground, art, reading, bedtime, routines faith community activities, sports, clubs

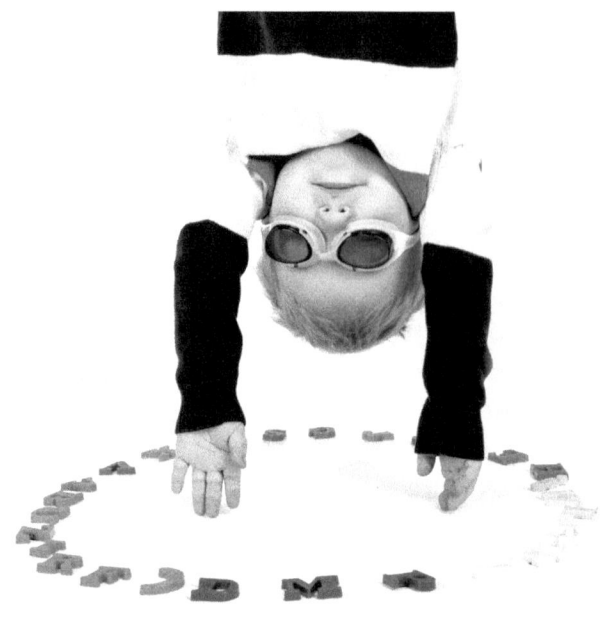

8 Comment more, question less

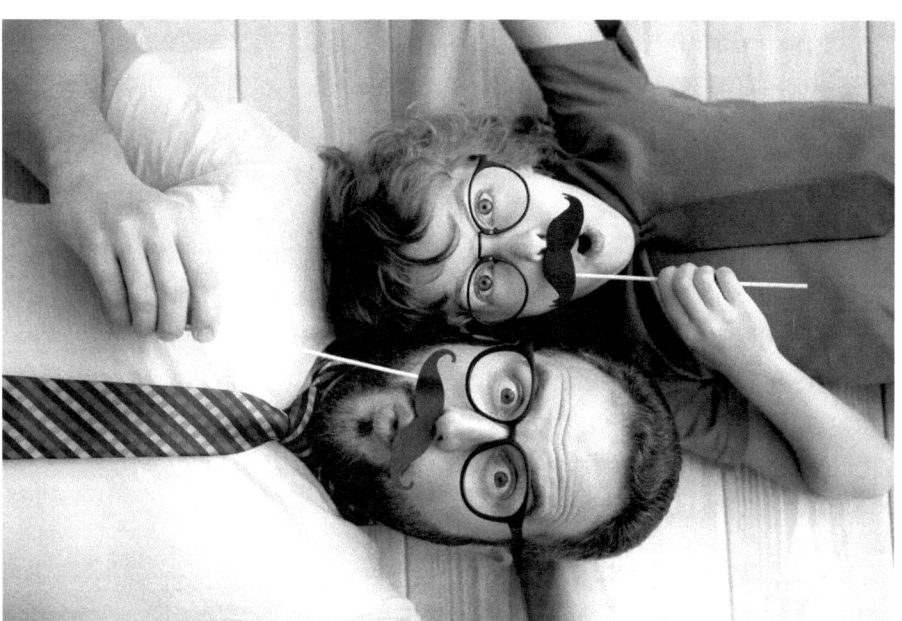

Comment more and question less is a fun way to talk *with* your child. Now that seems to make sense just fine. Let's talk about how. Try to limit the number of questions you ask. Instead take turns commenting on what you see, what you think, and what you feel. If your child needs support in commenting, offer a guided response that gives your child a springboard of ideas to work with to formulate an answer. It may be natural to follow up with a question to teach concepts at first and that is just fine. Work towards the idea that you can comment, and your child can comment. It puts you and the child in a world of commenting and sharing rather than questioning and answering. Here are a few ideas for commenting more and questioning less:

Question or Comment	Comment with a Guided Response	Outcomes Gained from Questions and Comments
1 Let's talk about what we see. You can go first, or I can go first.	1 I see a hat on the man. Your turn.	1 Literacy: book reading, looking at a magazine, looking at a scene in a nature
2 Let's talk about what we hear.	2 I heard the bird. You heard a bird too! Let's keep going.	2 Senses explored in the environment, vocabulary
3 Let's take turns turning the pages.	4 Let's take turns turning the pages.	4 Turn taking with the task involved in the activity
4 I will tell you how I feel about the birds flying then you tell me what you feel.	6 I want the bird to come back. Your turn. I want to see them fly backwards! Ha ha!	6 Expressing personal feelings and emotions
5 What else can we make fly? You find something and I will too.	7 I will pick the spaceship. You can pick the helicopter, plane, or make the book fly.	7 Enlarging categorical vocabulary category of what flies?

9 How many turns can we take?

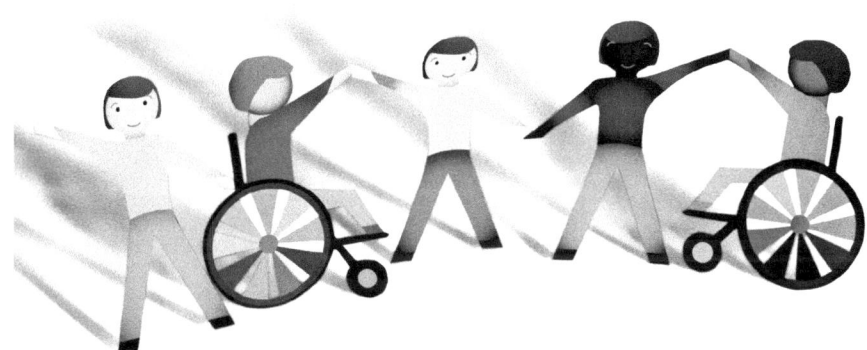

How many turns we take in a conversation helps us connect with each other and actions. It keeps a topic going. It improves our attention, memory, and motivation. It allows us more time to use and comprehend nonverbal gestures with or without communication boards or tools and verbal language expressed orally or with speech generating devices. See how many turns you and your child can take across different activities that involve communication. One cycle equals your turn and your child's turn. Choose an activity. Five options are noted but feel free to use activities or routines unique to you and your child. Note the number of cycles you and your child complete and celebrate them as you go!

1 Interactive game (e.g. peek-a-boo, ball roll/toss)
2 Commenting on images in a book or magazine
3 Pointing at things you see in the environment
4 Taking turns in playing a game or puzzle
5 Taking turns in pretend play

Getting Started with developing literacy

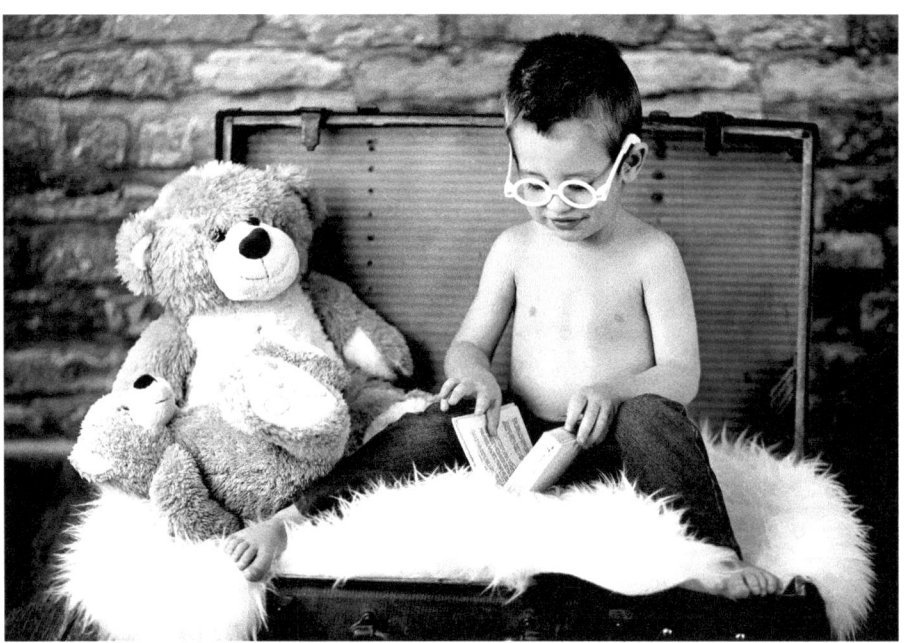

○ Opportunities in your environment

Reading

Literacy is the ability to read and write in a given language. The opportunity to read is everywhere. Since we are Getting Started with literacy, think about what you read in your daily environment and see how you can expose your child to your literacy experiences. All you really have to do is point out what you already know about the reading opportunities you use on a daily basis. You can do that! Soon enough, so will your child. Explore the options for literacy you have in your home. What do you read when riding in the car, bus, or train, or walking outdoors? What would you like to expose your child to more? *Getting Started* with assistive communication involves learning to read and write.

Options for what I can read!

What are we doing when we are learning to read? We are learning about how people, places, and things have names, how they relate together, and have a function through a story. We learn that we will be close together and have fun. We will learn to look at pictures, letters, words, and punctuation. By looking at the illustrations we learn about the setting and how characters feel. We will learn about the front and the back of the book, turn pages, pause, read and re-read. We will learn predictability. We will learn that we can control and begin to make sense of the world that is coming at us and that we can use what we see and hear to shape ideas, formulate an opinion, and state that opinion using multiple modalities of communication (e.g. verbally using voice or a speech generating device *Turn the page, Oh no! That's funny*, vocally, and nonverbally using gestures). Ask yourself: *Are reading options present in my child's daily life experience? What reading options will I work on today and what will I try next?*

- Books
- Mail
- Restaurants
- Books on CD
- Store Buildings
- Banners
- Digital books
- Restroom Signs
- Safety Signs
- Magazines
- Names of people, pets, activities, things

○ Writing

Just like there are many opportunities to read in our environment, there are many ways we can write. The best part is we get to start with scribbling and turn scribbles into meaning. Explore what options you have available to you in your environment and think about what options would be great to try today and in the near future?

1 Pencils, crayons, markers
2 Drawing chalk, sidewalk chalk
3 Wood dowels to draw in playdough
4 Fingers in shaving cream
5 Shape waxy string or pipe cleaners
6 Pencil grips
7 Adaptable pencils, markers, and crayons

Occupational therapists use many amazing tools to support the world of writing for children. Use the list here to get you started and speak with an occupational therapist for other tools, novel tools, for functional and fun ways your child can access and optimize writing and creating. Next, let's take a look at some skill sets you can consider while you build your child's literacy skills. Consider what skills the child has now, what skills the child sometimes uses and would benefit from more practice or exposure, and skills that would make for good next steps.

1 Hold a book right side up or look at a book in a mount
2 Use a switch to access a page turner
3 Swiping, scrolling, tapping, or other gesture to turn or move pages on an electronic device
4 Use a speech generating device or nonverbal cues to tell my reader to turn the page
5 Look and listen to talking photo albums
6 Observe and interact with objects paired with word labels
7 Scribble with markers, pens, crayons, or pencils adapting tools as needed
8 Make crafts related to a story
9 Use writing and reading technology applications to scribble on a tablet or touch screen

O Activities for Getting Started with literacy

View the literacy process as a partnered relationship between you and your child or your child and interventionists. Use the following literacy activities as a springboard of ideas to work with a child to develop beginning literacy skills. Consider the activities and recommendations a springboard for your own to grow each child's literacy path in their unique way.

Activity #1 Look at photos and photos with print

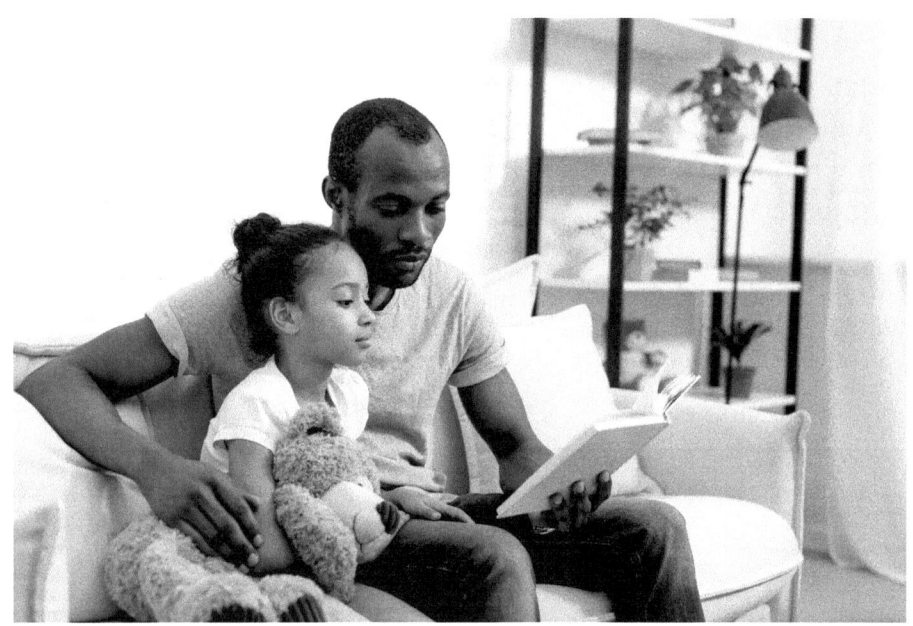

Collect or access photos of family members, friends, places the child likes to visit, favorite toys, preferred activities, and pictures that make you laugh. As you filter through photos on phones, tablets, or paper, identify the photos that your child enjoys the most with people in action or demonstrating emotions. Print them out on paper. Add a caption that can be as simple as labeling who or what is in the picture (nouns), stating the actions in the picture (verbs), and describing beginning attributes such as feelings, color, shape, and size (adjectives).

Activity #2 Make choices about books and other print materials like magazines or photo books

Choose four to six books the child likes. Choose books based on what sounds exciting to your child? What would be fun? What book teaches a concept you want your child to learn? Consider looking at magazines and other forms of print such as the daily mail even junk mail, catalogues. Feel free to use photo books as storybooks as they represent the family story, the child's story.

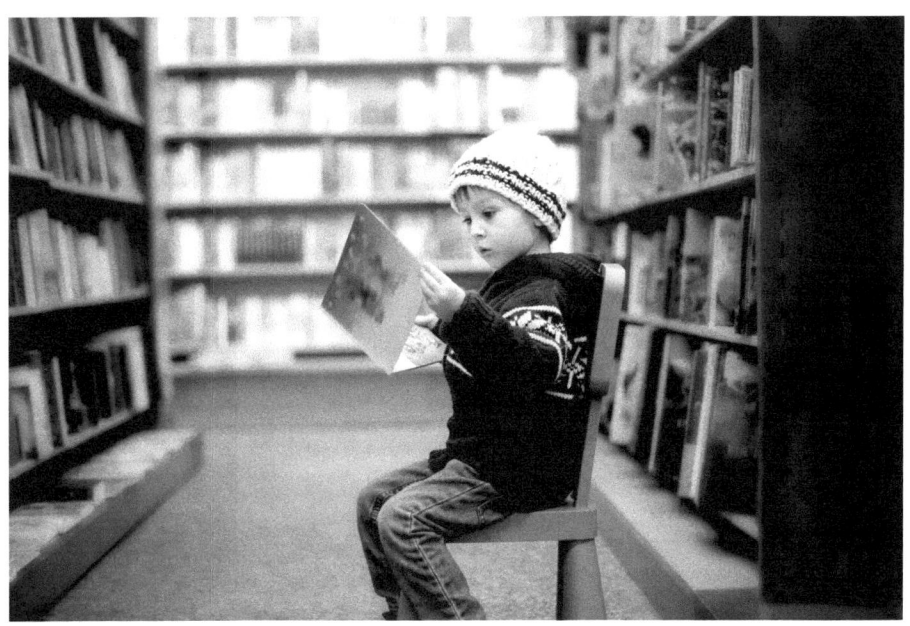

Activity #3 Listen to stories, repeatedly

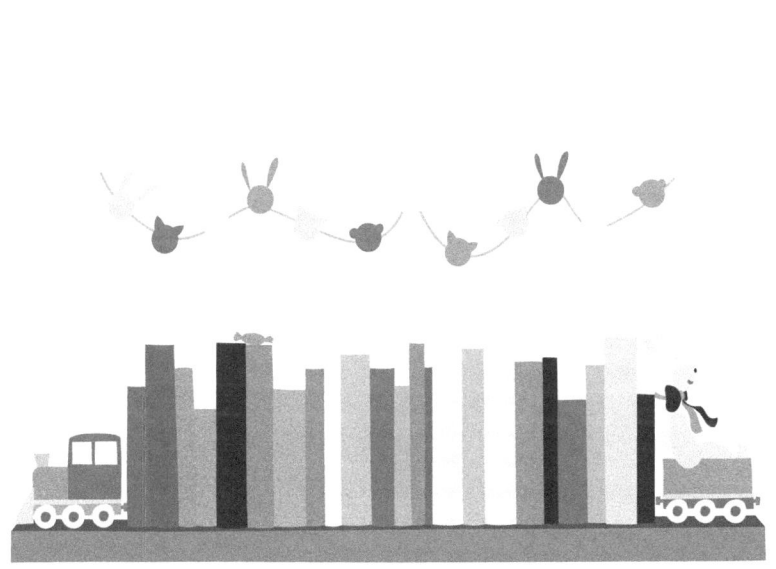

Re-read on consecutive days or cycle books then re-read, re-read, re-read, re-read and when you are done, feel free to re-read. Read with feeling and emphasis. Re-reading gives your child ownership of a story such as a working knowledge of text and pictures and excitement of the shared experience, anticipating what's coming, and security in the constancy.

Activity #4 Observe and interact with objects paired with word labels

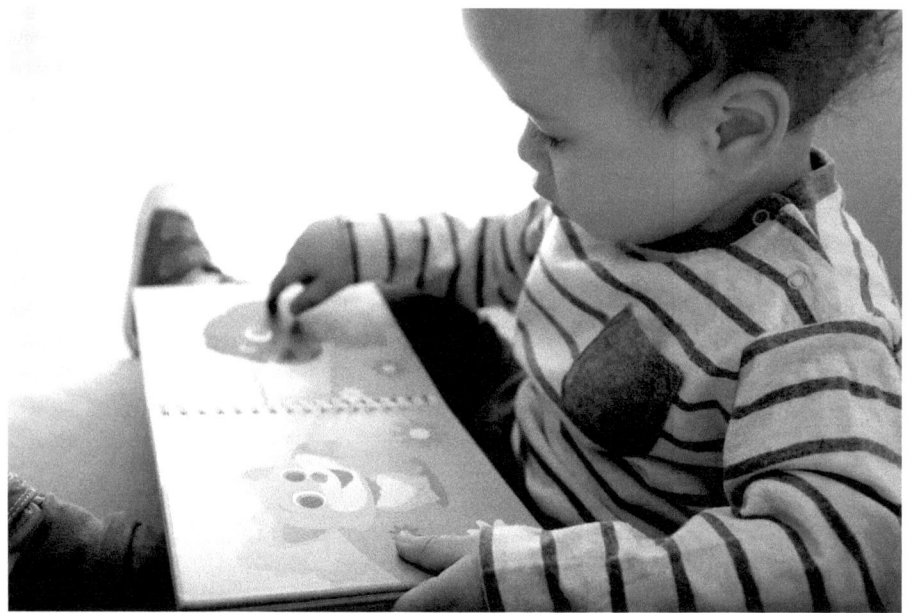

Take time to observe your child interacting with objects labeled with print. Observe your child as he or she looks at a book. If your child is engaged visually, allow that connection to continue even if you have completed reading the text. Let your child take in the words and images. Allow moments of silence and then talk. Consider the receptive language of the child as you label items in the home and name family members. After reading the text or providing a description of the scene or images, go back and label items, pair objects with actions, or give basic feelings, color, shape, and size descriptions.

Activity #5 Scribble!

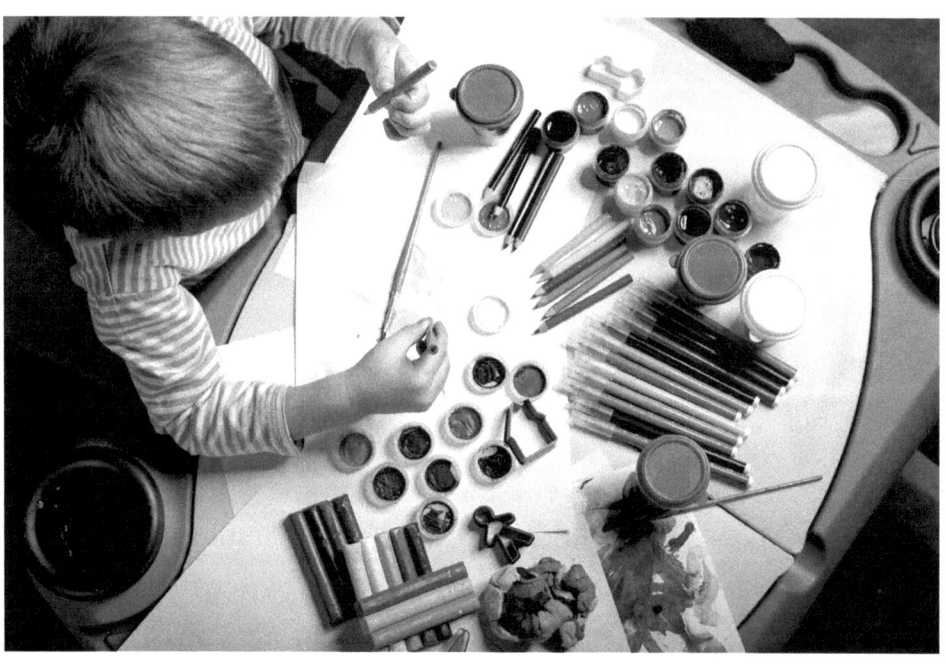

Scribble with markers, pens, and crayons with adapted grips as appropriate, play with dough, paint, build with blocks, bend pipe cleaners. Provide the child with lots of options to engage their fingers building fine motor skills. Each fine motor task helps build muscle tone. Model drawing lines, circles, and shapes. Turn them into simple drawings. Kids love to see adults draw, even stick figures. It is okay not to be an artist. Have fun in not being an artist. Have fun in the experience of trying.

Tips for successful interactions with literacy activities. Always keep your perspective on the child when choosing materials to engage your child. What is the most fun? Who does the child want to see in the photo? Where does the child like to go or be? What does the child like to play with? What inspires the child to be happy and excited? Then keep the making of materials simple. Print on regular paper if you do not have photo paper. Hand write captions or sentences. Use sheet protectors rather than laminating to save costs. Sheet protectors are easy to clean and you can change out photos.

Sensory considerations. How is my child accessing literacy? Does my child see print within normal limits, or do I need to consult with a vision specialist to discuss the best way for my child to visually interact with print such as glasses, providing a greater light source, enlarging or magnifying the text? What is the status of my child's hearing? Do I need to consult with an audiologist or speech-language pathologist regarding options to compensate hearing needs such as amplification options, reducing ambient noise in the environment, and helping my child learn to regulate competing noises?

What about communication access methods to literacy? Work with interventionists to consider access methods to literacy and communication. For example, direct selection with fingers or using the eye to make a choice. Other access methods can be a stylus, head pointer, or switch access to play books on CD or manipulate digitally based books or media.

Communication and social interaction. Complete a self-assessment to support the child. What is working when you read with your child? What can you try next? What did your child teach or show me when we read today, drew today? What behaviors did I observe the child expressing when we were reading?

- Feelings and emotions: Happy, no interest, sadness, excitement for characters
- Time on task: How long did my child engage with book? Denote the length of time and observe over time watching your child's attention span improve
- Awareness: How does your child show interest in and recognize pictures, words, and text in general. How does working with print improve behavior

- Communication: Expressing intent through non-erbal interactions such as giving, pointing, showing, and verbalizing using technology or their voice for word approximations, words, phrases, or sentences
- Types of engagement: Turning or requesting pages to be turned, holding a book upright, pointing, looking, commenting, and other requests; looking at video with text
- Cognition: Imagination, experience with connecting print and images to language and experiences, and experience with engaging with books, experience with the person(s) reading with your child, and the anticipation of future experiences with the same book, different books, and personal experiences (e.g. *We read about playing in the park. Tomorrow we are going to the park to feel the sand, slip down the slide, and fly like an airplane on the swing.*)

Getting Started with vocabulary

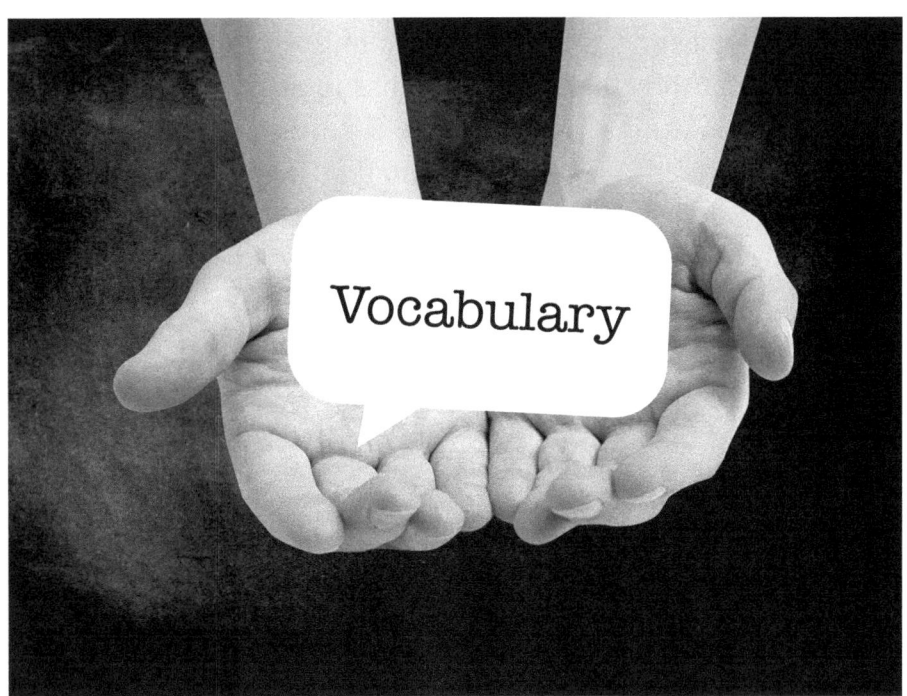

○ Supporting families and professionals in building vocabulary

Where do I start with vocabulary? Everyone asks that question. Every parent, every speech-language pathologist, every interventionist asks the same question. We are fortunate that a number of researchers and authors have developed lists to assist families and interventionists with the selection of vocabulary words that are published in articles (Banajee, DiCarlo & Striklin, 2003; Marvin, Beukelman & Bilyeu, 1994; Van Tatenhove, 2013). In *Getting Started* we will talk about the types of vocabulary to consider for a child that uses AAC. After you review vocabulary for *Getting Started* it is recommended that you read other chapters sections on vocabulary to get a feel for where to start and where you will be headed in supporting a child that uses AAC with vocabulary development. Let's start with core and fringe vocabulary.

Core vocabulary: Words that describe general, common nouns, or frequent ideas
    or concepts. Examples: *dog, man*, or *doll.*
Fringe vocabulary: Words that describe specific or unique ideas or concepts
    such as proper nouns. Examples: *Fido, Fred*, or *Fiona.*

What do we know at the *Getting Started* stage about the child, communication, and vocabulary?

1 We know that we recognize a child may express a concept many different
   ways, called *communication modalities*. The child may vocalize, verbalize with
   their mouth or speech generating device, give a word approximation, and use

nonverbal communication in the form of sign language, facial expressions, and body positioning.

2 We know that we want the child to use core words across environments for commenting, requesting, and other communicative intents.

3 We know we want the child to have access to and use fringe words so specific messages can be understood and expressed.

4 We know that we want meaningful communication between the child and communication partners thus emphasizing the importance of core and fringe vocabulary.

5 We know can model one to two words in the *Getting Started* phase both verbally and using AAC tools (e.g. communication board, single message speech generating device, multi-message speech generating device).

6 We know that children need to have experiences with objects, actions, people, animals, feelings, and the world in order to richly talk about what they understand.

7 We know that children need to have experiences across environments and that the modalities and types of conversations the child will have will vary across environments.

There is no right or wrong when choosing core or fringe vocabulary. Just remember that we use *core* words to talk about general people, locations, and animals and *fringe* words to talk about specific names of people, locations and animals. If you think about it, there are times you may talk with friends and say, *Hey let's go get a pizza.* Other times you may need to specify a location like *Uncle Kurt's Pizza.* For now, just think about what fits the communicative intent best. As the child's language knowledge increases provide access to more vocabulary so the child has options to express what they want to say using core or fringe words.

Getting Started with tools and access

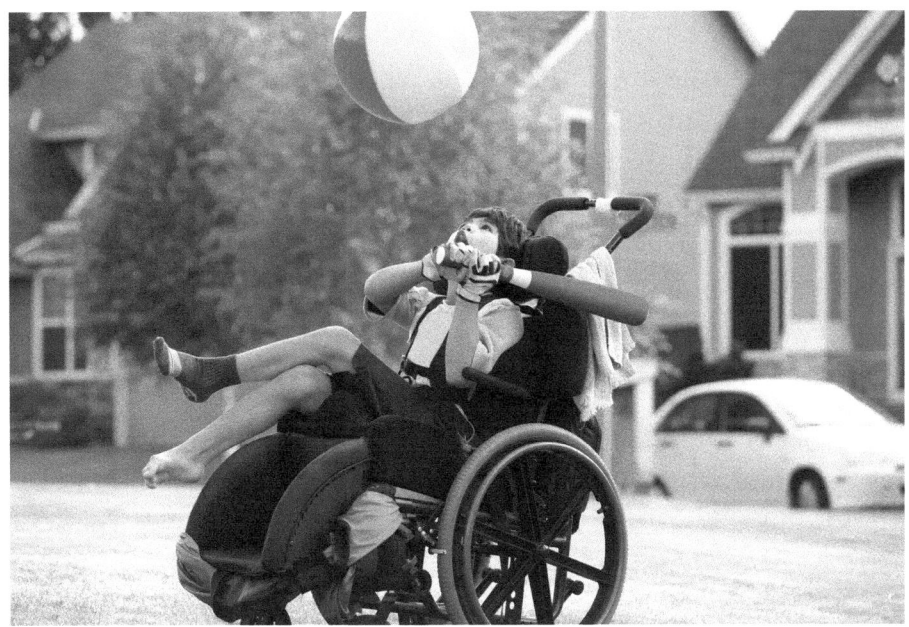

○ Mind and body at work

The purpose of *Getting Started with Tools and Access* is to give you direction in how to put the mind and body to work promoting joint attention with others and accessing tools to support communication and interaction in a given environment. We know to look at the many ways the body communicates and accesses tools to communicate. Sometimes when a child is *Getting Started* with communication, we need to start at the level of understanding that a symbol represents another object. Work with a speech-language pathologist to help you establish symbolic understanding at the appropriate level for your child. Remember to employ the Theory of Natural Consequences which states you will follow through with your child's request even if you know the intent does not match what you think your child wants. Circle back and give your child another opportunity to make another request. As attention and accuracy to symbol choices improves more symbols can be added to the AAC tools and devices. Other times, the right decision in *Getting Started* with tools and access for a child means trialing and implementing a high tech speech generating device and many other tools in between. The *right* decision is based on findings from a quality assessment. Look to each chapter to learn about tools and access methods to develop the right multimodal communication plan including tools and access methods for your child.

Communication board. Communication boards come in all sorts of shapes and sizes. What is the right size and shape for your child? The answer is many shapes and sizes depending on where you use the communication board and what messages the child will convey. Think where the communication board will be used. Will it be small enough to carry easily, attached to a ring, or attached with string or Velcro®? Think about how many icons, usually pictures with messages, will be needed on the board that match your child's scanning ability and provide relevant vocabulary. Will the board be specific to a situation within an environment (e.g. restaurant, park, school subject, recess)? Will the child point to icons with pictures and text? Will you have Velcro® options for the child to give to a communication partner? Again, yes there are a lot of questions, but they are great questions and help you see that communication is possible in so many ways.

Single message speech generating device. Single message speech generating devices are AAC tools that allow a person to express one programmed message that can express one word up to a few minutes in length of a message. The messages are digitized voices which means the person recording the message would hold down a button and speak into the device and record his or her voice. The beauty of single message devices is that they can be quickly and readily programmed for just-in-time messages. Just-in-time messaging means that when your child needs to express a word, sentence, or idea, the device can be programmed in the moment to meet the communication needs of your child. Just-in-time messaging applies to any device that meets the user's need in the moment it is needed. Single message speech generating devices are one way to meet that goal!

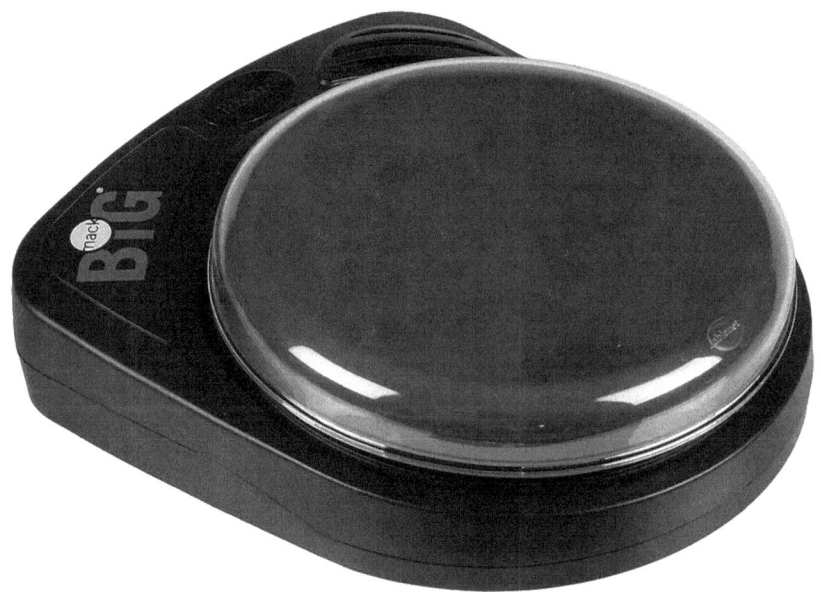

Have fun with combining messages. You can have single message switches set next to each other or purchase devices that can be linked together. The child would press one button to say one message, followed by another, followed by another. The number of linked messages is up to you and the child. Switch access is an option for single message speech generating devices. A switch can be used to activate an AAC device to state the message. The switch may have a wired connection or wireless such as a Bluetooth or LED (light emitting diode). There are many types of switches that accommodate a number of physical needs. Work with an AAC specialist to determine the appropriate type of switch for your child's communication needs.

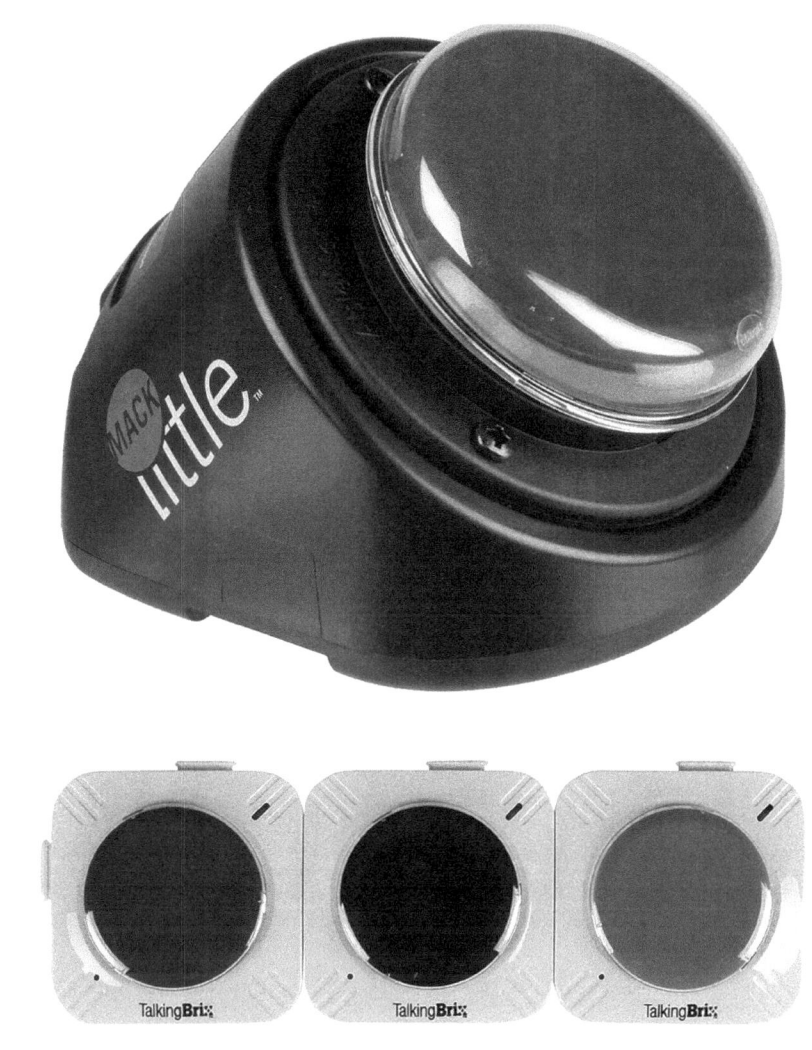

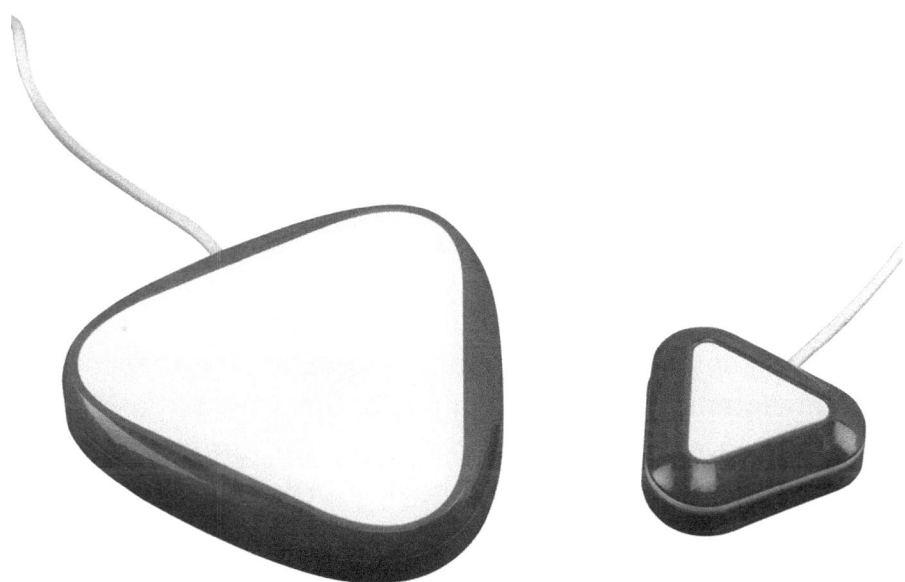

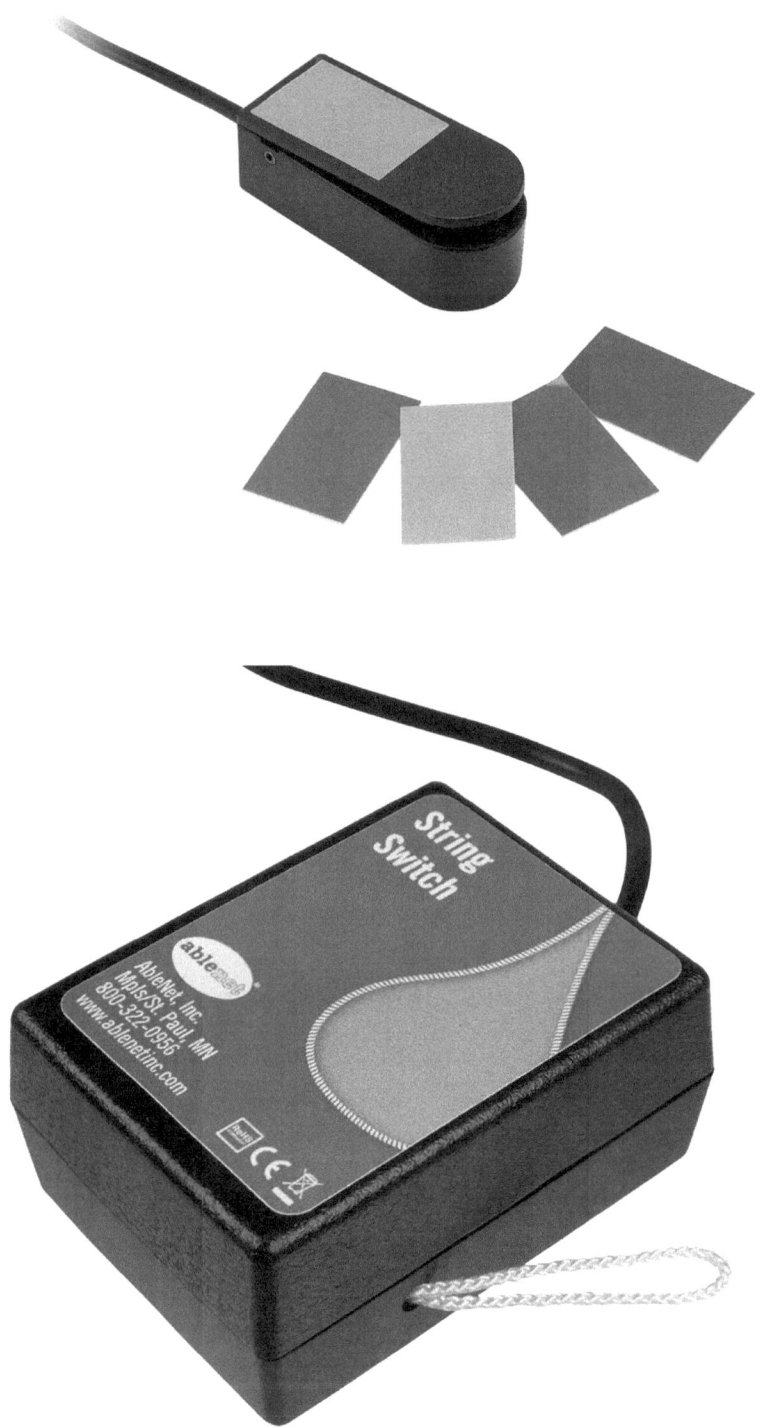

Dual message device. A dual message device is a speech generating device that has two buttons for communication. This is a great tool to use for communicators that have the symbolic understanding that they can make a choice or state intent from a choice of two options. As we head into technology remember there are communication devices for direct communication and switches that activate devices to speak a programmed message. Speech generating devices such as the iTalk2 Communicator by Ablenet is a great tool to use for expressing two messages. The beauty of a dual message speech generating device is the ease of programming that allows for quick access to communication readily adaptable to any communication context. Use a dual message speech generating device to state opinions such as *yes* or *no*, to state *read the page* or *turn the page* of a book, to state *my turn* or *your turn* while playing a game, to play *hot* and *cold*, to say *wait* or *keep going*, or any message that can have two choices.

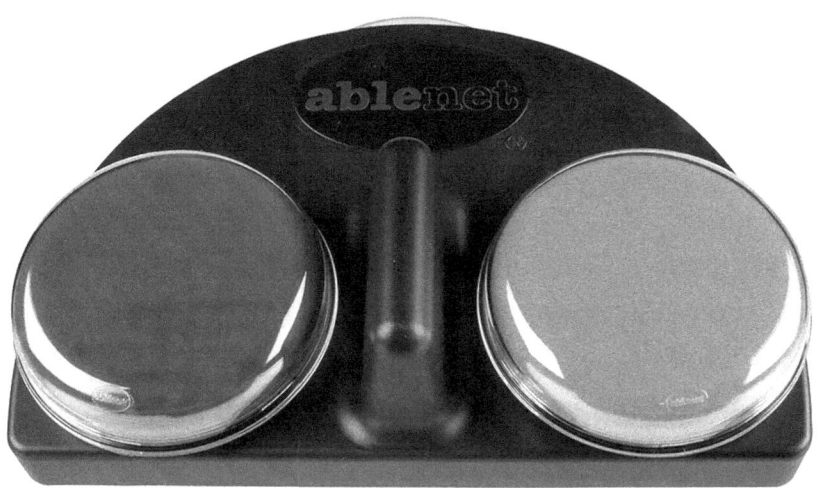

Access. Whenever the concept of access comes up you will think about the word *how*. How will my child access the speech generating device? That answer may be using his or her fingers, hands, eyes, knees, cheek or wrist. These are called direct selection. Other times a switch may be helpful to access the speech generating device. The Ablenet Blue2 Bluetooth switch is a good example of a dual option access method that will activate any Bluetooth compatible speech generating device. The white and orange plates of the Ablenet Blue2 Bluetooth switch serve like a computer left and right click. One plate can serve as a *shift* button and the other plate serves as the *enter* plate. The dual switch can be used to access environmental controls as well. Read on for more information on environmental controls.

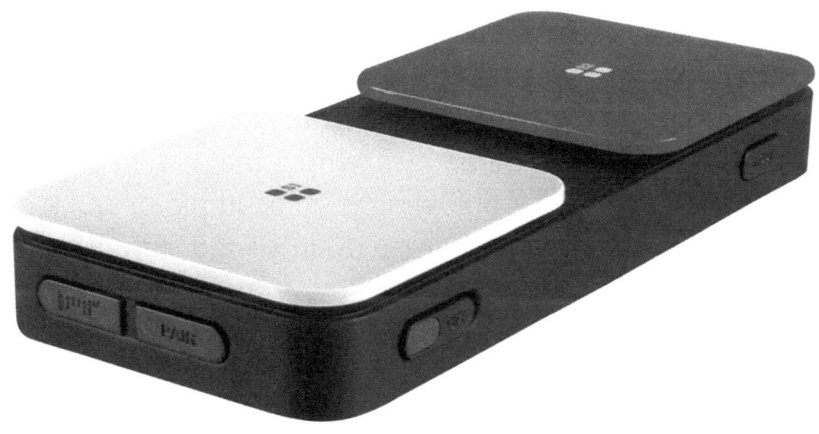

Visual scene display. Visual scenes on a speech generating device often have *hot spots* where a child can touch an area on the scene and a selection of vocabulary icons pops up. A visual scene is a picture of a setting providing a context for the child to communicate from, rather than one isolated and more abstract, icon. Visual scenes help both the communicator and the communication partner have a context for the message. Examples of visual scenes are pictures of rooms in the home, playground, classroom, or community-based locations your child frequently visits. A low technology visual scene can be a print out of a scene with icons of images on the sides of the board that can reflect nouns for choices (e.g. TV, music, game), action messages (e.g. *Let's talk, Let's play; I'm tired*), or descriptions (e.g. color choices for socks or shirts). When the user asks for an item, the communication partner will have an idea of the user's topic based on the scene (e.g. *She must want to listen to music on her player because she used her bedroom scene where her player is kept.*). Types of icons for visual scene displays include the following:

- Action oriented: Include people performing actions that may represent an object function such as a person opening a container or action verbs such as people drinking, eating, playing, walking, tossing, kicking a ball, etc.
- Topic oriented: The visual scene itself may imply the topic or add topic ideas on the sides of the scene such as toys, or emotions, friends, stories, etc.
- Item selection: Place icons with words at the sides of a visual scene to quickly express wants and needs or share information.
- Location: Use a visual scene with a number of smaller scenes that may be helpful for an outing to different parts of a park, town, beach, city, etc.

Environmental control. Environmental control systems for a child *Getting Started* with AAC? Sure! Why not? What are environmental control systems (ECS) anyway? An ECS provides the user with the ability to control things like turning lights *on* and *off* in a room or turn kitchen appliances like blenders and mixers on and off to make a favorite shake. For more mature users, opening and closing doors and windows, lowering or raising beds, and using telephones can be operated using tools such as infrared detectors, receivers, and transmitters. For our kids just *Getting Started* with environmental control consider using battery adapters to activate toys, infra-red switches to make a dog bark, walk, moo and more. Employ a switch that would allow a child to spin a spinner for art activities. The following is an example of an (1) environmental control switch, a (2) battery adapter, an (3) infra-red switch, and a (4) toy that can be activated using either the infra-red switch or other switch options with battery adapter.

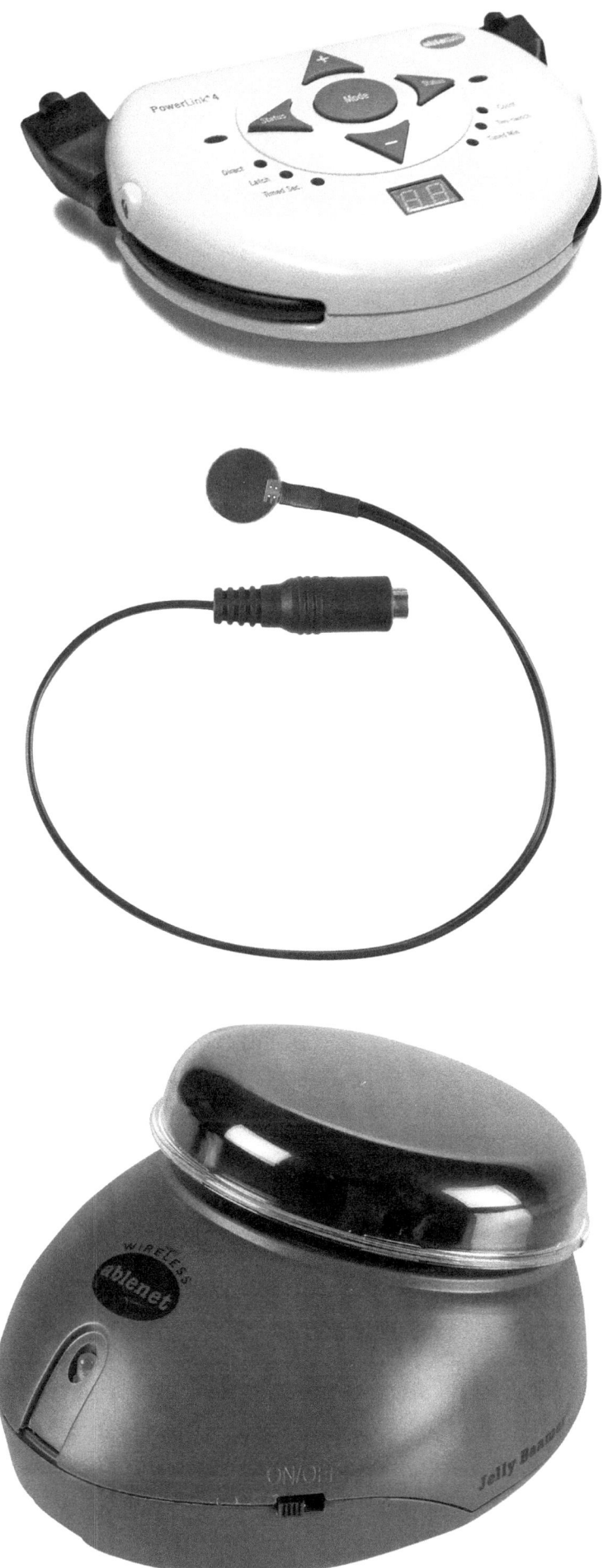

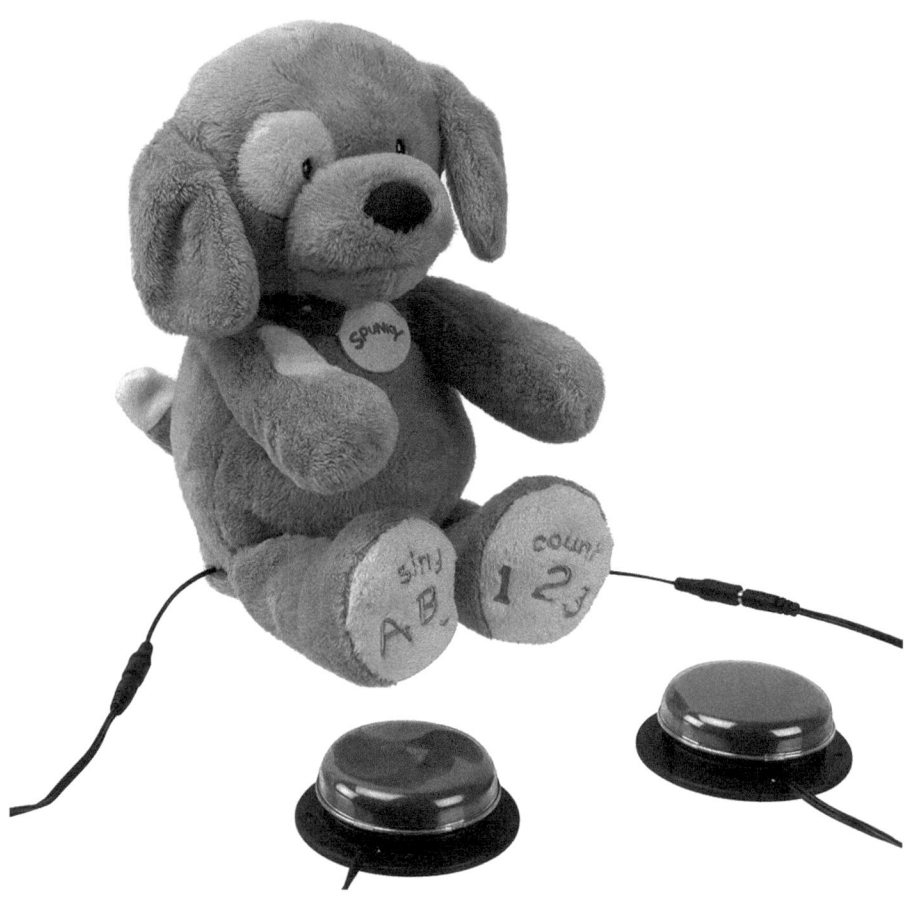

Notes: a few extra notes of consideration

1 Picture symbol systems – *What pictures should I use?* That is a great question and is a part of the *feature matching* in which AAC decisions on tools and devices are matched to the needs of your child. See *Bridging Skills* for a complete review of *feature matching* for speech generating devices. In the *Getting Started* phase of communication we select the right images for icons that best represent language. Some options include a photograph of an object, a complete or line drawing, or an image from a symbol set made by a company. Once again, visit Spectronics to compare symbol sets at www. spectronics.com.au/article/symbol-set-comparison. When considering which symbol system consider if the images are easy to associate with an object or concept or will my child have to work too hard to learn the associations between the symbol and the intended language target? Work with a speech-language pathologist or AAC specialist trained in symbol options when you have questions about what symbol system is best for your child when making communication boards. Most application and high technology devices will have dedicated symbol sets.

2 Tablet technology: Consider the button or icon size, the type of frame around icon, background of icon which makes it easier to see, how thick the frame is best, and the display size, meaning how many icons are on one display, the quality and likability of the voice, options for different voices, the option

to record voice. Consider if the features of tablet based AAC programs meet your child's communication profile. Work with a speech-language pathologist trained in AAC to support decision making.

3 Switch options: Switches allow a user to gain access to assistive technology that includes communication, games and toys, computers for learning, information, and fun as well as environmental control. As we think back to the idea of feature matching consider the child's physical parameters. Ask yourself some questions. Does the child need a switch that can be activated using minimal pressure or near proximity touch? Would the use of a body part aid access (e.g. cheek, elbow, knee, foot etc.)? Explore variety of switch access options (e.g. light pressure, head and cheek switches, ribbon, track ball switches, etc.).

4 If your child accesses the messages repeatedly, interpret the reasons why. Is it a sign that the message is very, very important to your child? Affirm the meaning. This repetition may be the only option to express a more complex message. Is the repetition occurring because the child is getting 'stuck' and is unable to move onto the rest of their intent? Prompting may support the child such as modeling the next icon. Is the repetition interpreted as a stemming behavior? Then bridge the meaning between the icon and the intent upon first activation. Follow through with an action so the child learns the message carries intent.

A summary for Getting Started

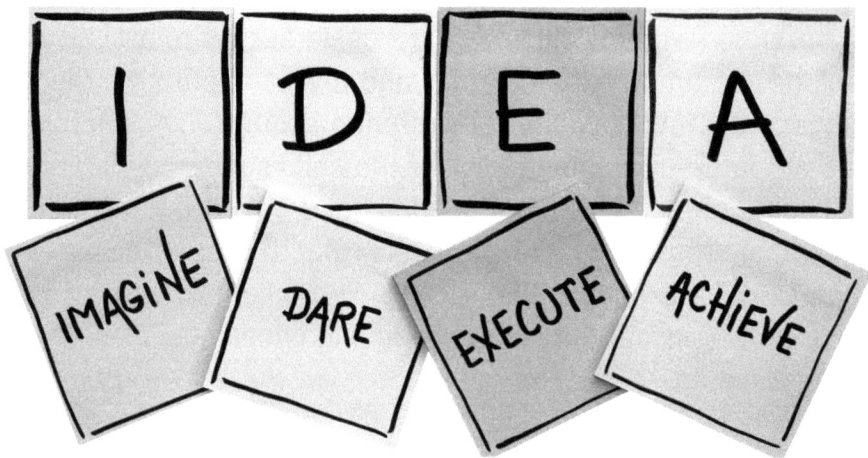

○ It's time!

Congratulations on *Getting Started*! You, your child, or your clients are on their way with communication using AAC. You know that *Getting Started* with communication is your time, your child's time, or your client's time to have their communication explicitly detailed and shared with communication partners! You gathered and detailed the child's verbal and nonverbal communication through the protocol, *Hear Me into Voice*. This necessary and informative first step provides you with a powerful tool that allows you to catalogue what and how your child is communicating in order to share that knowledge with others and use it to build more communication as a part of a complete assessment. As you start to think about the next steps for children that use AAC consider joint attention, memory skills, each individual learning style and strengths, and ways of showing communication. Just as important monitor your needs as a facilitator and what communication partners need to know to communicate with your child. Even though we are *Getting Started* with communication means we also want to be *Maximizing Participation* at each and every step and stage along the way. You are encouraged to review all of the chapters to gain an overview of communication across the stages. Remember to celebrate success at any stage from *Getting Started* to *Maximizing Participation*.

Before we go: let's make a communication board, card, or ring

People talk about communication boards all of the time. *It's easy! All you gotta do is . . .* Wait, what? Here is a list of the most often used low tech, specifically no batteries or internet required, options for communication including considerations, supplies, and tips. While the directions for putting together communication boards, and the like, is placed in *Getting Started*, people use low tech tools all the way through *Maximizing Participation* just like it may be appropriate for a person just *Getting Started* to use high technology speech generating devices. Communication boards are not necessarily a beginner's tool. They are a just-in-time communication tool. It may be the fastest most effective form of expression of a message for the AAC user and communication partners at the right time to express the desired purposes of communication. Remember to show others how they can talk with your child using communication boards too. Some children process messages more effectively when they can see their communication partners visually model messages that they also hear spoken.

Options: Low technology communication tools and why we use them

Communication board: Use a communication board for quick communication that will not run out of batteries because it has none. It also does not have a voice. It may be designed by a company, an AAC specialist, or self-designed. Make copies of card stock weighted pages on standard weighted paper for ease of folding for special outings or events.

Communication ring: Often used during active outings in the community or playground setting, the communication partner or AAC user flips icons with pictures and text hooked onto a clasped ring to express a desired message.

Communication card: Often smaller than a communication board, a communication card is used for specific communication purposes such as an insert in a book, used at a school center or station like art or math or fine motor, or used for transition between activities.

Supplies

Money: Some communication boards and icons for rings are available for download for free from AAC website. However, you still need the paper, a printer, or optional tools like scissors, Velcro® for removable icons, and laminating sheets or a laminating machine.

Time: Making communication boards takes time for planning the purpose and placement of the symbols and the materials.

Personnel: Are you making the communication board or can someone help you? Delegation is a beautiful thing.

Materials

Paper size: Standard stock size, half sheet, enlarged

Paper type: Standard or heavy weight, treated for easier cleaning, color options for vision impairment or learning differences or disorders, preferences, categorizing needs

Grid size: The number and configuration of the icons on the board

Symbols: Determine the languages and purposes of communication the language will meet. Determine the symbol images source: photos, symbol sets, computer images, hand drawings, line drawing, black and white, full color

Finishing: Lamination, page protector, placed in a folder or book, dividers

Additional board supplies: Scissors, laminating sheets or machine, ®

Tips from the trenches

1 Velcro®: Cutting Velcro® strips into squares rather than using ready-made dots is cost effective. However, when you cut the strips to the desired size, be prepared to clean off the Velcro® adhesive from the scissor blades every so often. Place the rough side, or the hook, on the icon. Place the soft side, or the loop, on the page or object the icon will attach to. Stay consistent!

2 Hot press lamination: A great way to increase the durability of boards and icons is through lamination. Do not laminate communication boards that will also have icons with a cold press machine or the sticky backing of Velcro will not stick. Laminate communication boards that will have matching icons with a hot press machine.

3 Extra supplies: Make an extra copy of vocabulary pages that are used to create communication boards in case of damage or loss. Laminating sheets are nice to have on hand to quickly repair or laminate a small number of icons so they may be added quickly.

Note: Check out the other *Before We Go* sections in the remaining chapters for helpful tools. See *Tips for Troubleshooting* in *Building Fundamentals*, a *Communication Wallet* in *Bridging Skills*, *Cool Things About Me* remnant book in *Making Connections*, and a *Let's Chat* talking tips page in *Maximizing Participation*.

References

Ablenet. (2018). Technology. Retrieved from www.ablenetinc.com/technology

Academy of American Poets. (n.d.). Poems for kids. Retrieved from https://poets.org/poems-kids

Adaptive Tech Solutions. (2017). Switch adapted toys. Retrieved from www.adaptivetechsolutions.com/cat-switch-adapted-toys.cfm

Banajee, M., DiCarlo, C. & Striklin, S. (2003). Core vocabulary determination for toddlers. *Augmentative and Alternative Communication*, *19*, 67–73.

Beyond Play. (2018). Products for early childhood and special needs. Retrieved from www.beyondplay.com/

Brady, N. C., Thiemann-Bourque, K., Fleming, K. & Matthews, K. (2013). Predicting language outcomes for children learning augmentative and alternative communication: Child and environmental factors. *Journal of Speech and Language Hearing Research*, *56*, 1595–1612.

Center for Literacy and Disability Studies University North Carolina Chapel Hill. (n.d.). *Project core*. Retrieved from www.project-core.com/

Donaldson, A. L. & Stahmer, A. C. (2014). Team collaboration: The use of behavior principles for serving students with ASD. *Language Speech and Hearing Services in the Schools*, *45*, 261–276.

Enablemart. (2018). Speech and communication. Retrieved from www.enablemart.com/speech-and-communication

Enabling Devices. (2018). Products. Retrieved from https://enablingdevices.com/

Flaghouse. (2018). Resources for sport, recreation, and special needs. Retrieved from www.flaghouse.com

Johnston, S. S., Reichle, J. & Evans, J. (2004). Supporting augmentative and alternative communication use by beginning communicators with severe disabilities. *American Journal of Speech-Language Pathology*, *13*, 20–30.

Kaderavek, J. N. (2015). *Language disorders in children: Fundamental concepts of assessment and intervention*. Boston, MA: Pearson Education, Inc.

Lund, S. K. & Light, J. (2007). Long-term outcomes for individuals who use augmentative and alternative communication: Part II – Communication interaction. *Augmentative and Alternative Communication*, *23*(1), 1–15.

Marvin, C., Beukelman, D. & Bilyeu, D. (1994). Frequently occurring home and school words from vocabulary-use patterns in preschool children: Effects of context and time sampling. *Augmentative and Alternative Communication*, *10*, 224–236. Retrieved from doi:10.1080/07434619412331276930

Nesbitt, K. (2019). Poetry 4 kids. Retrieved from www.poetry4kids.com/

Rehabmart. (2018). Communication switch accessories, adaptive switches, mounting arms. Retrieved from www.rehabmart.com/category/communication_switch_accessories.htm

Snell, M. E., Brady, N., McLean, L., Ogletree, B. T., Siegel, E., Sylvester, L., … Sevcik, R. (2010). Twenty years of communication intervention research with individuals who have severe intellectual and developmental disabilities. *American Journal of Intellectual and Developmental Disabilities*, 115(5), 364–380.

Special Needs Toys. (n.d.). Sensory toys and special needs toys. Retrieved from www.specialneedstoys.com

Spectronics. (2019). Symbol set comparison. Retrieved from www.spectronics.com.au/article/symbol-set-comparison

Van Tatenhove, G. (2013). Papers and resources. Retrieved from www.vantatenhove.com/papers.shtml

Woods, J. J., Wetherby, A. M., Kashinath, S. & Holland, R. D. (2012). Early social interaction project. In P. A. Prelock & R. J. McCauley (Eds.), *Treatment of autism spectrum disorders: Evidence-based intervention strategies for communication and social interactions* (pp. 189–220). Baltimore, MD: Paul H. Brooks Publishing Co.

Yoder, D. (2001). Having my say. *Augmentative and Alternative Communication*, 17, 2–10.

Building Fundamentals  with social interaction
Expanding communication

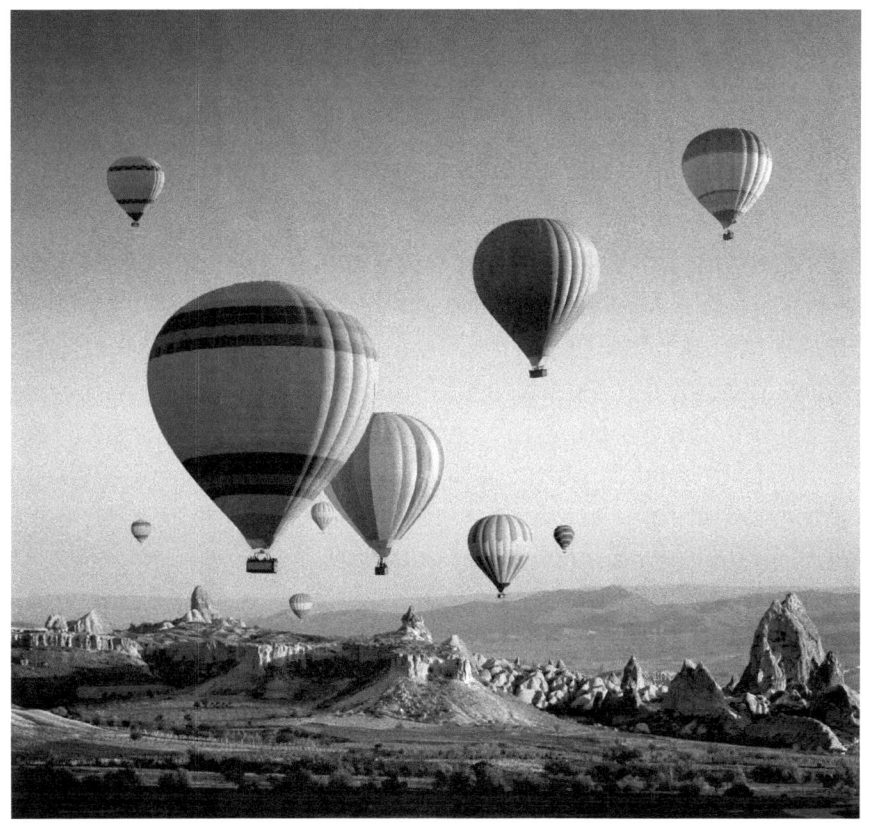

My contribution was to try to give the insight into the person of Moses and to highlight his need [for others] to see him as somebody who is loving and who expects love in return.

Parent (Rogers, 1999)

Building Fundamentals in communication takes all of your child's great communication skills identified in *Getting Started* and broadens that remarkable base to benefit the child's, the facilitators', and communication partners' interactions. We take a pointing skill and employ it to express communication across a broader array of visual options including symbols and icons for static communication tools and static or dynamic speech generating devices. Facilitators and communication partners learn new strategies to support children's communication by taking logical and natural next steps in AAC for supporting participation, teaching literacy, celebrating successes, and fostering multiple purposes of communication.

Defining key concepts in Building Fundamentals

Concept #1 Supporting participation: We support participation through a nuts and bolts look at your child's skill set using the protocol *Hear Me into Voice* and other formal and informal assessment measures that detail your child's communication and interaction. Each child's communication partners will translate everyday concepts that promote participation and provide the right opportunity to meet the important purpose of communication. The next step is to get your child's team members, the facilitators, and communication partners, on board with 1) understanding your child's skill set, and 2) using the skill set in the environments in which your child participates. This setting includes participation with other verbal and nonverbal peers across linguistic and cultural contexts (McLeod, 2018). Indeed, the intimate cultural interaction between the child and the child's environment may determine developmental change itself according to developmental psychologist Thelen (1991). Allow team members to embrace your child's communication skills set and engage them in talking about how your child can participate in class, on the playground, and in the community. Place the emphasis on participation. Help team members link questions to answers. For example, 1) What does participation look like in this activity and setting? 2) How can I use my child's communication within participation? 3) Where are the barriers, if any, to my child's participation (Beukelman & Mirenda, 2013)? The sooner team members feel they are a part of your child's solution to communication, the sooner you will see success and celebrate success.

Concept #2 Celebrating successes: Celebrating successes allows you to take a step back and say, *Hey, we are making progress with communication*! Success can be seen in your child with new responses, in facilitators when they bridge communication between a child and a peer or adult, and in communication partners when they reciprocate communication. A celebration is an occasion that carries with it an emotional connection, a validation of a job well done. The celebration is not just of your child but of the team working together and seeing that focusing on participation is the thread of success. It is a cognitive and psychological experience.

Concept #3 Fostering multiple purposes of communication: The third concept builds upon supporting participation and celebrating successes by revisiting the four purposes of communication (Light & McNaughton, 2014). Ask yourself, *Does my child have a way to express social greetings, have social etiquette with peers and adults, can share information, and express wants and needs?* Each purpose of communication requires vocabulary that may be the same and may be different. Some purposes such as social greetings may be learned faster than others and that is okay. Understanding and honoring the cultural differences enables the child to learn and grow using assistive technology in meaningful ways. Together the purposes form a complete communicative profile.

Now let's put these ideas to work. Review *Ideas at Work: Communication, Next Steps, and Goal Planning* for examples of ideas. Consider the ideas offered and work with a speech-language pathologist to catalogue communication behaviors you see in your child, the logical *next step* to the communication behavior, and a goal to measure progress. *Building Fundamentals* is all about beginning to use the rules of conversation through the purposes of communication such as greeting each other, taking turns several times, sharing information about actions and feelings with people and objects, being polite socially, expressing wants and needs, even ending a conversation and moving on!

○ Ideas at work: communication, next steps, and goal planning

Communication	Next Step	General Goal
1 My child squeezes my finger to make a choice or answer yes or no questions	My child will use a hand squeeze without my finger as a cue	Elaine will squeeze her hand to respond to five questions with 80 percent accuracy across two sessions as measured by charted data.
2 My child uses her eyes to look to the left and right to say no.	My child will turn her head left and right to say no.	Elaine will turn her head to the left and right to indicate no when answering five questions with 80 percent accuracy across two sessions as measured by charted data.
3 My child smiles inconsistently for communication purposes.	My child will use a purposeful smile to communicate intent	Elaine will use a purposeful smile to communicate intent when making choices in five trials with 80 percent accuracy across two sessions as measured by charted data.

Many children are learning to play with others in *Building Fundamentals*. It is typical for children to play independently, then next to a peer or sibling, and then use communication skills to make connections with peers as they build their communication skills. It is also important for the child to have group play and learning opportunities to help children learn to navigate social interaction, attention to the task, memory of the interaction, and engagement in communication.

A place to start with *Building Fundamentals*

Take a look at some important social and communication skills that can be fostered in the stage of *Building Fundamentals* of communication. These skills let the child and all communication partners know that language has an effect on others. In the left column are examples of target language skills. In the middle column are vocabulary recommendations for dynamic cultural and linguistic interaction. In the right column are gestural recommendations that support the language skill. It is more than encouraged to teach the vocabulary and gestural communication options to optimize the effective use of the language skills.

O Social language communication skills

Language Skill	Vocabulary	Gesture
1 Ask questions	*What's that?* or *Why?*	Shrug shoulders, point to an icon or, raise an eyebrow
2 Social greetings	Verbal or AAC device to say *hello* and *goodbye*	Wave hello or goodbye
3 Turn-taking	*My turn/your turn, you go/ I go, me/you*	Point to icons or the person to indicate a turn
4 Sharing information	Make a list of favorite objects and people's names	Point to favorite objects and people your child can initiate a conversation about
5 Initiating communication	Vocalization or words such as *hi, play?, go?*	Smile, giving a toy, showing a toy or icon of play such as swings or a play object
6 Self-regulation	*Wait, no, yes, I need a break, no more, one more, all done*	Look away, turn away
7 Agreement	*Yes, okay, yeah,*	Smile
8 Comment	*Oops, uh-huh, okay, yes, no*	Eye contact
9 Making choices	*I pick, I choose, I want*	Point to 2–8 picture icons to select a song in circle time, a book to read, etc.
10 Wants and needs	List/pictures of personal needs for self-care and hygiene, toys, preferred objects, and foods?	Verbalize, point to icons, or use a speech generating device to state wants and needs

Now let's meet Moses through a case study that details principles in *Building Fundamentals*.

Building Fundamentals case study: meet Moses

Moses, a six-year-old son, was born in Nigeria and is the eldest of three children. His mother is an outstanding English teacher whose students won awards of excellence and his father is a banker. After immigrating to the United States, his parents found a less homogenous culture where they experienced frequent misunderstandings specifically with their child's disability and eligibility terminology even though they are fluent in English. Little did they know that many native English-speaking parents are confused too by the laws regulating special education. His parents believe Moses will develop language and social skills with the right tools, techniques, and strategies including speech generating devices and literacy. They see him first as their son, who is so much more than the sum of his diagnoses of visual impairment and autism. Moses, who spoke as a toddler is now a limited verbal child.

His parents speak to him in English and Ibu, their primary language. His family and interventionists value his strengths. He pays great attention to those around him, wanting to interact in his unique way and follow directions spoken to him. They see his strengths as being a major contributing factor to his learning, communication, and participation. He is ready for *Building Fundamentals*. They asked themselves, What could happen when he has access to assistive communication so that he can participate, not just passively observe?

Building Fundamentals of communication for Moses means he and his parents, two siblings, and interventionists recognize the effect his communication has on others as he exchanges new information and takes turns in conversations. He strives to learn the fundamentals of participating using American English. How will he demonstrate he wants to be heard by others? How will he respond to others, initiate on his own, and express his specific interests? He expresses his own feelings and seeks solutions as a person and a communicator. According to authors Fryholm (2019) and Vygotsky (1986), language has history embedded within it. How will Moses articulate who he is and what he means when he has no history with this new language? *Building Fundamentals* is a time for the expansion of his language to articulate his ideas while he improves comprehension of his history with communication partners across environments.

○ Section 1 Social interaction: What are Moses' communication strengths and preferences? How does he interact socially with others?

Moses is described as *especially fast at learning* often reciting nursery rhymes as a toddler, his mother notes. When his mother comments on how obedient he is, she holds up her hand to give him a *high five*. He claps his hand with hers before he runs off. She goes on to state that, *People tended to like and admire him and extend their hands to him. Moses expects to love them in return. He appreciates good treatment. When he feels bad about being excluded, he tries to withdraw from the situation. He is very sensitive to other people. He always, in his own little way, expresses his appreciation, whenever he feels like he has been treated finely. He comes close to you, like he is about to hug you; but he wouldn't know how to grab out and hug. He likes sitting on our laps. He flies to his father to be near him when they are together at home.* His mother notes, *Of all the children [in the family], he is most peace loving. He has a lot of personality.*

What are Moses' communication strengths and preferences? Moses' mother recognizes how important communication is to him through his interactions. He enters into family conversations by moving his body closer to a person and smiling without verbal language to shape his intent. At school, he puts his face close to his teacher's face to get a response. Others notice he is extraordinarily bright child. He has interests and likes and dislikes, just like his younger brother Anthony and sister Chi Chi.

His smiles and gestures affirm that he prefers crunchy foods like pretzels, dried jerky like meat, pizza crusts, and lollipops. In fact, according to his mother, *Moses prefers eating as an activity. He seems to choose food by how the foods feel with his hands and teeth. Eating is his hobby!* However, his parents do not see a pattern to his early actions. Sometimes he accepts an object he seems to be interested in but other times he drops the object as soon as it is in his hand. Maybe his motor control did not allow him to hold the object. Maybe he lost interest. Now, Moses interacts using nonverbal language including smiles, pointing, moving closer to others, and gestures and actions to communicate with his parents, two younger siblings, and others. He may vocalize but rarely speaks a word. His mother may verbally models the word *bye* and pick up his hand to wave *bye* to which he repeats the word. He is beginning to use a static display speech generating device and communication boards with four symbols for social interaction to say, *Hi, How are you? Thanks!* and *Bye for now*, which are new steps forward and upward for him.

His mother comments that movement helps Moses focus his thinking while he uses his auditory skills. Even while he is moving his hands by flapping them in front of his eyes or looking away briefly, he is learning from the sounds around him. At school Moses generally sits for only 5 to 15 minutes at a time and then walks around the classroom. Educators observe that Moses pays attention for up to 30 minutes especially during the daily literacy lessons. Moses' mother reports that he thrives on compliments because someone *appreciates what he does.*

How does Moses interact socially? In Nigeria it is customary to show respect and humility with a communication partner by looking down at the ground. In the United States, Moses had to learn to establish and maintain eye contact by looking at his communication partner. Moses continues to look down with other adults as he had learned in his home country for many years. His mother reports, *His first instinct is to try to obey you and respect you, before his handicap nature stops him.* He is the first to follow his mother's every direction, even if his siblings remain unruly. She continues to say, *he does not stop just for a moment, he will* *not do it again.* When he promises to *behave well with others, he will most times.* His teacher reports that, *Moses is curious, interested, and observes others.*

When someone speaks to Moses in English, he takes his turn by replying with his own vocalizations sometimes with or without gestures. He may reply with a string of consonants and vowels, gestures like reaching for a person or object, or sometimes looking away. Strangers mistakenly interpret his communication as his speaking another language. Moses creates his own way of saying he was hungry by rubbing his stomach. The richness of Moses communication strengths and preferences serve as a wonderful springboard for Building Fundamentals of communication that allow connection for communication and participation.

⊙ Questions for Reflection

Section 1 Social Interaction Questions: What are Moses' communication strengths and ways he engages in social interaction?

1 Moses' distinctive communication strengths include all EXCEPT which one of the following:
   a Moses is a fast learner and capitalizes the use of his auditory skills
   b Moses expresses himself with smiles, body movements, and rare verbal speech
   c Moses pays attention to others and is motivated to interact with others
   d Moses has a visual impairment and stereotypical behavior associated with autism

2 Review the statements on social interaction. Choose words from the word bank to complete the statements.
   Word Bank: engages, proximity, auditory, gestures, turns
   a Moses is a curious _____ learner showing great interest in others.
   b Moses _____ with people and takes _____ with peers.
   c Moses uses physical _____ and _____ to engage or disengage.

Answers

1 Letters d. is the correct answers. Moses is more than his diagnosis of a visual impairment and autism. His strengths are in his nonverbal skills, auditory skills, and motivation to learn and be with others.

2 The following statements include the correct answers from the word bank.
   a Moses is a curious *auditory* learner showing great interest in others.
   b Moses *engages* with people and takes *turns* with peers.
   c Moses uses physical *proximity* and *gestures* to engage or disengage.

○ Section 2 Communication activities: In what communication activities does Moses participate in frequently?

Moses has an array of communication activities he participates in including music, familiar personal care routines, playing outside, sequences of events at home and at school, and going on car rides. The activities afford him the opportunity to communicate with his family and peers, teachers and interventionists, and less familiar people as well. Moses' family makes participation a priority for him across home, school, and the community.

Music: Often when Moses' dad turns on music from the radio, his brother and sister begin to clap and dance. Moses first smiles and watches them, eventually joining the dance. At other times, he is a reluctant participant. Moses may also sit down on the floor as if to say, *I do not want to dance.* Moses teaches us that sometimes we want to observe and sometimes we want to dance.

Personal care routines: Moses participates at home in a number of personal care routines such as hygiene, dressing, and getting ready to leave the house. These routines are familiar and important to him just like participating in community events and attending church. He follows the sequence for brushing his teeth, taking a bath, toileting, and other routines. His mother states, *He starts smiling when he is told that it is time for his bath. In wearing new clothes, he becomes the big man who walks with a special pride in his step. He is very neat and orderly. He is curious and intelligent, just not able to express it in words.*

Sequences of events: In a similar vein of understanding routines, Moses recognizes sequences of events that are common at home and school. His mother reported that on one occasion, *He was jumping up and down with excitement of having accomplished a task in helping his mother get a diaper for his sister. Then he laughed to make a joke as he took the diaper to his dad instead of handing it to his mother who had requested it.* He immediately gets up, picks up his chair, and goes to the door of his classroom when the teacher announces physical education time. Other sequences, like putting together puzzles, were not met with such vigor and satisfaction. While Moses completes a puzzle, his engagement is limited, perhaps because his restricted sight and use of his hands to place puzzle pieces correctly is challenging or maybe puzzles are just not that motivating for him.

Playing outside: Moses' parents know by the way he walks back and forth and goes to the door that he wants to go outdoors especially when he had been in the house too long. He walks to where his mother laid her house keys to encourage her to hurry up and leave the house. *Everything is in a hurry*, says his mother. His pacing, his sitting, then standing and running to the hall, then running back again to the couch, all in rapid succession were the signs to his parents that play time outside was in order. On days when Moses does not go to school, Moses opens the door, touches his mother, and goes to the door again as if to say, *Time to go out now.*

Car rides: Moses loves to ride in the car. He will sit straight in his seat and watch the cars as they go by. Moses is keenly aware of the family dynamics surrounding the car: Dad drives and Mom does not. He watches and waits to see if his Dad leaves the house first because this tells him that they are going somewhere in the car. However, if his mother heads to the door, he sees no need to be called to action because a car ride is not involved.

The beauty of the breadth of the communication activities Moses participates in creates a pool of ideas and serves as a spring board to new communication activities for routines, sequences, new hobbies, and community events for future participation and resulting communication.

Reflection Questions for Review

Section 2 Communication activities: In what activities does Moses participate in frequently?

1   Moses regularly participated in all of these activities EXCEPT:
    a   Music
    b   Riding in car
    c   Watching television
    d   Swinging

2   Review the statements on communication activities. Indicate T = True or F = False
    a   _____ The benefit of participation is that opportunities for communication are built in!
    b   _____ The opportunity to participate did not improve communication across partners.
    c   _____ Moses teaches us that participation in routines and sequences allow him to self-regulate, understand time and space, process ideas, and learn new information.

Answers

1   Letter d. is correct. Music, riding, and watching television are preferred activities for Moses. While swinging is a perfectly acceptable activity it was not in his repertoire.
2   Letter a. is True, with participation comes communication. Letter b. is False, as Moses communication did improve communication. Letter c. is True, the benefits of routines and sequences support self-regulation, understand time and space, process and learn.

○ Section 3 Facilitator strategies: What strategies do Moses' communication facilitators and partners use at home and at school?

Home: Moses' most familiar communication facilitators and partners at home are his parents and siblings. Moses' parents serve as communication facilitators when they help others understand his smiles and actions. Moses' parents are also his communication partners as they interact throughout the day. His family feels his hearing is sensitive so they use the strategy of speaking softly to him. His family reported, *He could hear noises seemingly for miles and miles away.* His mother speculates that *lacking full vision makes his hearing more sensitive. As an infant, if you made any noise around him, he would squeal. Now he is interested in every sound, seeming to be all ears and to ask, 'What is that sound?'* His family is keen to follow routines that allow Moses to understand what the task is, when he is supposed to do the task, and why. Moses was not above highlighting violations to routines. One time, Anthony sat in the right-hand corner of the couch, Moses made it clear that place was his and he nudged him gently as if to say, *This is my place, move please.* His family provides Moses with the gift of time to process information. This strategy allows Moses to take advantage of his strength with auditory processing and then work with his sensory regulation to accomplish a task or process input from the environment.

School: Moses is assigned to a class of young children with complex communication and physical profiles, ages 5–12 years. Moses is patient and cooperative, but functional communication interaction with other classmates is limited. Most of the children use unique nonverbal communication to express themselves. Moses' teacher and aides are his primary facilitators and communication partners. Moses recognizes the class routine and follows visual schedules made for him each day. The visual schedules allow Moses and interventionists to anticipate specific academic tasks and events such class time, recess, physical education, or snack. A psychologist recommended that his classroom placement be in a language rich environment that follows a strong academic curriculum. As of yet, no reassignment is made.

Many of Moses' interventionists and paraprofessionals are keen to monitor his need for input and to help him initiate movement with verbal prompts or touching his arm. He communicates with his eye gaze, smiles, physically moving toward preferred activities and is ready to make choices while his educational team supports his communication. The team learns to support AAC access strategies such as eye gaze at icons, pointing, and vocalizing to initiate communication and to lead others. The IEP team employs the strategy called aided language stimulation in which adults and peers model messages on Moses' communication boards and speech generating devices. The modeling supports Moses' ability to learn the sequence of steps to express a message. The IEP team recognizes that one key next step will be to add more icons so he can express his feelings and emotions. His current AAC tools and devices include communication boards, visual schedules, and multiple types of single message speech generating devices. The IEP team provides Moses with a LittleMack© and BIGmack©, single message speech generating device to participate in circle time and to make choices. He also wore an AbleNet TalkTrac Wearable Communicator© speech generating device on his wrist that allows him to express four programmed messages for social greetings and responses. To accommodate his vision needs the team enlarges visual symbols and selects contrasting background colors.

Reflection Questions for Review

Section 3 Facilitator Strategies: What strategies do Moses' facilitators and communication partners use at home and school?

1 All of the following facilitator strategies were successfully employed in Moses' home EXCEPT which one of the following?
   a Giving clues in a soft voice
   b Building skills within routines
   c Providing instruction through drill
   d Offering positive reinforcement such as high-fives and verbal praise 'good job'

2 What strategies do Moses communication facilitators use at school? Match the strategy to the example.

Strategy	Example from Moses
a Aided language stimulation	_____ Touch cues at the forearm support Moses' initiation of a motor plan
b Prompts	_____ Communication boards, single and multiple message speech generating devices
c Recognize communicative intent	_____ Modeling communication by creating messages using Moses' AAC tools and devices
d AAC tools	_____ When Moses rubs his stomach, it means he is hungry

Answers

1 Letter c. is the correct answer. Providing instruction through drill is not a strategy that was employed. Giving clues in a soft voice, building skills within routines, and offering positive reinforcement are strategies used to teach and communicate with Moses.

○ Section 4 What were Moses' reading and writing experiences?

At home Moses is expected to engage in writing activities while his sibling complete their writing homework. Moses works on drawing lines and circles on paper independently. Usually he holds a crayon or colored pencil. This task is a challenge for Moses as often his independent movement of his arms and hands create random drawings and often he drops the pen.

At school, educators, aware of his literacy needs, read books aloud to Moses and the other students daily and note his interest. Educators see him respond when they spell the letters of his name M-O-S-E-S. When it is his turn, he heads to the front of the class to pick up his name card with the letters and return to his seat. Moses' teacher includes him in the afternoon 30-minute daily phonics lesson that incorporates a visual and kinesthetic component to support his strong auditory skills. The literacy class is comprised of similarly skilled children from different classrooms. In the lessons, Moses' teacher holds up an 8 ½ × 11" card with a single consonant or vowel. Then the educator models the hand and arm motions associated with the letter and says the sound it makes when read. Moses with the other students follows the hand and arm movements and says the sounds. The letter sounds are then blended to form words. He begins to establish decoding and sight word reading. He begins to develop friendships with the other children. For Moses, writing is more art than seeing letters and hearing sounds, it is a time to make friends. His teacher describes his participation in reading and writing tasks. He notes, *Moses is truly curious and interested in what is happening. He will sit and observe others.* He looks forward engaging with his peers and literacy.

Moses keeps working on his goals at his educational level to gain the most benefit. The team has fought past outdated attitudes that promoted low expectations and thoughts that literacy should take a back seat to 'other priorities' for people with severe disabilities. The team at his previous school advised Moses' mother not to expect to *do reading and writing* since Moses had *a hundred other problems.* However, a simple observation of Moses by his new educational team detailed that he had interest in photos, engaging with books, and drawing with interesting utensils. They see literacy ability in Moses and expect these and more skills to develop. The literacy program allows Moses to be actively engaged in his learning incorporating multiple modalities of his hearing, limited vision, need for movement, and application to literacy.

⊙ Questions for Reflection

Section 4 Literacy: What are Moses' reading and writing experiences?

1   How does the reading program selected for Moses' align with his strengths as a learner?
    a   Incorporates movement, visual, and auditory modalities
    b   Focuses on letter and sound association, sound blending and word recognition
    c   Includes peers he could engage with during the reading and writing process
    d   All of the above

2   What outdated attitudes did Moses' IEP team need to fight to promote the best literacy program for Moses?
    a   A child has too many other problems to focus on literacy.
    b   A child must have a certain level of intelligence to work on literacy.
    c   A peer is not a model so access to a variety of types of peers is not necessary.
    d   All of the above

Answers

1   Letter d. All of the above. The literacy program selected for Moses aligns with his strengths as a learner including movement and multiple sensory modalities taught in a natural progression along with peers that make the literacy experience rich.
2   Letter d. All of the above. There are many outdated policies and practices that inhibit children's literacy learning, communication and participation. Moses' IEP team changed their practices to promote literacy skills for children that use AAC.

○ Section 5 Vocabulary: What vocabulary does Moses comprehend and use to participate?

Moses has a rich comprehension of social language and is learning to build fundamentals of expressive language at home and school. He understands the verbal instructions his parents and teachers give him that contain social and academic vocabulary. *He proves to me he understands me by following through with what I say*, his mother notes. The communication tools and devices give Moses access to quick communication and include messages for social greetings, social closeness, requesting wants and needs, commenting, and negation. Quick phrases with social greetings allow Moses to say, *See you soon!* and share information to state, *Let me watch too! Just a minute*, or *I need a break.*

Expressing feelings and emotions with family when he is hurting, happy, or frustrated is a priority for Moses. On rare occasions his mother describes that words seem to *fall out of his mouth.* One morning his mother tried to put on his sock and his toenail got caught. The toenail hurt and Moses pushed his mother and told her, *Go away.* Feelings and emotions words are especially helpful when he has an *immense demand on his heart and mind.* She believes he is telling her, *Allow me to express myself. I have a right to express my feelings. You must find a solution.* He also needs to share his happiness and to reject a request or delay, *No, not now, I will in a minute.* At times he prefers to get up and move for a few seconds, so requesting, *I need to walk now*, or, *I need a break* would make this change of pace welcome to his communication partners. The quick phrases are and continue to be motivating words that will bridge with more complex language as it develops for Moses.

The IEP team gave his mother the idea to take advantage of his stylistic prowess and not only gave him opportunities for choice making during dressing (e.g. blue shirt, brown socks) but to add other relevant describing words (e.g. too scratchy, nice and soft, too tight). He loves turning the music *on and off*, finding where the car keys are *on the chair*, asking to *go out or come* in. While Moses was off to a great start with AAC, he needs to express social etiquette through phrases that supported his communication activities like, *Please move over, I want to help you; Thank you for helping me*, and *You're welcome.* His mother and team incorporated question phrases associated with food preparation such as *What are you fixing now? When will the dinner be ready?* The educational team explores vocabulary that allows Moses to express his comprehension of stories read to the class focusing on the characters, setting, problem, and resolution. This vocabulary supports his thinking, expression, and participation and allows other to hear his voice. They recognize that reading for social studies and scient content requires vocabulary and understanding relationships of events that are complex.

⊙ Questions for Reflection

Section 5 Vocabulary: What vocabulary did Moses comprehend and use to participate?

1 Moses' comprehension of vocabulary is evident in which ways. Indicate T=True or F=False.
   a _____ Moses follows directions given his academic vocabulary.
   b _____ Moses responds to social communication regularly.
   c _____ Moses understands complex abstract communication.
2 According to the case study what AAC expressive vocabulary would Moses benefit from? (Choose three options)
   a Greetings and closures (e.g. hello and goodbye, see you later)
   b Requests (e.g. When dinner will be ready)
   c Sharing information including feelings and emotions
   d Yes and no

Answers

1 True responses are correct for the first two statements. Moses follows conversations socially and at his academic level. However, at the age of nine, Moses does not yet understand most complex abstract communication. It is important to distinguish that this challenge is due to his age and not his disability.
2 Letters a., b., and c. are categories of vocabulary that encourage appropriate interactions for Moses with family and people at school. The ability to say yes and no is important. In Building Fundamentals, we want a child to express the intent behind a statement of yes or no.

○ Section 6 Tools: What AAC tools and devices help Moses with Building Fundamentals in his participation at home and school?

AAC tools equip Moses with multiple modes of expression. Moses' educational team knows from research that using a speech generating device will not interfere, or deter the use of, his occasional spoken speech. His participation with language using communication boards and single and multiple message speech generating devices supports classroom activities such as taking his turn during circle time and making choices. Educators use a single switch speech generating device with a recorded message and simple line drawings to name four sequences in an activity. Moses presses the dual message device to greet others in the morning (*Hi, How are you*?) or request items *(I like that, I don't like that)* such as food or toys and answer academic questions. When Moses has difficulty initiating a motor movement to activate the message programmed on the device, an assistant provides a touch cue. To build fundamentals of language, Moses accesses quick phrases and specific vocabulary. Moses' language development grows at home with his siblings and at school with his classmates when he independently participates by stating, *My turn*! They also recognize that he is physically active and mobile which means that his displays must be mobile. Some speech generating devices require technology that he can carry easily or wear. The watch style device, TalkTrac Wearable Communicator©, is perfect for him to state quick messages for social greetings and quick social responses. Moses and the students in his class benefit from access to assistive technology and play a key role as contributors in *Building Fundamentals* of language development and communication.

A proverb of Moses' native country of Nigeria is *Before shooting one must aim.* Moses' family and intervention team take aim at the goal of communication and language development that leads to greater participation by taking purposeful steps to inform his decision making. They completed the protocol *Hear Me into Voice* to best detail his present communication. They discovered the next steps to foster Moses' communication by augmenting with verbal speech and promoting his participation by developing a multimodal intervention plan with AAC tools and devices to best meet Moses' communication needs and support required for his communication partners.

Questions for Reflection

Section 6 tools question: What is the impact of AAC tools and devices on Moses' communication?

1 Which statement reflects the impact a speech generating device has on spoken language?
   a Speech generating devices do not deter verbalizations and improve participation.
   b Taking away speech generating devices would force Moses to speak.
   c Speech generating devices are not necessary if Moses can use nonverbal communication.
   d Speech generating devices for a limited verbal child are not necessary.

2 How can using AAC tools and devices aid with Building Fundamentals for communication and participation? Select the best answer.

    a AAC tools and devices provide access for the user and communication partners to communicate and participate by using and combining vocabulary that achieve the purposes of communication.

    b AAC is not used for comprehension.

    c AAC is only a tool for the AAC user not communication partners.

    d A device with 'yes' and 'no' and 'please' and 'thank you' suffices for a child Building Fundamentals because communication partners can ask more complex questions that require a one-word response from the child.

Answers

1 The correct answer is a. Using speech generating devices do not deter a child's verbalizations and do improve overall participation. It is outdated thinking that denying a child a speech generating device will force the child to speak or are not necessary for a limited verbal child.

2 Letter a. is the correct answer. AAC tools allow a user and communication partners to participate and communicate. AAC is not just a user experience. AAC is for comprehension and production of rich language.

Case study closing thoughts

Moses is a child whose parents and interventionists honor his interactions with others. *Moses is very curious and intelligent, just not able to express it in words*, his mother states. In *Building Fundamentals*, expand upon your child's established skill set in using familiar routines and vocabulary and move forward using single, dual, four message sequence for greetings, choice making, and describing activities. Keep up the great work in fostering joint attention and add in fun connections with intent, participation, turn taking, question asking, greetings, regulating person and other's behaviors, agreement, and yes, rejection too. Now that's a lot! The great part is that communication is happening so dive into the communication behaviors you see now. Use skills and behaviors you know now in *Getting Started* and consider the logical next steps as your child and team members are *Building Fundamentals*.

Building Fundamentals with communication activities

○ Core words and quick phrases

Now that we have a social and communication skill set established let's add more communication activities. While we head into *Building Fundamentals* activities keep in mind, we will continue to foster joint attention, memory, cognition, and communication. Address the following questions to get yourself started as you help your child build fundamentals. *How long is my child maintaining joint attention for one task and across tasks? What does attention look like for preferred tasks and non-preferred tasks? What types of communication modalities does my child employ with or without facilitator support across different tasks and people? Does the use of gestures meet the communication needs of the interaction? Given the environments my child's participates in what vocabulary needs to be accessible? Would a single or multi-message speech generating device be best? Would a complex dynamic display speech generating device be a better match? Would a low technology board meet the need?*

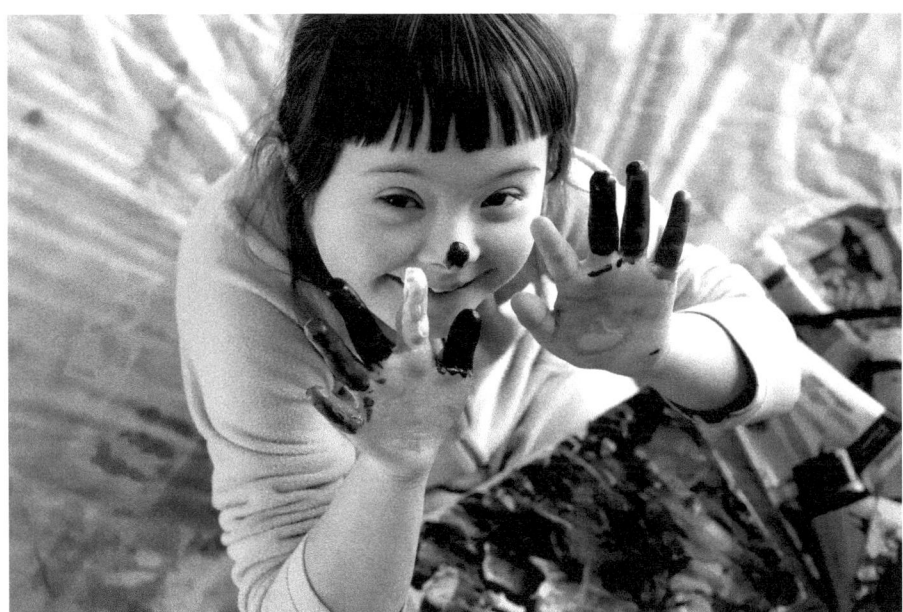

Building Fundamentals communication activities

1 We're Talking Screen Time
2 Groovin' with the Music
3 Cascading Communication – Playing with Pals and Siblings
4 Do It! Giving Commands with Spatial Objects
5 Images of Me: People, Places, and Things
6 What's the Morning Chatter?

Activity: We're talking screen time

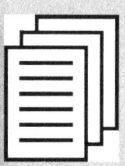

A place to start

Screen time becomes communication time! Children and adults have fun with TV time, tablets, and console games, coined *screen time*. Now we add communication as a part of the fun in the interaction. Continue to follow your family and classroom rules on screen time quantity and quality and add new communication to screen time routines. The pause button may become your new best friend. Let's talk about how.

Communication partner: what I am doing with my child

Make a choice board with the available types of screen options. Talk to your child about how using screen time for you both to comment about what is happening, to indicate turn taking, and work on language targets that may be core words such as *game, music stop*, and *go* or fringe words such as names of specific games, television shows, or tablet applications. Then let your child know that you will be pausing the device at times to allow for talking time. Talk about the idea of commenting, asking questions, and making requests. If you are not sure if your child comprehends the message you are saying, err on the side of caution and proceed! Keep talking! Numerous stories are told by families of children with complex communication profiles that once their child begins to communicate using AAC they are amazed at what their child knows and the level of vocabulary used. The lesson here is to continue to talk to your child.

Vocabulary targets: TV, tablets, and talking

Yes, No, Ohhh no! Play that again, That was so awesome, That's good, Let's try a different . . ., No way, Ooopsie, that happened, I don't know, Wait a minute, Are you kidding me? That's hilarious, funny, silly, scary, boring, no good, so-so.

⊙ My Tool Box

- ◎ Screen time option (e.g. Show, tablet application, gaming system, movie)
- ◎ Core and fringe vocabulary on a communication board or speech generating device
- ◎ Transition tool such as a schedule board or a timer that indicating breaks for commercials, time to comment, comfort breaks, and to transition to another activity

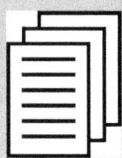

What my child is doing with me

Make sure you and your child are actively engaged with the media form. Use a communication board to make choices about which media form to watch. Recognize that what interests you in a show or program may not be the same as what interests your child such as the story or the music and that is okay. Think about the number of exchanges you would like to have with your child to build attention to a task. You can say something like, We will talk about the show three times (or five times) and then you can share if you want to continue the show or take a break.

Activity: Groovin' with the music

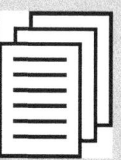

A place to start

According to the National Association for the Education of Young Children (www. naeyc.org), music sets the tone for learning. In addition to listening, moving, dancing, and tapping to the music, children are engaged with each other through melody and poetry. These principles of learning cross all ages and generations. Engagement breeds opportunity for participation cognitively, linguistically, and physically and that is what we want. Music is fun for most people including parents and interventionists and is supported as a powerful tool (Show, 2012). In fact, you may have so much fun with music you may feel like you are not teaching communication when in fact you are simply living communication . . . and interaction . . . and having fun. You might be thinking, didn't we go over using music as a way of *Getting Started*? Yes, we did. Now we are going to progress our communication options with both vocabulary and music song choices. As you head into *Building Fundamentals* skills think about how choice making can be blended with a comment or request. Make choices for the type of media and genre for the music. Then provide the opportunity for commenting on the music. We want your child to take the next step in recognizing that he or she has control within the interaction, with a purpose and intent. Enjoy each interaction.

Communication partner: what I am doing with my child

Make music a choice. When music in an option at home and in therapy sessions, the child is likely to choose it because it's fun! Country, classical, singing, jazz, you name it. Music can be a main activity, used at the start or end of a session, or may just be spontaneous when family and friends are around. WOW think of the opportunity for fun, interaction, and participation for the child if language is a part of the musical experience. Talk about feelings generated by the music (e.g. *This music is exciting. I feel relaxed now. This music is scary!*). Have a communication board or speech generating device with programmed options including music. Then have another communication board for requesting and information sharing. Play music and pause after the chorus, comment, and support requests to change songs or genres.

My Tool Box

- Any music source such as a car radio, music player, phone, tablet, CD player, etc.
- A way for the adult to change or control the playing of the music
- A way for the adult and the child to manipulate the music (e.g. volume controls, switch access with a battery interrupter for music players, on and off dials or buttons) →

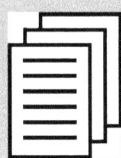

- ◉ Multiple communication options for your child

    - ◉ Nonverbal communication modalities (e.g. eye gaze, head nods, hands, feet, etc.)

    - ◉ Communication board options

    - ◉ Speech generating devices

What my child is doing with me

Your child is hopefully having fun with music physically and emotionally and now will have a way to communicate during music and that communication will be honored. Honoring communication does not mean that the child always gets his or her way. It does mean that the communication is acknowledged. Therefore, if your child makes a choice to choose a different song, you may choose to change the song immediately or you may opt to say, *I hear you. We will change the song after your choice of this song is complete.* If your child is just learning that their voice matters for the first time, you may elect to change the song immediately.

Vocabulary targets: groovin' with the music

Yeah, Nah, Next song, I don't like this song, That's fun, I like this one, Play it again, This is a boring song, Change it, No wait go back to that one, Stay on this song.

Activity: Cascading communication – playing with pals and siblings

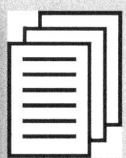

A place to start

Up to this point we have talked a lot about participation and how to recognize, catalogue, and build communication. Now let's look at how to play. Better yet, let's look at how to play with pals and siblings. Help your child learn to transfer those great budding communication skills with other communication partners across tasks and across settings or environments (Kaniel & Feuerstein, 1974). Remember that communication grows and spreads like a wonderful explosion cascading into new settings like classrooms and playgrounds and with others like pals and siblings. Your place to start is picking a setting and a person other than yourself to cascade communication.

Communication partner: what I am doing with my child

Expanding your child's communication partners and environments is such a powerful and amazing step. Not only do you open up your child's world, you open up your world and role in three distinct ways. First, you step into a new role of helping others understand your child's modes of communication. Fortunately, you already know those modes because you completed *Hear Me into Voice*. Select one way your child most consistently expresses a preferred message. Secondly you model what communication looks like for peers and siblings. Third, you serve as a communication facilitator that supports effective communication between your child and peer or sibling and others without directly influencing the course of the interaction. Look to My Tool Box for materials and communication options.

My Tool Box

- Play materials: Bubbles – too baby-ish? Never! Try larger bubble wands, balloons, Mr. Potato Head, blocks, toy cars and planes, dolls and action figures, card games to play Go Fish, UNO, matching, board games, puzzles

- Multiple communication options for the child

  - Nonverbal communication modalities (e.g. eye gaze, head nods, hands, feet, etc.)

  - Speech generating device with a single message option

  - Communication board option

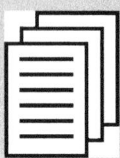

What my child is doing with me

Interestingly the heading for this section was almost changed to, *What My Child is Doing*, sans *with Me*, but while we are interested in expanding *your* child's repertoire, you are an active figure in the communication. What your child is doing with you is looking to you to facilitate interaction. Your child is having fun in a social context and may lose sight of the task of communication. This opens up the opportunity to 1) make sure your child is actively communicating, 2) you serve as an active participant, and 3) you validate your child's communication within the context of the group dynamic. We are in the *Building Fundamentals* stage so baby steps with social interaction with peers and siblings is expected. Therefore, keep an eye on core vocabulary that would allow that next step in participation to happen. If the first step is to have the opportunity to be a part of a social dynamic, then the next step is to determine key core vocabulary that will support communication in the social dynamic. The following core vocabulary offered is a start, a launching pad. Consider developing a choice board of activities or use a core board of activities already developed from other activities.

Core vocabulary targets: cascading communication-playing with pals and siblings

Hi, bye, that's good, cool! Go, yes or sure, no, let's make a different choice, no way, stop

Activity: Do it! Giving commands with spatial concepts

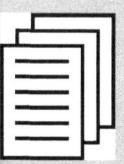

A place to start

Kids like to give directions! Have control, take control, set your child up to give commands in a world that is often out of their control. Giving commands allows a child to know and experience that he or she has an impact on another person's behavior. In *Getting Started* there is a big emphasis on joint attention that is built upon in *Building Fundamentals* by focusing on communication impacting other's behavior. Giving commands does exactly that and while we are at it, let's build vocabulary skills in the area of spatial concepts called prepositions.

Communication partner: what I am doing with my child

Teach vocabulary such as: *on, off, in, out, over*, and *under* with most games or activities. While some prepositions are offered, please feel free to use prepositions that make sense to your child and the context. Consider making a game using toys. You can prompt *Where should I put the car?* Your child can respond with the appropriate preposition such as *on or off* the track, board, box, or etc. You may also your child apply commands using drawing materials. *Draw the line up, down, over, on.* Another fun game is to use tangrams and receive directions on where to place shapes to make an object using circles, squares, rectangles, and parallelograms.

My tool box options depending on the task you choose

- Variety of cars, small toys, blocks, etc. Collect a grab bag of miscellaneous toys
- Container, box, sorting tray
- Drawing materials
- Games like tangrams, board games, dice, and more
- Multiple communication options for the child

    - Nonverbal communication modalities (e.g. eye gaze, head nods, hands, feet, etc.)
    - Communication board options
    - Speech generating device with a single message option

What my child is doing with me

Your child is giving commands and your child is learning prepositional concepts. Best of all your child is learning that he or she makes an impact on your actions, your behavior. Your child can be prompted to give command at this stage using a communication modality such as pointing, a communication

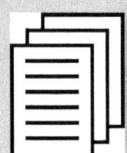

board or a speech generating device to indicate which person to follow and confirm communication with a *yes, no, that's not what I meant, you are good to go.*

Vocabulary targets: do it! Giving commands with spatial concepts

On, off, in, out, over, under, yes, no (Feel free to work with fewer or other prepositions).

Activity: Images of me: people, places, and things

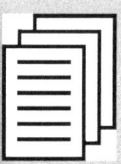

A place to start

Put your child's world into pictures and print. A child using AAC will benefit greatly from having his or her world favorites shown in pictures with print. This means generating pages with relevant pictures and the word or words describing the people, places, and things. Having images of people, places, and things accomplishes multiple objectives: 1) Having the images and words available to talk about is accessing memories and sharing experiences; The images represent a form of the child's identity that may be fluid and changing as your child matures; 2) The pictures and images are an opportunity for self-expression when they are available on a communication board, a speech generating device; 3) They allow your child's communication partner to have a common ground in which to talk and interact with your child. How incredible! We want our children that use AAC to initiate conversations and we want others to know they can initiate interaction with a child that uses AAC. Now let's talk about how.

Communication partner: what I am doing with my child

Create a list of preferred people, places, and things. Do not feel the list has to be exhaustive. In fact, you can keep the list shorter with three to five items so communication partners do not feel too overwhelmed in knowing what to choose to talk about. What you can do is have a running list or picture page of possible options especially if you are worried about limiting your child. If you are just *getting started* with *Building Fundamentals* (no I am not apologizing for the unintended pun) go easy on yourself in trying to *do it all* and just get the project off the ground with a few images. Create pages and organize these people and places on a communication board, a folder, binder, or book, or a speech generating device. Once your pages are created show the pages to the intervention team so they can use them in therapy and better yet expand to new communication partners. For example, have the classroom teacher show children in the classroom what your child likes to do, where your child likes to go and has gone. Make a grab and go page of topics and things people can comment on when your family is in a public place like a park or at sibling activities, or sporting events, art classes, or music concerts. A lot of modeling is occurring at this stage but that is great because you and your child are *Building Fundamentals*.

My Tool Box

- Pictures: Family with printed names, friends with names, people in the child's life with names and titles as applicable, places the child likes to go on a fairly regular basis, special places the child may visit or

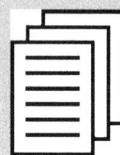

> has visited, special toys, objects, favorite things, colors, pets; favorite activities they each like to do.
>
> ◎ Communication board, folder, binder, book, static speech generating devices or other ways to present the images with vocabulary for commenting and sharing
>
> ◎ Create a quick communication page or tip card to attach to a backpack or wheelchair
>
> ◎ Optional: Create a 'library' page of people, places, and things for anyone to draw from, to add, or take away from a communication board when talking with specific people.

What my child is doing with me

Your child is learning that he or she can strike up a conversation with inviting images and words to interact with children and adults. This is a powerful tool that supports your child as much as the communication partners. It is fun. It is quick. It is effective. Your child role play interaction with the pages you make for your child.

Vocabulary targets: images of me – people, places, and things

Yes, no, That one, look, That's my favorite, hi, bye, What do you like? Where do you like to go? Give me time to pick what I want to tell/show you, I need a minute, Ask me another question, Let's pick together. Let's talk about another picture. Show me what you like to do!

Activity: What's the morning chatter?

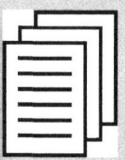

A place to start

What's the morning chatter? For adults this time may be checking in with social media, the morning news, a greeting at the cafeteria or office break area. We all have a way to get our day set, our social greetings, and a plan for the day. So, let's make sure that happens for our children that use AAC. Circle time centers of many early education offer routines in which children respond to their name, talk about the day of the week, work on time, the weather, names of classmates present in school, the activities for the day, and other fun events. For AAC users, let's have the daily schedule set so expectations are clear and communication hits the ground running.

Communication partner: what I am doing with my child

While many options are offered in the *My Tool Box* section, do not feel pressure to do them all. Pick something that works for you to integrate into your child's communication repertoire such as talking about events at different times of the day, reinforcing the names of people that will be a part of the events of the day, include expectations for weather, the day of the week, the joke of the day, tasks that must be accomplished, and more. Talk about what communication may be needed when so your child can anticipate how to use AAC.

⊙ My Tool Box

- ◉ Core communication board for commenting
- ◉ Communication board or speech generating device page with weather words
- ◉ Communication board or speech generating device page with day of the week cards
- ◉ Monthly calendar (traditional home style, school style, communication board or device)
- ◉ Digital and analogue clock
- ◉ Names of family members, friends, and other adults the child will closely interact with in the day such as therapists and academic staff
- ◉ Nonverbal communication modalities (e.g. eye gaze, head nods, hands, feet, etc.)

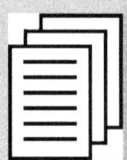

What my child is doing with me and others

Remember what are we doing in this stage of communication? Right, we are *Building Fundamentals.* By engaging your child in the morning or daily chatter of life, you are building the fundamentals of what people know about or find out about in their day. Discussing these chatter topics gives your child a sense of the world he or she is in. It can help explain why he or she needs pants instead of shorts, why it seems to be cold or hot outside, a sense of when class, therapy, and play time will occur, and who the child will interact with during the day. Discussing these topics will support the child's self-regulation. Use these topics to help your child comment and ask questions about his or her day.

Core vocabulary targets: what's the morning chatter?

Yay, no, really, today, tomorrow, Say it again, I need to say something else, Uh oh, good, wait, what did you say? Tell me that again. Who is coming? Who will I see? No way. Hold on.

Building Fundamentals with facilitator strategies

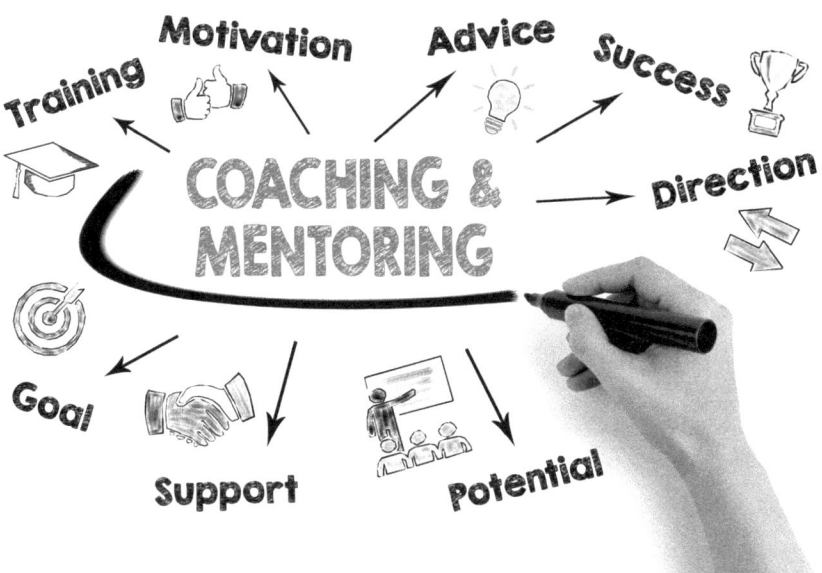

○ Grab and Go Coaches' Corner

This *Grab and Go Coaches' Corner* for *Building Fundamentals* is dedicated to supporting facilitators, communication partners, and children with learning language, playing, trying new tasks, discovering opportunities, shaping ideas for communication, and just having fun with interaction. It is a terrific stage. Let's look at some ideas that can support you, support your child's language, communication, interaction, and participation development.

1 How Many Icons Should I Pick?
2 What Size Should the Icons Be?
3 How Do I Pick Appropriate Games to Play?
4 Literacy, Hide and Seek, and Flashlights Too!
5 Play Opportunities: Thinking Multi-Sensory
6 Fostering Your Child's Initiation of Communication
7 Honoring the Child's Communication and Therapeutic Communication
8 Communicating So My Communication Partner Understands

○ *Facilitator tips for* Building Fundamentals *with communication*

1 *How many icons should I pick? That's the question.*

Answer Part A: Focus on skill development not quantity: We want your child knowing how he or she is successful with the communication process. The more motivating the items, the more likely the child will want to communicate. If you think about your favorite things, the list is not going to be super long, so it is okay to keep the number of items on the lower end to emphasize the priority of learning to make a choice or select an item to express an intent.

Answer Part B: Two to 12 icons should get the job done. In the stage of *Building Fundamentals*, children should have the option of choosing between two and 12 (or more) preferred objects or pictures. Remember in *Getting Started* we begin with learning that symbols represent objects or concepts. Then children learn to differentiate between a preferred and non-preferred symbol. Now we look at adding more symbols. Know that two symbols are just fine! Your child is increasing comprehension and symbolic understanding at the same time. Keep your priorities firm. Here are some more questions and ideas you want to keep in mind.

1 Monitor the difference between too many choices and the ability to scan choices.
2 How many items will impact my child's ability to attend to a choice?
3 How many items will overwhelm my child?
4 Does my child have symbolic understanding of the symbols offered?
5 Does my child still need to learn other concepts represented in the image?

Are you seeing a change in how long it takes for your child to respond? Are you seeing any shut down behaviors? Is accuracy impacted? Work with an speech-language pathologist to get you started in answering all of these questions. This is what they are good at! Consider the time it takes for your child to respond. In some cases, the time delay may be a clue that symbolic understanding of an object or idea is not solidified. Time delays may also represent processing or motor planning delays. In some cases, such as autism, waiting may be the necessary and right thing to do or providing support in initiating a response. For children with intellectual delays or differences, working on decision making skills may be a necessary step to success.

2 What size should the icons be?

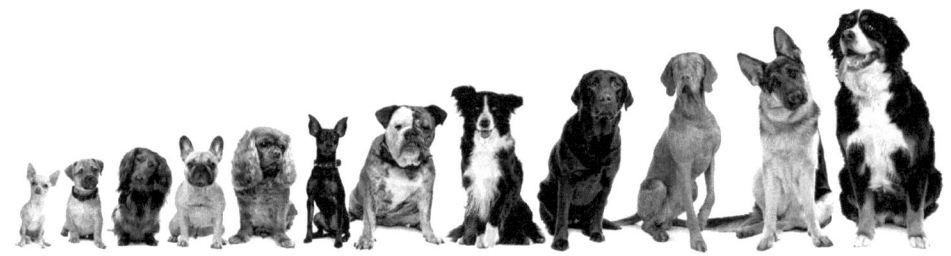

Answer: The short answer is, assuming your child has symbolic understanding of the icons containing pictures with words, you want to consider your child's vision and fine motor skills. Ask and answer the following questions to guide your decision making. I know that is not a direct answer but just keep reading.

1 What size do my icons (pictures with words) need to be in order for my child to see the images?
2 What size do my icons need to be in order for my child to point to them?
3 What size do my icons need to be in order for my child to pick them up?
4 Does my child have the strength to pull an icon off of a Velcro© board?
5 Are the icons best represented on the selected grid size of a speech-generating device?

Answer: okay here we go. What size do my icons need to be?

Typical or corrected to normal vision: If your child does not have a vision impairment then you can probably make icons smaller than you think. Typically, icons are 1 inch to 1½ inches in size. Some communication apps have ½ inch by ½ inch icons. See which size your child can access most easily. Size matters and it is a secondary decision at this stage because we are not managing a lot of icons at one presentation to your child at this stage in the game. Worry less about size.

Vision impairment: Work with a vision specialist and a speech-language pathologist to decide how large the icons should be, how far apart the icons should be placed, what color and thickness the border lines should be, and finally what is the best background color.

Speech generating devices: Static speech generating devices will have a set sizes for the images and the sizing will work for most users. The size of the icons can be one square inch up to three square inches or more. Dynamic display options on speech generating devices will vary so size is a *feature consideration*. See *Feature Matching* in *Chapter 5 Bridging Skills.* Some tablet applications and all high-tech speech generating devices allow adjustments to icon size in addition to background color modifications and border size. Other advantages of some apps and most speech generating devices are the options to have auditory scanning, visual scanning, or auditory and visual scanning of the icons. Be aware of set vocabulary with apps or high-tech device for how salient it is to your child. Work with a speech-language pathologist to answer your questions. Use what makes sense!

3 How do I pick appropriate games to play?

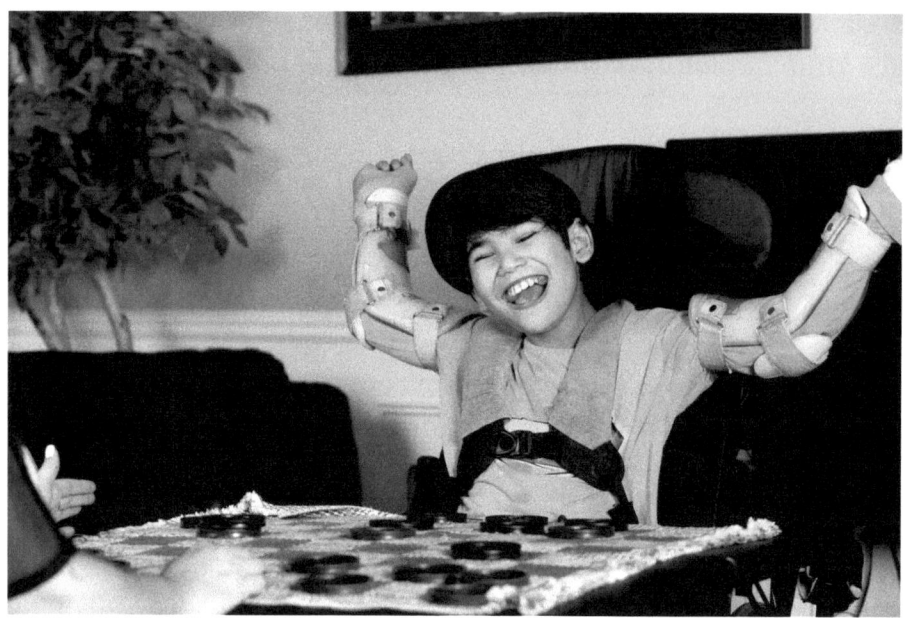

Good news! Many games work across ages. Purchase common children's card games. Pick up some balls. Acquire a 12-24-300 piece or any size puzzle and your child will construct. Use board games and support your child as needed with turn taking that provide classic good fun for friends and families. Consider team board game playing rather than playing one person against another. Your child's participation with peers and adults may include spinning a wheel, throwing dice, counting spaces, moving markers, stacking wood, telling you what to do, and many more options. Focus language development on engaging phrases on a single or dual switch such as *Build the blocks higher!* and *Knock 'em down!*

4 Literacy, hide and seek, and flashlights too!

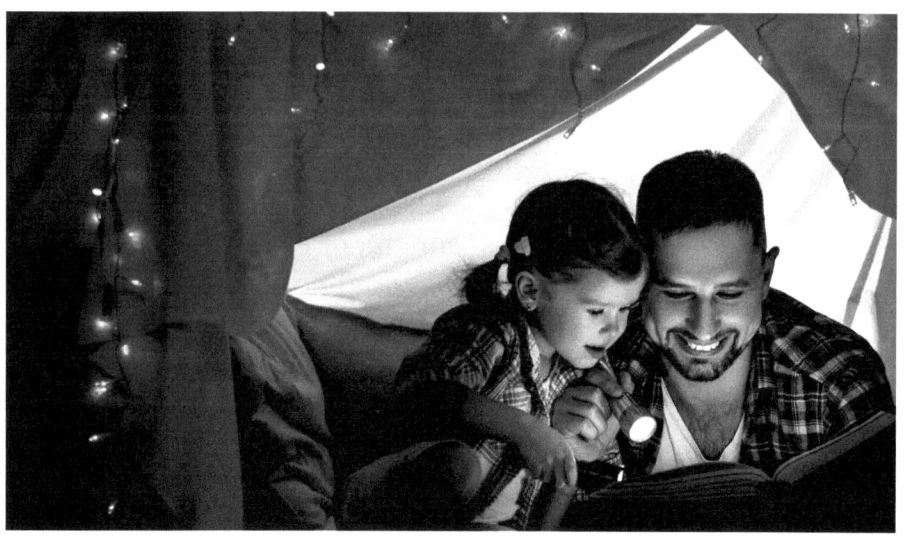

Think of one of your favorite stories that you enjoyed reading again and again just for the fun of the story and interaction. Do that now with your child building anticipation and familiarity with a story, redundancy in hearing and seeing language with each reading, deeper learning, and engagement. Choose one of your child's favorite books that engages your child because the story is captivating, the pictures are vibrant, the popup or flap book is fun, or maybe you are sharing one of your favorite childhood books. Then, each day choose something different to do with the same book using the following ideas as a springboard to even more ideas.

Day 1 Select and read a favorite book.
Day 2 Hide the book in the room and find it together.
Day 3 Use a flashlight and read the book in the dark or a dimly lit room.
Day 4 Put the book in a box or bag and 'unwrap' the book.
Day 5 Record your voice reading the book and play it back while you follow
  along.

5 Play opportunities: thinking multi-sensory

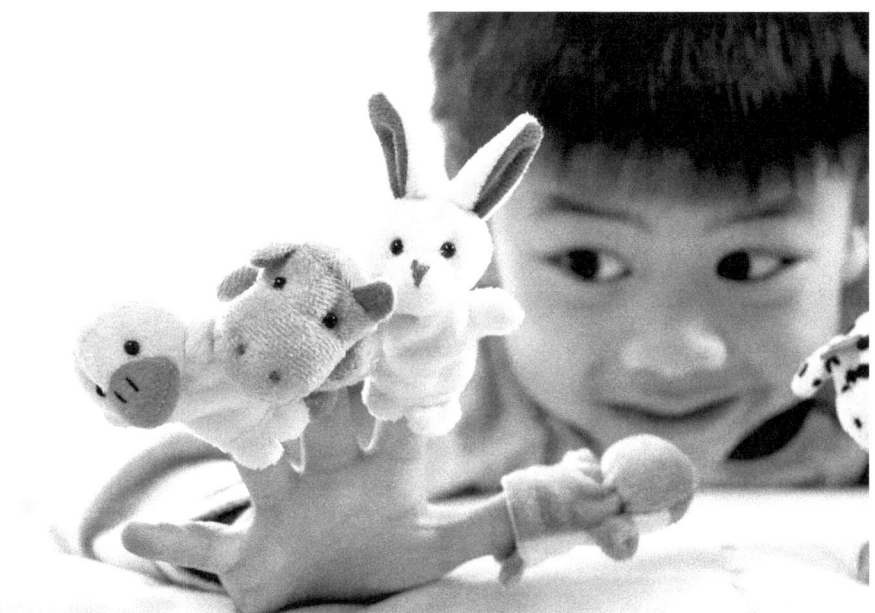

A messy kid is a sign of a good day! Finger puppets, paper bag puppets, play dough, shaving cream, painting, sand, seashells, uncooked pasta, slime, mud, blades of grass, leaves, sticks, straws, Q-tips, pipe cleaners, craft feathers, rocks, coins, flowers, spices … and just keep going! Google 'messy crafts' and hundreds of activities and website will populate on your computer screen. Many crafts contribute to the development of writing skills. Don't worry the interaction does not have to be messy but it does have a great opportunity for language development. Access spin art with a switch to activate a battery-operated art spinner. Children that use AAC often have physical limitations and guess what? They love to play too even if it means getting some motor help to interact with mud and paint. The fun with interaction and language is priceless. You may discover new favorite activities and means of effective communication with multi-sensory play.

6 Fostering your child's initiation of communication

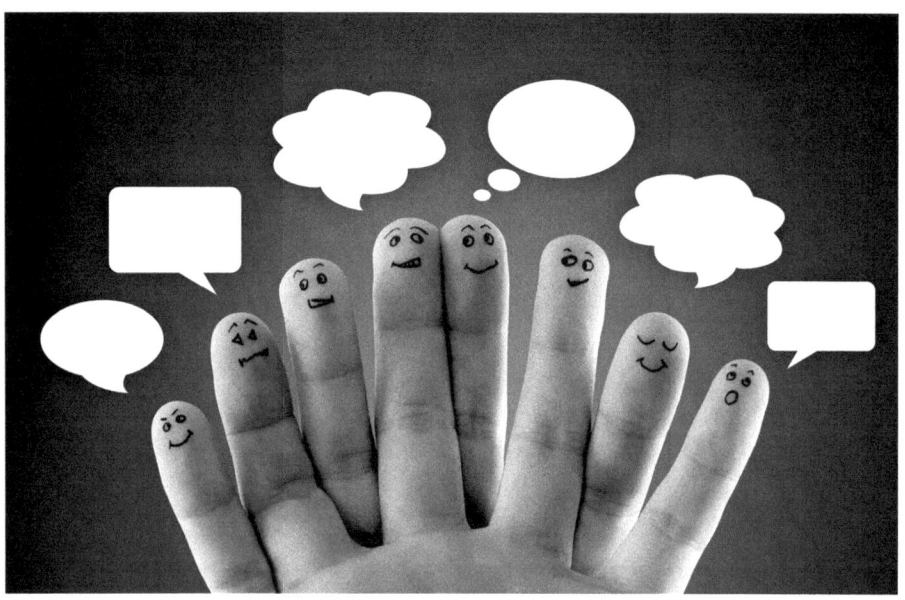

Tell me 2 ways...

Tell me 3 ways...

Moving your child beyond making a choice is a common desire voiced by interventionists in the world of AAC. There is nothing wrong with asking your child questions and offering choices. We want to create many types of reciprocal communication including initiation. Keep your child's communication tools and devices in his or her reach. Offer many opportunities for your child to comment. Remember to question less and comment more with your child. When your child initiates a request or message, treat this request or message as valid and follow through with granting the request and sharing information back. Let your child know his or her initiation of communication matters.

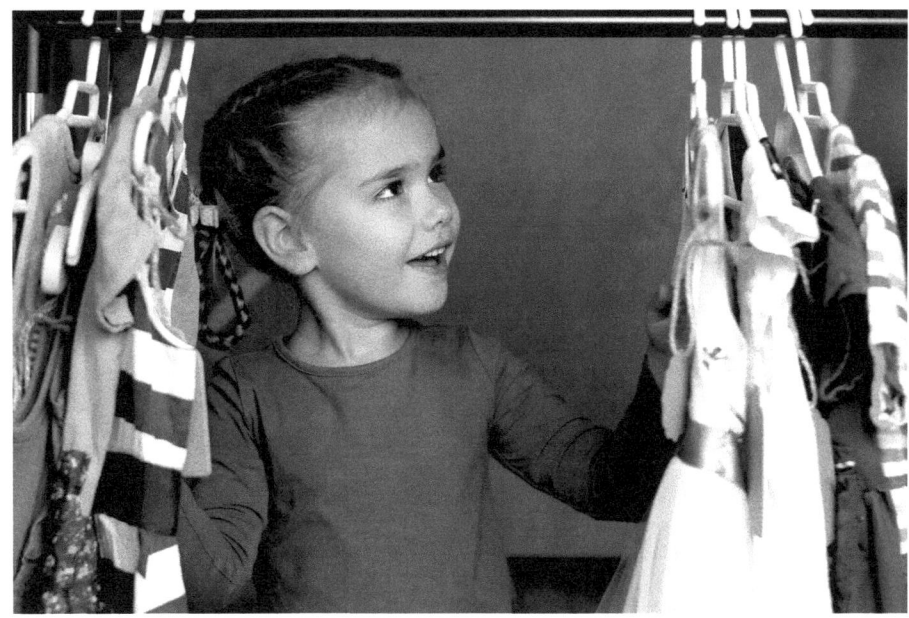

What's the difference? In the *Getting Started* stage you as a parent or interventionist gathered the ways or modalities your child communicates. Now in the *Building Fundamentals* stage you want to reinforce those ways your child communicates a message in two ways. The first way is honoring your child's communication by responding immediately as in a typical conversation. The second way is therapeutic communication. Simply stated, talk to your child and say, *Okay for the next 15 minutes I want you to practice telling me your message in as many ways as you can. You can use your head turning, your eyes, your hands, your voice, or your speech generating device.* For example, your child can indicate they want to continue an activity. If your child uses eye gaze, acknowledge that communication with praise and say, *Okay, great now tell me two ways.* If your child uses a speech generating device acknowledge that communication with praise and say, *Okay now tell me three ways!* Even if your child has more than three communication modalities, sticking to two or three ways so you accomplish both practicing communication modalities and eventually honoring the intended message. Increase or decrease the number of modalities depending on whether your child is having a good day, needs to expand his or her repertoire, or is having a challenging day. *Praise or comment for each way your child chooses.*

8 Communicating so my communication partner understands

Teach your child to use a different way to express a message depending on the communication partner's understanding of your child's intended message. Best case scenario is that the communication partner is informed of the ways or modalities your child uses to communicate. This is the opportunity for your child to put the last tip to work. Practice what to do if the partner asks your child to repeat or gives an inappropriate response. A facilitator or parent will

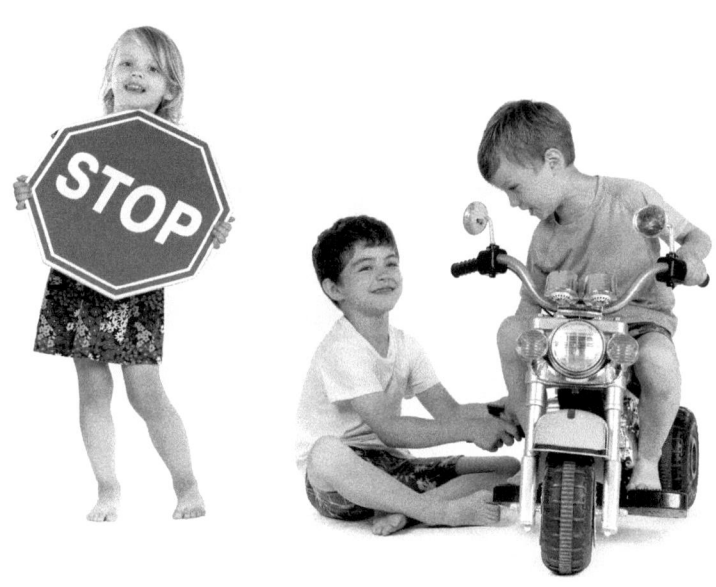

support your child and communicator by saying to your child, *Tell him your message another way. You can use your head nod or speech generating device.* As your child progresses with skills you will reduce the level of cuing. The reduction of cuing in this circumstance is representative of the skill level that is discussed in *Making Connections* and *Bridging Skills*.

Building Fundamentals with literacy

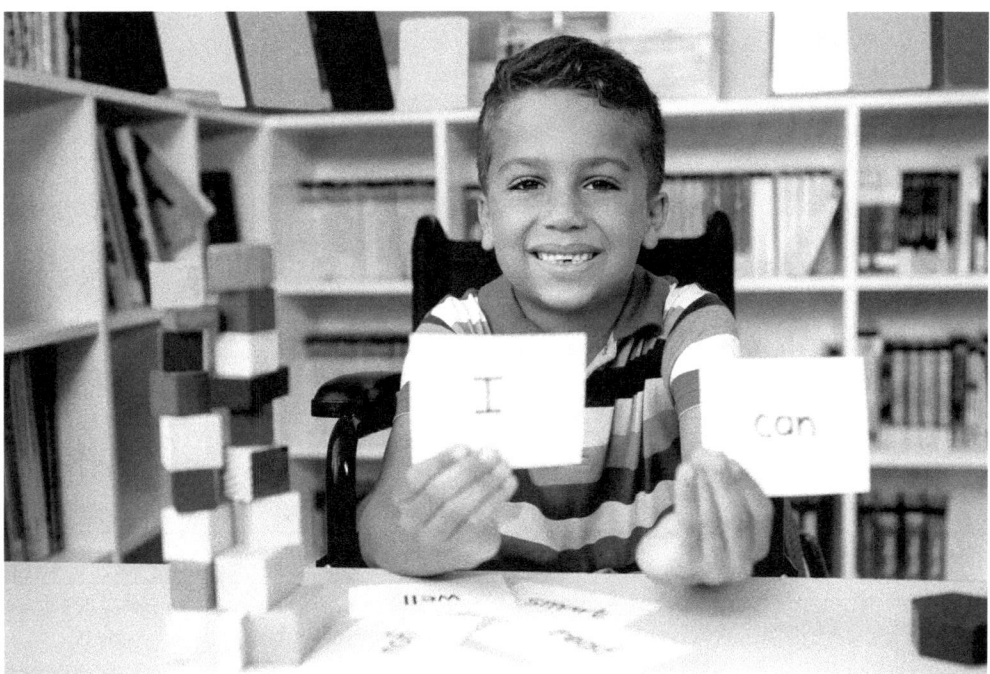

○ Reading and writing my way

Options for literacy

We learned in *Getting Started* that literacy is the ability to read and write in a given language. Multiple options for what can be read are offered including books, magazines, and community signs such as safety signs, stores, and restaurants. We also talked about many tools for writing including novel ideas such as chalk, waxy string, and dowels to draw in play dough. Finally, we talked about ways your child and adults can build literacy. Visit *Getting Started* to re-familiarize yourself with the charts and options then continue on with the following ideas to develop fundamentals with literacy.

Reading

As we are *Building Fundamentals* with literacy, think about what you found to be successful in *Getting Started* both for your child and yourself. This means you have identified an array of literacy options your child likes to read (e.g. books, labels, community signs), writing tools that work for your child, and a literacy skill set (e.g. interest in books, attends to the story, likes to turn the pages) that is established, being built, with projections for future options. You have a list of ideas to help you help your child be successful with literacy such as consistent exposure to reading and writing and simplifying or summarizing a text to keep your child's interest strong. Remember to have fun in the literacy development process! If you are having fun, then your child is having fun. Now take those successes in reading and move to even greater success using the following expansion ideas. Remember these relevant *Getting Started* questions: *What are you working on now that is supporting literacy? What literacy skills would you like to expose your child to more? What literacy skills would you like to expose your child to in a different way?* You may have other questions to ask for a child with combined vision and hearing loss. Visit the website Literacy for Children with Combined Vision and Hearing Loss at http://literacy.nationaldb.org/. The site offers valuable information on reading, writing, vocabulary development and more. As you dive into resources decide the steps that make sense for your child with the intervention team.

Options for my reading: what I am working on and what I will work on next

Reading Opportunities	How I Work on Reading and What I Will Work on Next
1 Books and magazines	• *People read to me often.* • *I point to pictures.* • *I match words using the best communication method for me.* • *I complete repeated phrases I see read to me.* • *I turn pages in a book with my hand or a page fluffer.* • *I have switch access to play a book on CD.*
2 Mail	• *I sort the mail by names in my family.*
3 Safety signs	• *I say stop, go, or wait.* • *I read safety signs like exit.* • *I read restroom signs.*
4 Restaurant signs	• *I make a choice between two or more restaurant signs.*
5 Store/Building signs	• *I know I made it to our destination by pointing to the building sign.*
6 Restroom signs	• *I can read the door sign to know it is a bathroom.*
7 Singing songs with lyrics	• *I sing vocally.* • *I sing using my speech generating device.*

Writing for expression

Writing allows others to hear our thoughts. Augsburger (1982), a psychologist, states that *to be heard and to love are so similar that most people cannot tell the difference.* Being heard and loved supports our children's communication in writing. Multiple ways to write and to have fun with the experience of writing include drawing in sand or shaving cream. We want writing to be fun. Now let's add in some functionality to writing expanding the idea of writing to include a communicative message.

Options for writing: how I work on writing and what I will work on next

Writing Tasks	How I Work on Writing and What I Will Work on Next
1 Writing/typing names	• Switch access keyboard • Traditional or big keys keyboard • Wrist cuff stabilizing a pencil, stylus, or other utensil
2 Tracing my letters, words, phrases, sentences, and ideas	• Physical support as needed to trace or write on paper, tablet • Wrist cuff stabilizing a pencil, stylus, or other utensil
3 Labeling items in drawings	• Physical support as needed to trace, write, or draw • Wrist cuff stabilizing a pencil, stylus, or other utensil
4 Writing numbers and number words	• Physical support as needed to trace or write • Wrist cuff stabilizing a pencil, stylus, or other utensil

A few tips for facilitator's role in literacy building narratives

1 Engaging the child by repeating short phrases and sentences with great feeling from text, pictures, and the context. Children hear, see, and respond to emotions called for in the text. They listen to the rhythmic, rhyming verbal productions. This rich experience lays the groundwork for engagement with others, engagement with text, engagement with fun, and engagement with the motivation to read.

2 Allow child to select books and talk about characters, actions, setting, feelings, conflict, solutions.

3 Play with sounds, such as sound to letter correspondence with AAC tool support such a messaging option on a speech generating device that allows the child to match sounds to letters, to blend sounds in words together, and recognize rhyming words.

4 Point out key words in books, magazines, brochures, and appropriate print media. Generate a connection between the words your child is learning, and words represented in other texts across environments such as words on menus, coffee table books, and doctor's office books.

5 Talk about the illustrator who designed the pictures and the author who wrote the text. Talk about the physical size of the book (e.g. big, medium, or a small book), with or without pictures, books with a few words or many, and a short or a long book!

6 Stabilize books and other materials to free your hands up to interact more with your child communicate ideas more effectively. Use a bookstand or a recipe book holder. Consider books on tablet technology with a mount. For drawing or writing consider using a slant board or binders with Velcro for stabilizing materials like books, papers, tablets, and more.

Building Fundamentals with vocabulary

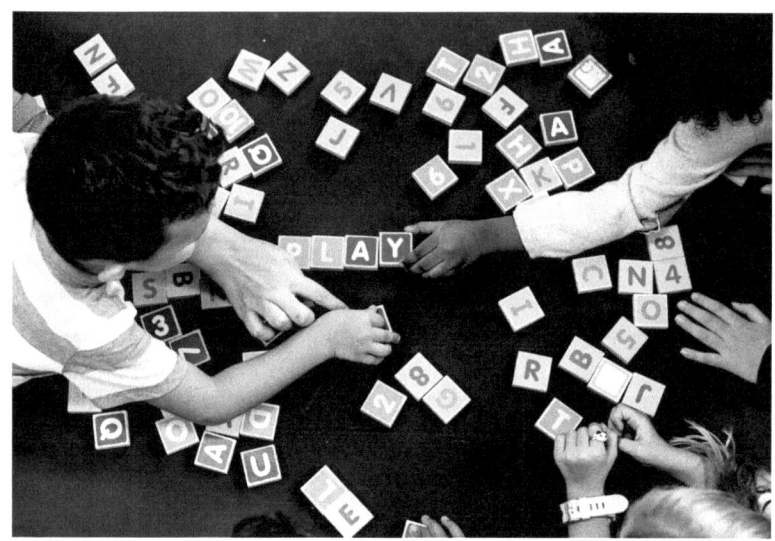

○ Words and word images that are important to me

Vocabulary becomes multi-faceted in *Building Fundamentals* as we note the growth in quantity or size and its many word combinations. It is an exciting time of growth and development. Your child already has a start with vocabulary from *Getting Started*. In *Building Fundamentals* we want to focus on expansion and visual memory. By expanding single words representing core and specific fringe vocabulary your child can combine words to produce a novel phrases or simple sentence and more quick messages. Think of expansion as either a lateral move by broadening the types of color, number, shape, nouns, verbs, and others typically in your child's environment or the quantity of new descriptive words and more nouns and names that build on your child's existing and expanding knowledge base.

Visual memory, a form of muscle memory, helps people recall where icons are located on a communication board or device. Children need to know that icons will be in the same place each time they want to use them. To illustrate this point, think about how you have the applications organized on your phone organized. Then, think about how you feel when you see the icons jiggling and with one false move they are moved around, or worse, deleted. Panic! Frustration! Relief when order resumes. We want to make good choices about organizing vocabulary and limit reorganization. It is quite typical as vocabulary is building that shifting will occur. Just make informed decisions about adding and organizing vocabulary to minimize the impact on your child's visual and auditory memory demands.

Decision making with vocabulary

Let's tackle vocabulary. Consider word choices and phrases. Ground your thinking in participation to help you think through vocabulary options. *What environments and people will my child socialize with? What academic goals does my child need and want to accomplish? What vocabulary is required to meet both social and academic objectives?* Researchers (Banajee, DiCarlo & Stricklin, 2003; Van Tatenhove, 2013) provide great insight into where to start in building vocabulary for children. See Top Words Used by Toddlers and AAC Clinical Application and how Van Tatenhove (2013) adapted the list for AAC clinical application. Remember, think participation first and then you have participated in informed vocabulary decision making.

Top Words Used by Toddlers and AAC Clinical Application

Top 22 Words Used by Toddlers *Banajee, DiCarlo & Stricklin (2003)*		*AAC Clinical Application Word Usage* *Van Tatenhove (2013)*	
All done/finished	No	Again	Mine
Go	Off	All done	More
Help	On	All gone	Not/don't
Here	Out	Away	Stop
I	Some	Down	That
In	That	Go	Up
Is	The	Help	Want
It	Want	Here	What
Mine	What	I	Up
More	Yes/yeah	It	Yes
My	You	Like	You

Vocabulary is more than expanding mean length of an utterance, it is connecting words to action and understanding. Prizant (2015), in his book *Uniquely Human*, suggests that a sequence of actions or behaviors become scripts to help us follow time sequences and reach a deeper meaning. Words that help children and adults understand and produce a message contribute to the shape of the script, the sequence, and the meaning of the communication and interaction.

Take a look at some quick message options as a springboard for messages that work for your child and his or her social, cultural, and linguistic community.

My phrases

Social Greeting	*Sharing Information*
1 *Hi what cha' doin'?*	1 *I have something to say.*
2 *Hey what's up?*	2 *Give me a minute to put my message together.*
3 *Hi, how are you?*	3 *Give me three choices to answer you with.*
4 *See you later.*	4 *I know what you mean.*
5 *Catch you later.*	5 *I don't know what you mean.*
6 *I need to go. Talk to you later.*	6 *Can you say that again?*

Social Closeness/Etiquette	Wants and Needs
1 Can you sit next to me?	1 Can you help me with my . . . (e.g. lunch, AAC)
2 I need a hug.	2 I am feeling ____ today.
3 Go away.	3 Hand me my toy/book/other.
4 Not now.	4 I need a snack.
5 I want to be alone.	5 I need to use the restroom.
6 Please that would help me.	6 I want to know what that is?

Vocabulary tips for facilitators and communication partners

1 Is the word meaningfully relevant to my child? If so, include the word.
2 Do you have fringe words specific to your child such as important names of people, places, and things? Do you have core words that allow commenting and discussions of topics?
3 Create multiple opportunities for the child to learn and use new vocabulary. What may take one to four opportunities for one child to learn a new word could take 60–70 opportunities for another child to learn the same word. Have fun and do prevent drilling when your child learns vocabulary more quickly.
4 One way to increase the opportunity count is to make learning multi-sensory. Can the child say, see, hear, draw, smell, touch, or eat the represented word? Is the word in written form or represented in an image or both on an icon on a tool or device?
5 Allow the usage of new vocabulary occur across contexts at home, school and in the community. Take learning from the clinic or home into school and the community.
6 Aided language stimulation: Practice modeling core vocabulary on the child's communication board or speech generating device.
7 Add photos and names of new peers, locations, events and more to communication boards, books, tools and devices.
8 Play word search games to improve timing and accuracy of locating vocabulary on tools and devices.

Use the following list of ideas as a springboard of vocabulary. Choose vocabulary that is relevant to your child.

Building Fundamentals: vocabulary springboard

◉ Pronouns: I, that, me, mine, you, your
◉ Transportation: Car, wheelchair, bike, wagon, scooter, truck, van
◉ Feelings: Happy, sad, angry, silly, frustrated, bored, excited, shy
◉ Clothes: Shirt, pants, shorts, dress, skirt, shoes, socks, sandals, Dafo braces, underwear
◉ Action Verbs: Look, stop, go, like, love, want, walk, jump, run, kick, hear, see etc.

- Sizes: Small, little, tiny, itty-bitty, big, huge, ginormous
- Shapes: Circle, square, triangle, rectangle, hexagon, octagon, trapezoid
- Toys and Objects: Books, action figures, dolls, building toys, puzzles, crafts, sand/park/bath toys
- Quantity: More, less, numbers
- Sports: Ball play, soccer, T-ball, tennis, football, swimming, gymnastics
- Entertainment: Music, TV, movie, park
- School: Names of teachers and interventionists, key administrators and staff relevant to the child, classroom numbers, playground equipment, daily schedule, calendar, clocks, and timing words

As you review the list of options for vocabulary words just remember that success is starting with one word. Moving to combining two or three words is great too. The earlier word lists may be too much or too little. Think expansion: What word can I add to my child's repertoire that will grow categorical vocabulary and thinking? How can I expand my child's language comprehension and expression by combining words? If you are comfortable with these two ideas then you understand how *Building Fundamentals* with vocabulary will support your child.

Building Fundamentals with tools and access

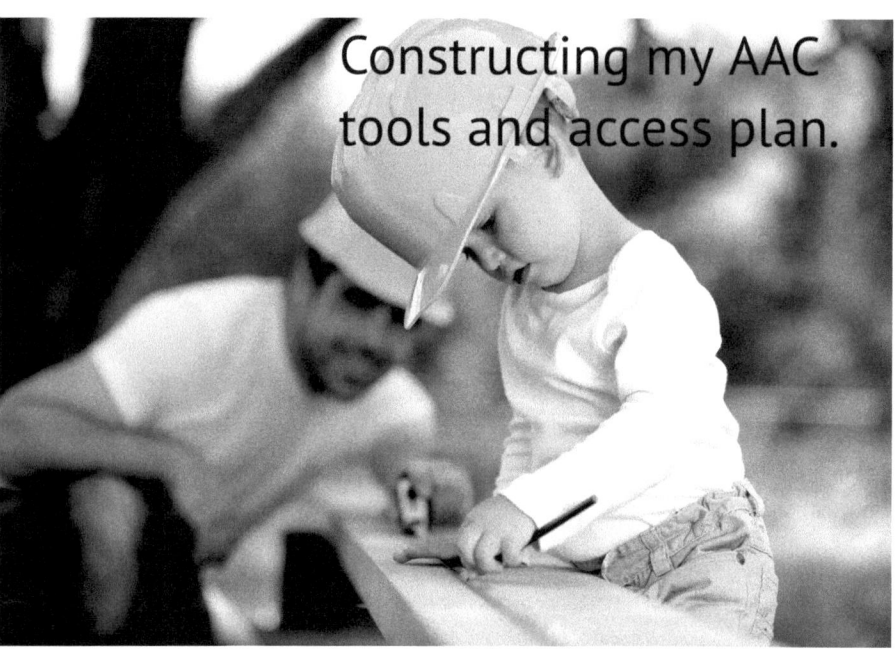

Constructing my AAC tools and access plan.

○ I have AAC options!

It is time to get excited! Why? We are building your child's AAC tools and devices library! The purpose of *Building Fundamentals with Tools and Access* is to give you direction in ways tools and devices support child with complex communication profiles in the environment that promote interaction. A selection of tools and devices introduced in *Getting Started* continue to be relevant for a child who is *Building Fundamentals* and onward into *Making Connections* (for children using language to connect to peers and express more complete ideas), *Bridging Skills* (for children ready for a degree of independence with supported communication as needed), and *Maximizing* Participation (for children requiring limited or no communication support across communication contexts and communication partners). A list of the tools and access options from *Getting Started* is listed here.

Option #1 Communication Boards: While discussed in *Getting Started* the vocabulary options may increase dramatically making communication boards relevant at each stage.
Option #2 Single Message Speech Generating Devices
Option #3 Dual Message Devices
Option #4 Visual Scenes
Option #5 Environmental Controls for *Getting Started*: Accessing and activating toys

Now, read through the options for *Building Fundamentals with Tools and Access* and consider how useful each option is to your child. These same questions were asked in *Getting Started*. You will see them in each chapter because they are consistently good and relevant questions to ask. Why? A couple of things could have happened. Either your child developed and is ready for a new tool, the tool or device remains relevant as a primary or secondary option, or the right person or motivation came along, access is possible, and your child is now experiencing success.

- *Have I tried the option before? Did it work? How well did it work?*
- *Should the team try the option again?*
- *Should we get another professional perspective on the option?*
- *Should we look to another option?*
- *Should we combine more options?*
- *Could one option help another option?*

Remember that each question and technology option at any stage do not have to reflect a right or wrong decision, rather a possibility that the option is worth a look, or not. Base your answer on your child's communication profile today and what your child's communication profile may be tomorrow. *Building Fundamentals* will pick up where the options list in *Getting Started* left off including the option numbers with technology that will broaden vocabulary, a little or a lot, and combine words for novel messages and quick phrase messages.

Option #6: Environmental control for Building Fundamentals

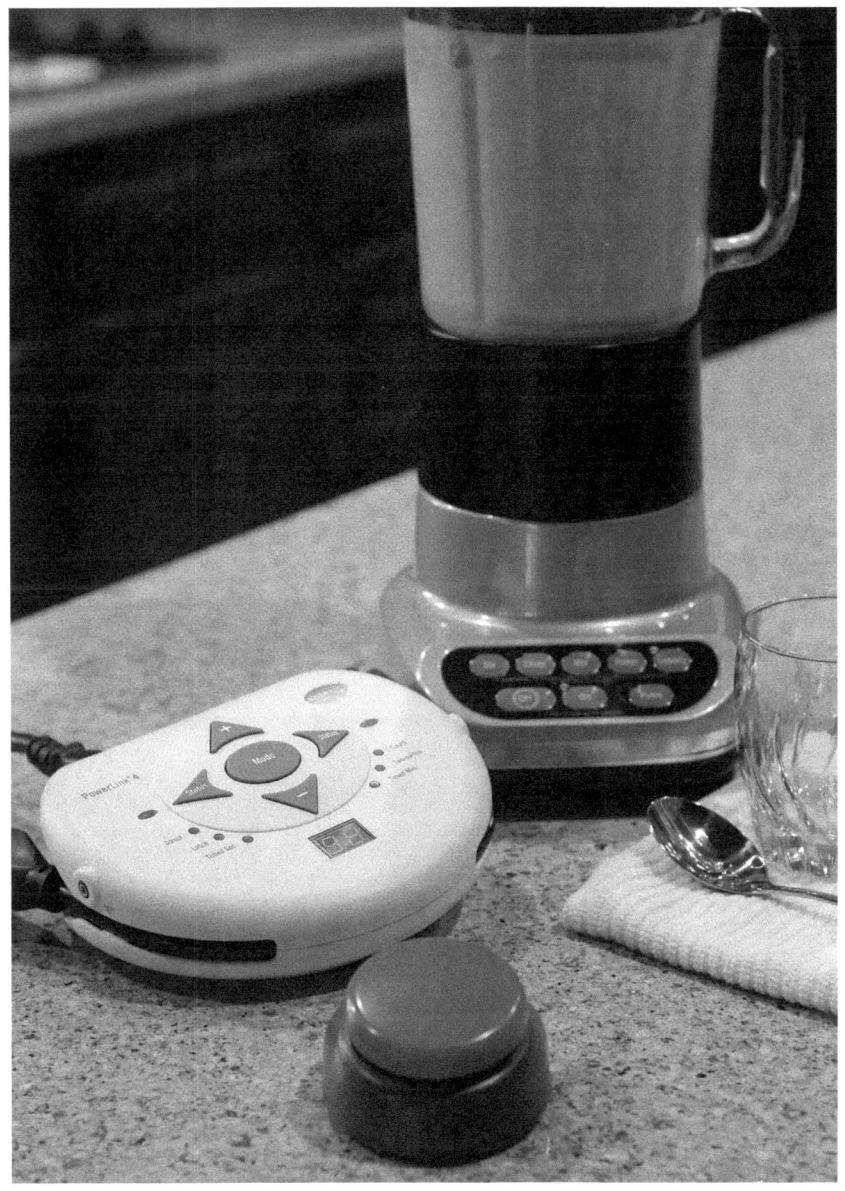

Talk about fun! Talk about being practical! Talk about empowering! Using environmental controls does exactly that. Your child gains control of turning electronic devices *on* and *off* including lights for a room, CD players, and starting and stopping a blender to make a snack. The company, Enabling Devices, calls environmental control switches, *capability switches*.

Option #7 Talking photo albums

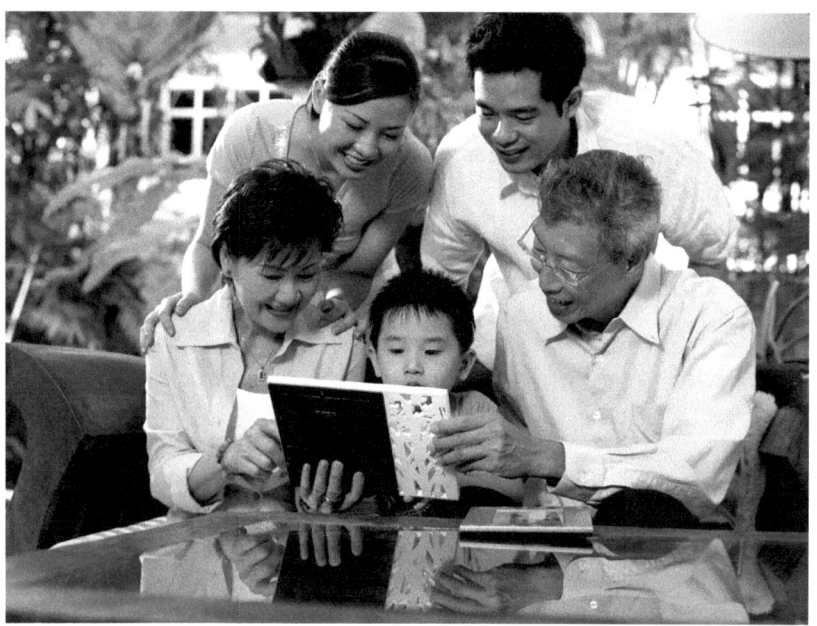

A number of talking photo albums are available on the market that allow familiar and less familiar communication partners to hear your child share information about family, friends, favorite toys, activities, hobbies, events and more. Albums, whether talking or not, are fun, inviting, and a great conversational piece. Make sure you program a question at the end of the message for communication partners to share pictures or stories of their related experiences (e.g. *Tell me about somewhere you have been lately*!)

Option #8 Static display speech generating device

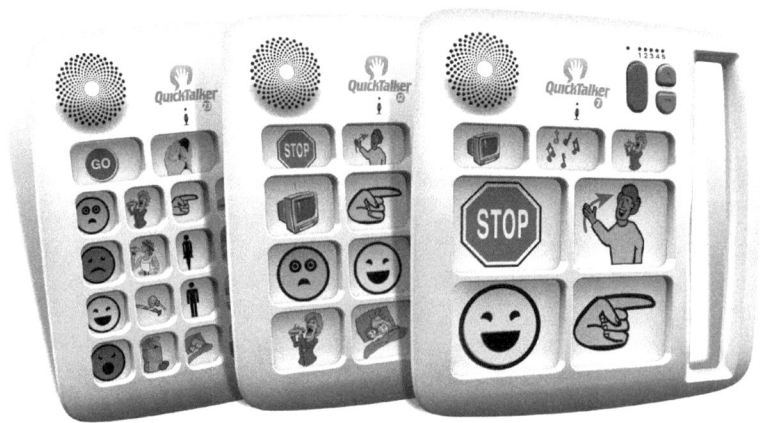

AAC INTERVENTION PLAN WITH CASE STUDIES

A mid-tech voice output communication board like products from GoTalks by Attainment (https://www.attainmentcompany.com/technology/gotalks) or Ablenet Quick Talker (provide a child with the option for words and quick messages to be programed in isolation or in a sequence for the purpose of novel messages. Images with words are printed on paper called an overlay. Often there are a number of levels of messages that can be programmed with speech. A facilitator may slide in the picture overlay, select the level associated with the picture overlay and the user can begin to communicate with the icons. If other vocabulary is required on a different page, the picture overlay is replaced, the level is adjusted, and the user can proceed with communication. Often overlays can be made for setting specific communication such as centers at school, common activities or routines, and to share all purposes of communication. Be sure to back up the overlays to have on hand as a replacement if lost or damaged and for emergencies.

Option #9 Tablet or phone technology

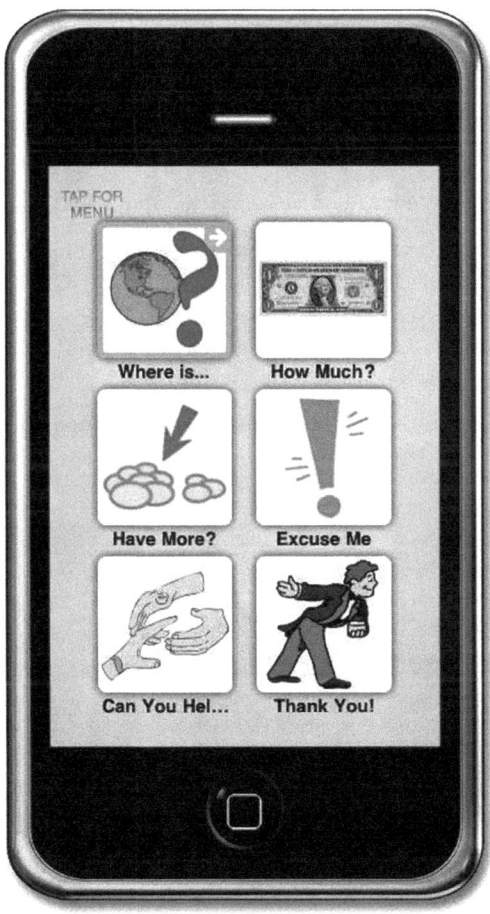

Would an app on tablet or phone technology work for my child? Definitely! Remember we want a multimodal communication program to maximize communication and participation. The use of application technology can be great as a primary communication option, a supplementary communication option, or the best option in context such as quick communication, a way for managing daily schedules and transitions, and academic learning.

Tips for tablet, phone, and application technology:

1 Consider the full spectrum of *feature matching* (e.g. size of the button options, the symbol system used, the adequacy of the volume, etc.) to make sure the application meets the needs of your child. See the *Bridging Skills* chapter to consider all of the factors involved in feature matching. Make sure you and your child's intervention team are making feature decisions for maximum participation and not just financial decisions.

2 At times tablet or phone-based technology is employed to supplement communication. In this case make sure the applications you choose have the same or similar symbols for the icons. Make sure the supplementary tools are functional and meaningful to your child. Ease for communication partners may not represent ease for the AAC user.

3 If you would like to use an app for quick communication, there are free apps such as Sounding Board from Ablenet (https://www.ablenetinc.com/soundingboard) that can support this need, along with many others with a range of low to high costs. Work with an AAC specialist to sort through the application options as there are many.

4 If you would like to use an application for self-regulation, scheduling sequences, or participating in school activities, there are many options. Work with special educators including AAC specialists to make sound application decisions for your child. In many cases, a no tech option may be the best option however a technology-based option may fit a need or lifestyle of your AAC user. Employ technology for the best fit for your child.

Option #10 E-Tran boards, plastic, plexiglas, or sheet protectors!

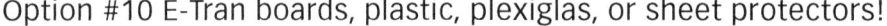

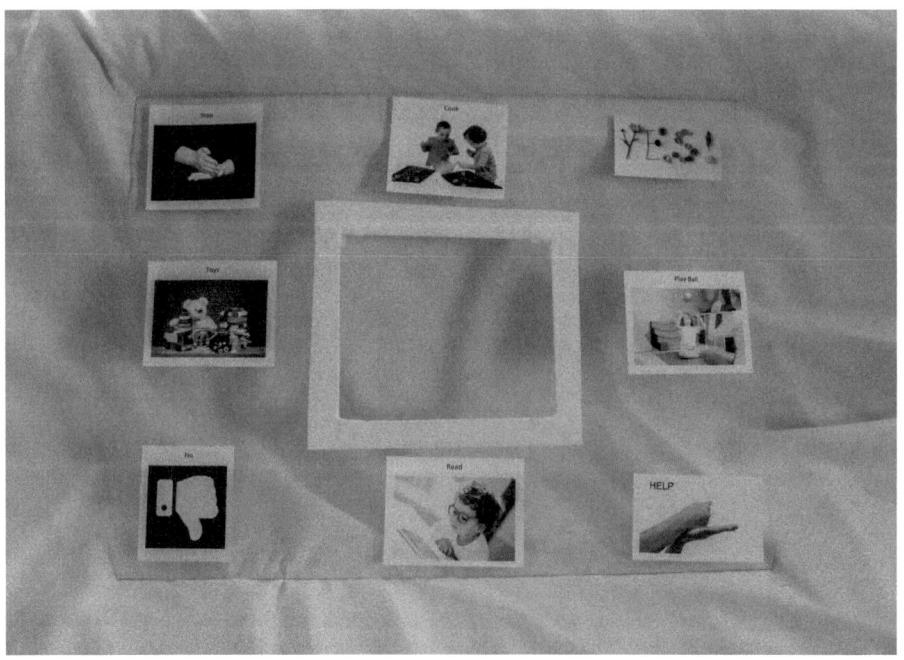

Clear plastic becomes a communication board! The formal name for a clear plastic or Plexiglas communication board is an e-Tran board. Place icons on the sides of the Plexiglas so the AAC user can use eye gaze to select the message while the communication partner follows the child's eye gaze. You can use a product from a company like Enabling Devices or make your own eye gaze or pointing board using something as simple as four sheet protectors that overlap! Start by placing icons in corners, left, right, top, bottom to make it easier to see where the child is looking. Gradually add others to fill in empty spaces.

Option #11 Dry erase board

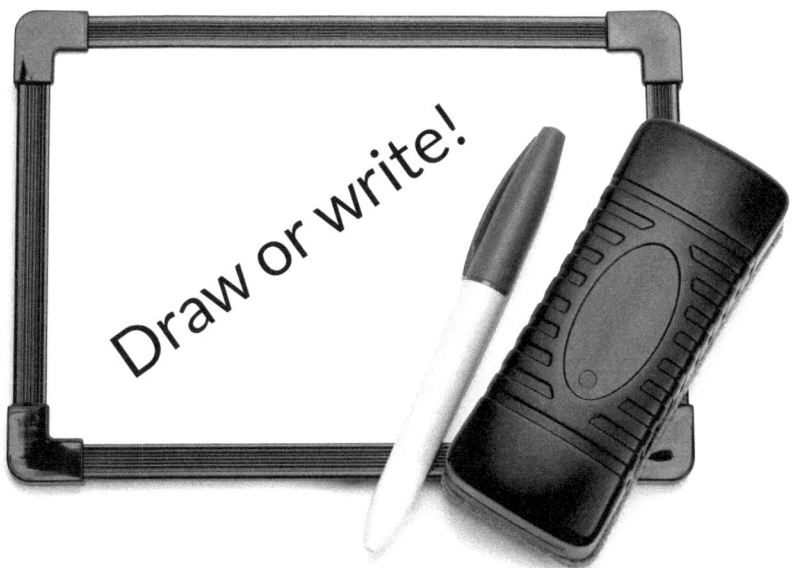

Keep a dry erase board on hand for quick communication messages. If you are an artist you can draw images. If are not an artist (a.k.a. Dr. Mayne and Dr. Rogers), then simple line drawings or better yet, simple words can be written for quick communication. You can also use the back of the dry erase board as a communication board by attaching icons with Velcro© for a choice board or masking tape for pointing only. Now you have a quick communication board for written choice communication and icons for expressing messages.

Option #12 Access tools: stylus or wrist cuff

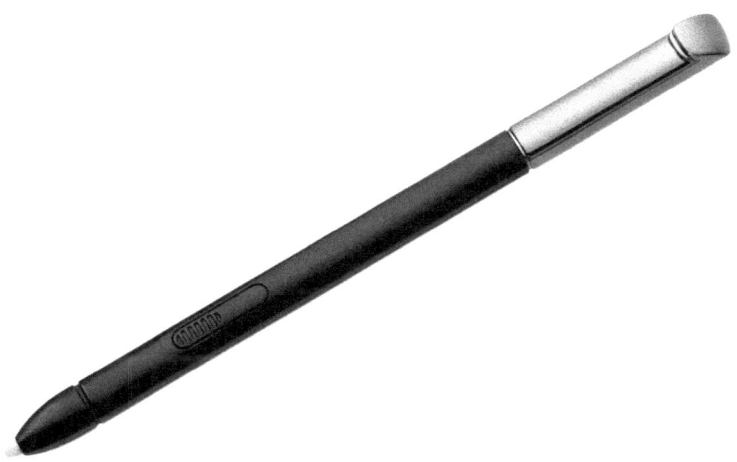

A way to improve physical access to communication boards or devices is to consider if assistive technology tools may assist the child. A stylus is a tool that can help with choice making for low- or high-tech communication, as gripping may be more accessible than pointing at an icon. Consider a hand or wrist cuff and place a stylus or pencil in the cuff to improve access if holding a stylus is a challenge. Work with an occupational therapist and AAC specialist to locate and work with access tools.

Option 13 Book readers: page turners vs. audio books

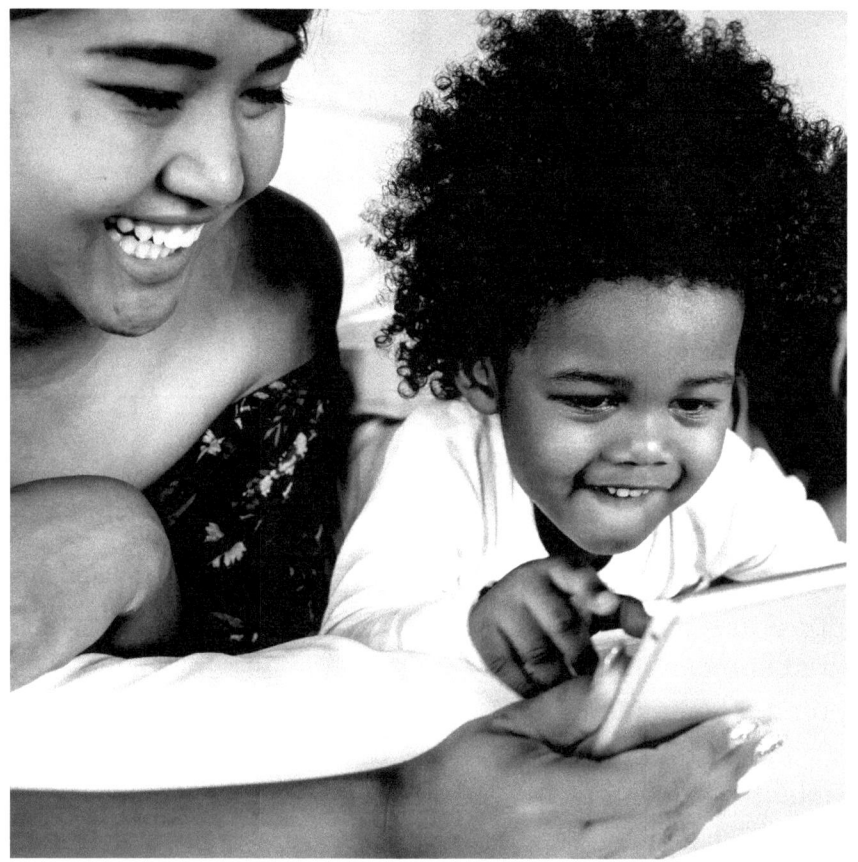

Book readers are available in many formats and offer varying features. Some book readers allow the child to read each page of a hard- or paperback book or magazine and determine when to turn the page. Audio books read a book out loud to the child either through a speaker or ear buds. Decide which features of the tool or device match your child's access needs to books. Would your child benefit from seeing a complete book in an electronic format with the pictures included? Can the book be read out loud? Can the size of the letters be increased? Can words, sentences, or paragraphs be highlighted? Is there a dictionary available? Can you adjust the lighting? Do you need schoolbooks? Look into Bookshare (www.bookshare.org/cms/) and apply for a free account for students with a documented disability that will allow the student to hear and see texts and books. There is also a Bookshare tablet application called Read2Go (www.bookshare.org/cms/help-center/reading-tools/read2go). Some applications offer monthly subscriptions. Other applications offer books to be bought on a book-by-book basis. Some books are free. Work with a local library to help you through the options for books in an electronic format.

A summary for *Building Fundamentals*

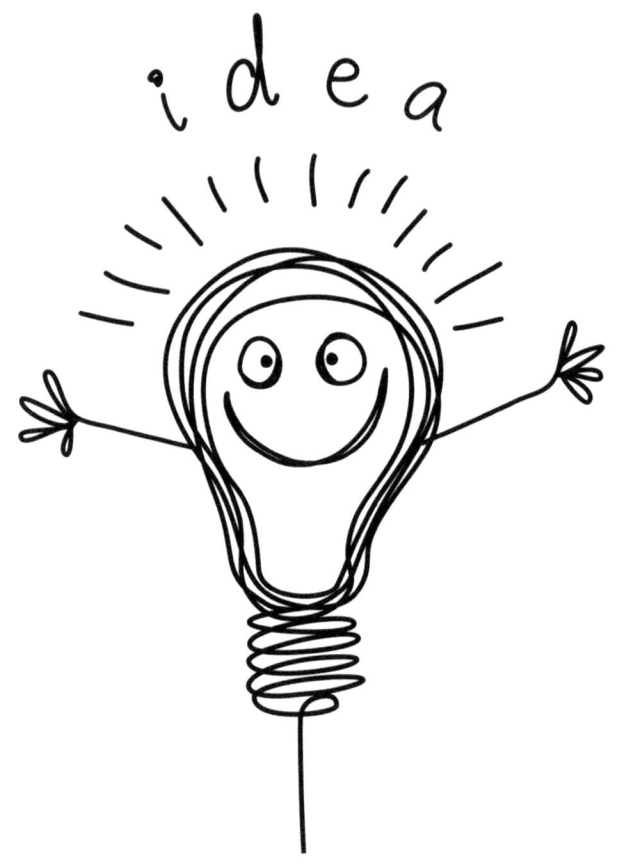

○ Ideas in action!

Building Fundamentals is about expanding communication using technology and adding vocabulary for participation! A communication skill set is established. Success! It is okay if all of your child's AAC communication skills determined from the *Hear Me into Voice* and work completed in the *Getting Started* stage are nonverbal such as using gestures, body positioning, and vocalizations. It is also just fine to have a combination of nonverbal, vocal, verbal, low technology communication boards, and single or multi-message speech generating devices. Your child has started communicating. Now we take this great start and build on it by expanding language forms, looking at how communication can be used across environments, looking at the needs of communication partners, and making sure your child is transitioning well to a more advanced level of communication. One way to monitor this transition is to keep an eye on joint attention, attention to task and learning, memory, motivation and skill level of both the child using AAC, facilitators, and novel- and known communication partners. Much of the chapter on *Building Fundamentals* is focused on the next steps. It is great to have some established communication skills but all too often taking the next step can be as challenging as the first step. The content in *Building Fundamentals* provides you with charts and tools to help you. The ideas serve as a guide, inspiration, and a springboard to ideas that work best for your child. Visit sections as needed from *Getting Started* and look ahead to *Making Connections* to make the right plan of action for the AAC user and communication partners. Review the remaining chapters for a complete working concept of AAC from *Getting Started* through *Maximizing Participation*.

Before we go: troubleshooting the environment, nonverbal communication, and device use

Troubleshooting is the bright side of frustration. Let's face it, breakdowns happen. Here is the good news, if you are troubleshooting you are trying! In this section we explore improving communication success through AAC with the environment, adjustments to support nonverbal communication, and tips for device use.

○ Tips for troubleshooting the environment

Place yourself in a similar position as the child with the AAC tools and devices and observe how light and sound impact you and thus your child's ability to communicate.

- Check for light or glare <u>in the eyes</u> from bulbs, the sun, or other sources of light.
- Check for light or glare <u>on the device</u> from bulbs, the sun, or other sources of light.
- Monitor the number of objects, toys, and other distractors.
- Observe how conversations with people in the room or outside of the room impact your child's ability to attend to communication for learning or social interaction.
- Ask yourself: To what degree is ambient noise from trucks, cars, carts, weather conditions, and subtle sources of noise from projectors, lights, and others impact communication?
- Temporary visual distractions happen. Adjust the setting and make a request for children to play elsewhere or for adults to limit walking in and out of the room.
- Turn temporary auditory distractions from children, adults, television, music, and toys into an opportunity for the AAC user to comment, *It's a little loud in here!*

○ Tips for troubleshooting nonverbal communication

- Line of sight: Apply a 45° angle or less rule between the communication partner and the AAC user in order for both parties to communicate nonverbal messages.
- Physical proximity: Have communication partners accommodate for vision needs by standing close enough or far enough away. What is the optimal distance? Include distance information for communication partners on a tip card.
- Clothing comfort: Is there something bothering the child physically such as a shirt fold on the back, a bothersome pocket, problems with a sock, tags, or other?
- Positioning comfort: Adjust ankle, knee, hip, shoulder, neck, elbow, and wrist positioning in relation to field of vision, mobility, and ease of access to AAC tools.Would a change in seating and positioning optimize the interaction for all communication partners?

- Alertness level: Is the child tired, excited, distracted (see attention)?
- Sensory needs: The child is bothered by a texture or basic need like hunger or rest.
- Attention: There is something much more interesting going on that your child is seeing, hearing, or both that is distracting the motivation to use nonverbal communication.
- Motor: To what degree is a physical disability impeding the ability for your child to communicate nonverbally. Consider fatigue, time of day, medications, motivation.

○ Tips for troubleshooting interaction

If the child provides no response or rejects AAC tools or devices, not related to operational competency or technical difficulties, try the following.

What the Child Might Indicate	What You Can Try
What? I don't understand.	Reduce or change what you are saying to the child. Are the statements or questions too long? Is the vocabulary too complex? Is the word order too complicated? Are you speaking too quickly?
Say that a different way.	Provide language input in a different way such as typing the message while speaking a message or just typing the message.
Ho-hum, I'm bored . . .	Change the activity. Offer choices for a change in activity.
How much longer?	Let the child know how much longer at task will last; how many repetitions or items are remaining.
Give me a minute.	Pause for greater time for processing.
Hold on.	Pause for motor planning time to respond.
Let me try again.	Provide numerous practice opportunities multiple times a day in different settings and with different people.
Let's get silly!	*I am a kid after all.* Let's have fun with communication: jokes, board games, Simon says, crafts, silly pranks, and more.
Show me how on my device.	Provide aided language stimulation = have the communication partner model generating a message on a communication board or device.
You lost me.	Work at the success level of the child on a given day. Some days are great for working on grammar and other days it is okay to reduce the complexity of the expected length or type of response to make sure communicative intent is met.
(. . . silence . . .)	Silence may have multiple intents: agreement, disagreement, nonplussed, over stimulated, or just plain finished. Each requires more information to confirm the intent. Offer follow up questions and choices including the opportunity to say, *I need a break.*
Happy, Sad, Angry	Talk through feelings and emotions including the positive and negative emotions. Provide the vocabulary, aided language stimulation (modeling), and independent practice. Talk through emotional situations to help your child understand what they and others are feeling based on a challenging event.
Let me see, let me see . . .	Include choices, expect initiation, and confirm choices.
I'm feeling off . . .	Check the sensory experience of your child: cold/hot, hungry/full, overstimulated/under-stimulated, external noise or light, textures, physical discomfort, fear, triggers, illness.

Do you want more ways to empower communication and participation including troubleshooting with AAC? Then read what is coming up next in *Making Connections.*

References

Ablenet. (2019). Retrieved from www.ablenetinc.com/

Attainment Company. (2019). GoTalks. Retrieved from www.attainmentcompany.com/technology/gotalks

Augsburger, D. (1982). *Caring enough to be heard*. Harrisonburg, VA: Herald Press.

Banajee, M., DiCarlo, C. & Stricklin, S. (2003). Core vocabulary determination for toddlers. *Augmentative and Alternative Communication*, *19*(2), 67–73.

Beukelman, D. R. & Mirenda, P. (2013). *Augmentative and alternative communication: Supporting children and adults with complex communication needs*. Baltimore, MD: Paul H. Brookes Publishing.

Bookshare. (2019a). Retrieved from www.bookshare.org/cms/

Bookshare. (2019b). Read2Go. Retrieved from www.bookshare.org/cms/help-center/reading-tools/read2go

Bookshare. (2019c). Read your way. Retrieved from www.bookshare.org/cms/

Fryholm, A. (2019, July). Writing the unspeakable. *Christian Century*, *136*(16), 32–33.

Kaniel, S. & Feuerstein, R. (1974). Special needs of children with learning difficulties. *Oxford Review of Education*, *15*(2), 165–179.

Light, J. & McNaughton, D. (2014). Communicative competence for individuals who require augmentative and alternative communication: A new definition for a new era of communication?. *Augmentative and Alternative Communication*, *30*(1), 1–18.

Literacy for Children with Combined Vision and Hearing Loss. (n.d.) All children can learn to read … let us show you how. Retrieved from http://literacy.nationaldb.org/

McLeod, S. (2018). Communication rights: Fundamental human rights for all. *International Journal of Speech-Language Pathology*, *20*(1), 3–11.

National Association for the Education of Young Children. (n.d.) *Planning for powerful guidance: Powerful interactions make a difference*. Retrieved from www.naeyc.org/resources/pubs/tyc/dec2013/planning-for-positive-guidance.

Prizant, B. M. (2015). *Uniquely human: A different way of seeing autism*. New York, NY: Simon & Schuster.

Show, J. (2012). *Teaching your child with love and skill: A guide for parents and other educators of children with autism, including moderate to severe autism*. Philadelphia, PA: Jessica Kingsley Publishers.

Thelen, E. (1991). Motor aspects of emergent speech: A dynamic approach. In N. Krasnegor, D. Rumbaugh, R. Schiefelbusch & M. Studdert-Kennedy (Eds.), *Biological and behavioral determinants of language development* (pp. 339–362). Hillsdale, NJ: Lawrence Erlbaum Associates, Publishers.

Van Tatenhove, G. (2013). Papers and resources. Retrieved from www.vantatenhove.com/papers.shtml

Vygotsky, L. (1986). *Thought and language* (A. Kozulin, Ed.). Cambridge, MA: MIT Press.

Making Connections  4
with social interaction
Communication counts

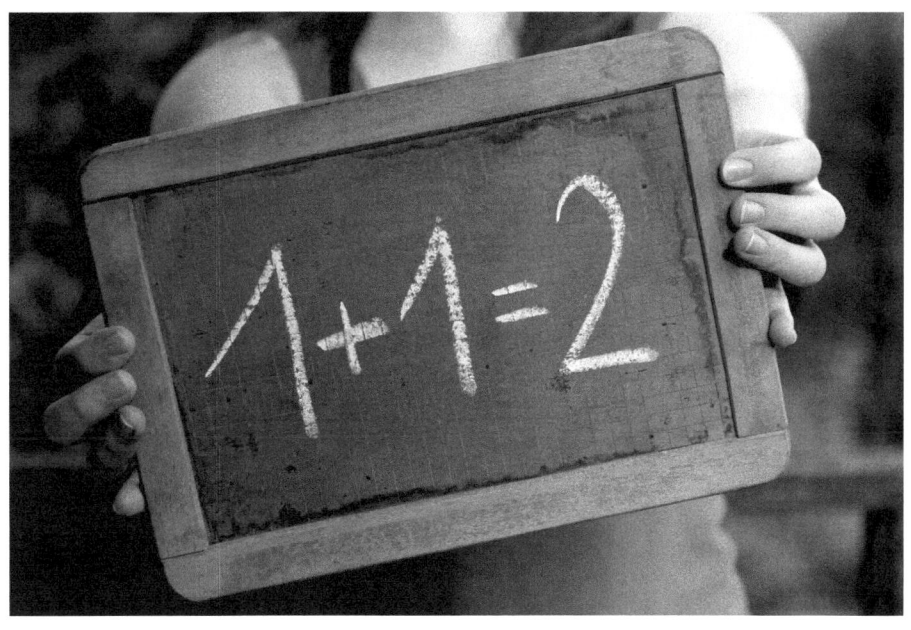

I expect to see the child's perspective. I want to know what would really, really help her in her whole life?

Speech-Language Pathologist (Rogers, 1999)

Making Connections with augmentative and assistive communication skills means that we see children, families, and interventionists who understand the idea that quantity and quality communication matters in our use of language, our participation, and in our friendships as communication partners. We look for communication everywhere. Fleischman and Fleischman (2012), the father and daughter authors of *Carly's Voice* write that children using AAC are learning how to look for communication opportunities with friends and communication partners are learning how to interpret their friends' nonverbal and verbal communication. 'In a world of silence, communication is everywhere; you just have to know how to look' (Fleischman & Fleischman, 2012, p. 197). Children achieve communication concepts through comprehension and production of phrases and sentences using multimodal means including nonverbal communication through their bodies, vocal and verbal communication, aided by communication boards, and speech generating devices. That sounds like a lot.

It is, and that is a good thing. We want our children to be *Making Connections* between their intent, their messages, and new communication partners. We are stepping into the purposes of communication.

We spent time in *Getting Started* and *Building Fundamentals* talking about concepts like joint attention, words and their combinations, and seeing that communication causes an effect on others. In the *Making Connections* stage, we want communication to count by making an impact for the child and communication partners with active language and interaction. We will use what stands as the pillar of shaping communication interaction, the four purposes of communication established by Janice Light in 1989 and addressed again by Light and McNaughton (2014), including wants and needs, information sharing, social closeness, and social etiquette. These purposes are being met simultaneously as appropriate to the context of the situation. At the earliest age, an eye gaze may share information of interest and a smile be a response to social closeness. Your child impacts communication partners and social groups by expressing a message that influences group members including friends. Now we add feelings and emotions, using language to contribute to others, understanding consequences and implications, following directions, and developing friendships. Wow! What an amazing transition we are making from joint attention and word productions using any modality, to communicative intent with words and phrases and now *Making Connections* using these great communication skills.

Making Connections: intervention plan: concepts, goals and strategies

As we head into the intervention plan for a child *Making Connections* let's take a look at a few key concepts. These ideas are not every possible idea to consider but do help you shape a plan and can serve as a springboard to other ideas that best match your child's and communication partners' needs. Look back to Part I of this book for a model of how to plan an intervention session.

○ Concept #1 Developing friendships – purposeful play

Help your child develop friendships through purposeful play. Day care, school, and community experiences offer a melting pot of potential friends. Ask teachers to help identify potential friends. Plan activities such as art and physical activities such as playing with foam balls, making or playing music while dancing and parading. Allow for spontaneous play but a few planned activities can set and keep the play in motion. Check out Hasbro's Toy Box Tools: Making Play Accessible (https://toyboxtools.hasbro.com/en-us) for ideas to improve play for children with autism and other disabilities. Parallel play with crafts, playdough, or individual puzzles can be a place to start. In other cases, plan cooperative play where children engage with each other to play a game or build together. Set a time of how long the playtime will last to allow for self-regulation. Include quiet activities, bathroom breaks, a snack break. Designing a plan can be a first step help your child develop friendships that will lead to less planning and intervention on your part later as friendships grow. Now let's look at a number of activities on the following pages that will support your child as he or she is *Making Connections* with communication and participation focusing on language development including feelings and emotions.

○ Concept # 2 Expressing feelings and emotions

There are six basic emotions. Surprise and disgust expand the original four core emotions of happiness, sadness, anger, and fear. Cowen and Keltner's (2017) research, through a review of 324,066 individual responses to 2,185 emotionally evocative videos, yielded 27 different emotional experiences with many gradations of emotions. They state that while commonalities exist between people, individual cultural experiences shape interpretation of emotional experience and semantic space or the words people use to describe emotional states. Therefore, include socioemotional communication words on communication boards and speech generating devices so children have the opportunity to express feelings and emotions.

○ Concept #3 Using language to contribute to others socially

We all have a variety of roles we play in different groups. Sometimes we are leaders and sometimes we contribute but do not actively lead. Consider what social participation looks like for your child across groups given the four levels by Beukelman and Mirenda (2013).

1 Socially influential: Socially influential children have friends that include their peers with and without disabilities and assume leadership roles in their peer groups. The children initiate activities and have a direct influence over group decisions and social choices.
2 Socially active: Socially active children have friends and are involved in peer groups but have less direct influence over the social climate of the group or group patterns.
3 Socially involved: Socially involved children have a smaller circle of friends and exert less influence in social situations, are passive participants or observers in social situations.
4 Social non-participants: Children that are social non-participants have limited or no access to peers without disabilities. Social non-participation is generally undesirable.

○ Concept #4 Understanding implications

Consider the following tenets for you, as a facilitator, to help your child learn the implications of his or her communication.

1 Provide cues: Guiding your child to the relevant parts of the task.
2 Study perception: Identify the critical or distinguishing features and differences between stimuli (what your child sees or is engaging with such as toys, books, pictures, etc.). Engage descriptive words such as color, shape, size, quantity, composition, function, and question forms of *who, what, when, where*, and *why* to add to your child's experience with language.
3 Activate knowledge: Label vocabulary, talk about how people interact (e.g. actions, feelings, responses) using previous and related experiences to stimulate new knowledge.
4 Executive functioning: Teach children how to be flexible thinkers to solve problems.

○ Concept #5 Following directions

What does it take for your child to follow a direction? Think through the following I statements:

1   *I need to perceive that I was asked to do something whether I get that message from sight such as reading or seeing someone's nonverbal cues including lip reading, from hearing a message, and/or through the sense of touch.*

2   *I need to have time to process and know what I was asked to do which means I understand the vocabulary, context, and timeline in which the direction should be followed.*

3   *I have access to the tools to follow a direction and if not I need access to the tools to follow the direction.*

4   *I need to recognize if I need help to follow the direction.*

5   *I need a facilitator or communication partner to recognize what help or support I need to follow the direction.*

6   *I need to maintain attention and memory to complete the task managing engagement when someone is giving me support and recognizing when not to interrupt me.*

7   *I need to anticipate change and manage problem-solving using decision making skills required through executive functioning to complete a task and self-regulate behavior.*

8   *I need to know what finished looks like. I need to know when I have completed the job.*

9   *I need to know if I met the objective of the person that asked me to follow the direction including if a reinforcement is given or not, such as verbal praise, a thank you, a monetary exchange, etc.*

10 *I need to know if I am finished and I can transition to another activity or if I have more or other directions that need to be followed.*

Each of these steps takes time to be processed, organized, and executed. The giver of the commands needs to understand that the time across steps may take microseconds or minutes.

With the concepts of socioemotional language on the forefront of our thinking read and reflect on Alexa and learn from her through this case study. Explore how Alexa, her friends, family, and other communication partners connect activities, feelings, thoughts, and plan for her participation. As you read the case study consider the following questions. Who is Alexa and *how is she Making Connections with learning, comprehending, and expressing language including literacy using multimodal AAC?*

Making Connections case study: meet Alexa

Making Connections through participation is the opportunity Alexa, her family, and the intervention team are waiting for. They are taking advantage of expanding language and ideas and developing friendships. Alexa, a much loved eight-year old daughter, diagnosed with Rett syndrome, depends on her sister, parents, and caregivers to help her with her physical difficulties as she walks, uses her hands and eyes, experiences respiratory complications, and the near absence of expressive verbal language. Her eyes look for details in her environment and connections with others. Her mother, a school administrator and her father, a family counselor at a church, are the efficient managers of Alexa's daily schedule, educational plans, and after school activities. They dress her every day in clothing color coordinated with terrycloth bibs about her neck for involuntary drooling. Her friends sense that Alexa appreciates them for who they were. She laughs, comments with her voice sometimes, and subtly cries when in distress. Her parents and sister Lillian are continually aware that she has *something to say* and interpret her many communication messages such as, *I love music, I'm interested*, and *I would like to go outside*. She works with her speech-language pathologist to develop communication and literacy through nonverbal means and speech generating devices.

○ Section 1 Social interaction: What does Alexa want us to know about her communication strengths and needs?

Results from the administration of the protocol, *Hear Me into Voice*, yielded 44 ways Alexa communicates with her family. Alexa's communication strengths begin with her eye gaze to direct communication partners' attention. Alexa uses her eyes, voice, sighs, and cries as the most easily accessible nonverbal modalities of communication. She will gaze out of the front window of her grandparents' home, look at her parents, then back outside, until they take her to the beach. Alexa shows frustration by rubbing her eyes or massaging her hair and scalp, saying *I am bored. Please help me learn something now.* She smiles and shakes her head *no* especially if she is asked to do the same repetitive activity. She frequently wrings her hands and puts the fingers of one hand into her mouth whether giving her comfort or perhaps for incorporating sensory information. Other times she taps one hand on her lap. Alexa works hard to coordinate the muscles of breathing, vocalizing, and moving of her lips and tongue in her mouth. Her mother states, *I think she does try to move her mouth in certain ways. You can hear sounds when she sings with her dad.* Day in and day out Alexa learns as her family and friends listen, interpret, and respond to her communication. They wait the 15–60 seconds it takes sometimes for her to respond.

At home, Alexa has many interests with music, cooking, and books at the top of her list. She sits on the piano bench as her mother plays and her dad strums the guitar. She reads books with her family and caregiver and accesses books online with them. She loves to take walks and go swimming with her dad. She smiles when pretending she is at a tea party while drinking from plastic cups. Alexa and her mother peel and chop vegetables for their supper. Her parents feel that Alexa jokes with them when she shakes her head *no* for a favorite activity and then smiles once they acknowledged her ploy. She welcomes their asking, *Are you teasing us again?* as she looks out the window because she is too tired or wants a change of activity.

At school, Alexa uses a wheelchair for the majority of her transportation. She uses a walker for short distances and with sufficient support, she is able to walk short distances in the community. She enjoys adaptive bowling and riding an adaptive bike during physical education with her friends at school. She can hold writing utensils for brief amounts of time before seemingly flinging them away. Socially, Alexa thoroughly enjoys outings such as participating in library activities and going on community field trips with other typically developing peers and her friends with disabilities including Tim, Jared, MJ, and Adam. Her father and mother acknowledge that Alexa has a way of being with other people and friends stating, *She just accepts them and loves them, and they feel that. Other people have expectations and are very judgmental. She is not. She is happy when somebody is with her. She just pushes for simple acceptance. She doesn't have any requirements, any expectations. Everybody wants to contribute to society. Many times, people do not give her a chance to communicate or they don't listen to her.* Alexa greets guests by looking at them and smiling broadly. A tip card in her pocket or on her wheelchair helps less familiar people talk with her. Her mother comments, *You can't get to know and love a person until you have listened to them. Then you learn to love them.* Her mother marvels at her friends saying, *Kids just love her, come up and talk to her, and want her to sit by them.* Her mother summarizes Alexa well stating, *To know me is to love me.*

⊙ Questions for Reflection

Questions for Section 1 Social interaction: What does Alexa want us to know about her communication strengths and needs?

1. Match the people Alexa socially interacts with to the corresponding number.

   a _____ Family

   b _____ Friends

   c _____ Community People

   1. Learn how Alexa communicates verbally and nonverbally from reading her tip card
   2. Know 44 ways Alexa communicates; Participate with Alexa during music, cooking, reading, parties, and walking
   3. Believe in Alexa, enjoy her friendship, feel her empathy and know their lives are enriched because of interactions with her

2. Answer T=True or F=False for the following statements about Alexa.

   a _____ Alexa communicates only using her eyes

   b _____ Alexa plays jokes on her family

   c _____ Alexa has the diagnosis of Rett Syndrome and wants social interaction

Answers

1. Letters a.=2, b.=3, c.=1 Each set of communication partners, whether family, friends, or communication partners, benefits socially and emotionally because of Alexa, her communication skills, and her participation with them.
2. Letter a. is False: While it is true that Alexa uses her eyes to communicate, she also uses her body, voice to vocalize, and is Making Connections with a speech generating device. Letters b. and c. are True. Alexa has the diagnosis of Rett syndrome. While she works hard to communicate, she plays jokes on her family, looking out the window when she is tired or wants a change of activity. She has a strong intellect and loves to connect with people emotionally, share information, and be a part of the action. She thrives on participation.

O Section 2 Communication activities: What activities did Alexa participate in with her family and others at home and in the community?

Families whose daughters were diagnosed with Rett syndrome told Alexa's parents that music therapy enhanced their daughter's learning, so they asked school administrators to integrate music at school and in her community program. The educators responded. The music therapist collaborates with the classroom teacher to play music and get the children moving each day. The after-school recreation director sings, plays the guitar, and creates music sessions. Alexa and her friends learn and enjoy participation, clapping their hands and humming along. Alexa taps rhythms with her hand and contributes by playing a tambourine in the school music class.

Alexa needs the activities that the occupational therapist (OT) targets to maximize the use of her hands. The OT fit Alexa's hand with a splint to quiet one hand so that her other hand has more purposeful movement. However, the funding agency refused to pay for OT services because Alexa had made *insufficient measurable progress.* Alexa's mother reasoned that stopping occupational therapy solidified that self-fulfilling prophecy – she did not make progress because she did not have therapy. Physical therapy (PT) was authorized when Alexa developed scoliosis, an excessive sideways curvature in her spine. Her physical therapist understands the importance of communication, so she integrates communication into the weekly visits to Alexa's classroom. *Look at me if you want to go to the computer*, her physical therapist says, and Alexa looks at the PT. Together they walk to the classroom computer where Alexa selects a named picture by turning her head toward the PT. Alexa pays close attention to each display and creates her own story. Though some days are better than others, Alexa continues to make significant progress in physical therapy. One of Alexa's long-time interests is horseback riding at the equine therapy program. During her hippotherapy, a combination of physical, occupational, and speech-language therapy while riding horses, Alexa rides the horse named Wrigley. She takes pride in participating in Wrigley's feeding and grooming as well as caring for some of his equipment.

Alexa also participates in events at the community church. Alexa's father addresses the needs of people with disabilities in his ministry. He invites parents, organizes committee meetings, and designs educational events to promote inclusion of people with disabilities. Friends with and without disabilities sit together, enjoy and sing music, and engage in activities during the education time. The church leaders ask for volunteers to be *spotters* so that each child with special needs will have a facilitating companion. Zarah, an 8th grader, has volunteered and has been Alexa's *spotter* for more than a year. Zarah pushes Alexa in the wheelchair across the ramps from the church to the education building where they meet the class of 20 other children. Alexa and Zarah tap out the rhythms of the hymns. Zarah holds the single message speech generating device so Alexa can say the verses recorded by her mother. Through participation across therapies, community, and religious activities in everyday environments, Alexa is *Making Connections*.

Questions for Section 2 Communication activities: What activities did Alexa participate in with family and others at home and in community?

1 How did participating in music and physical therapy affect Alexa's participation?
   a   Music motivates Alexa's mind and body as she claps her hands, hums, and smiles.
   b   Physical therapy was discontinued because Alexa was unmotivated.
   c   Equine and physical therapy are unrelated disciplines that do not impact Alexa's communication or participation.
   d   All of the above

2 Indicate T=True or F=False regarding Alexa's participation in communication activities.
   a   _____ Participation across environments is Alexa's responsibility alone to initiate.
   b   _____ Freedom of movement in horseback riding awakens Alexa's physical abilities and taking responsibility in grooming horses gives her a source of pride.
   c   _____ Engaging with a peer-mentor at the church allows Alexa to participate with music enriching the experience for Zarah as well.

Answers

1 Letter a. is the correct answer. Music therapy activates parts of the brain providing motivation for Alexa to clap and tap. Physical therapy was not discontinued and all therapists connected communication to their goals to support participation.
2 Letter a. is False and letters b. and c. are True. Participation is a group experience. With peer mentor and adult need training, gains in communication and participation benefit everyone. Equine therapy provides both physical stimulation and emotional support.

○ **Section 3 Facilitator strategies: What strategies do facilitators and communication partners use to promote participation with Alexa?**

Alexa's parents are her most reliable communication facilitators and partners. They recognize their daughter's physical differences and understand that her inconsistent behavior due to Rett Syndrome is expected because she has difficulty with her motor planning and not because she does not understand. They facilitate their daughter's communication partners by interpreting her nonverbal communication and making people aware of their child's ability to participate. Her parents know when to pause and wait, watching for her smiles, her eye movements, head, and body positioning. They also understand her intentions when she speaks with her speech generating device. Her father states, *When you are a parent living with these kinds of things, you know that you do so much better if you don't let yourself be limited by what a diagnosis tells you. My child is there in a greater sense than what the diagnosis tells me.*

Alexa's parents appreciate the educational aides who know how to be good facilitators and communication partners with Alexa. They listen to her communication, have high expectations, follow through consistently on her educational goals, and make connections for communication between Alexa, her peers, and adults. However, not every classroom aide experience served as a positive experience. Alexa's parents observed that, *Sometimes the classroom aides were more protective. They didn't expect her to grow, to improve. They just kinda mothered her. They would not give her a chance to communicate or they wouldn't listen to her. They already had an idea that this was a child who was developmentally delayed and very behind. She was so sweet and so cute. She was like a little baby.*

Facilitators like her family and friends are critically aware of her abilities, communicative intent, and the support she needs for participation. Friends who became her communication partners wait patiently while Alexa organizes her thoughts and programs her body and communication device to respond. They also recognize that verbal cues help her. They know Alexa stands up more quickly if they first count, *1-2-3, stand.* Empowering communication partners with strategies empowers Alexa to participate. That is why the tip card in her backpack, on her walker or wheelchair is so important. Other communication partners who come to her home or work with her after school watch Alexa and asked her family to help them know the ways she expresses herself and what they can do to optimize communication when they interact with her. *I think communication partners should listen to the parents. I know things about Alexa that I am convinced of, but I don't think anybody else is hearing me. When teachers say to the parents 'step aside, I'll take over now,' they miss a gold mine of information and help from the parents. If communication partners just watch the parents and listen to them, they can understand how and what the child is like. If people know and watch parents, that's information.*

⊙ Questions for Reflection

Questions for Section 3 Facilitator strategies: What strategies do facilitators and communication partners use to promote participation with Alexa?

1 Indicate True or False: What are the roles of the facilitator and communication partners?
   a _____ Facilitators can also be communication partners.
   b _____ Facilitators seek to foster communication between all communication partners.
   c _____ Facilitators offer communication and participation support as a last resort.
   d _____ Communication partners and facilitators basically do the same activities.

2 Identify the INCORRECT reason why communication partners should wait for Alexa to respond.
   a Alexa has something to say and she will say it if we give her time to locate and gaze at her message.
   b Stopping Alexa before she communicates stifles her intent and limits her participation.
   c Waiting is an opportunity for the facilitator to program Alexa's device and speak for her.
   d Communication partners know that Alexa's body requires additional coordination time.

Answers

1 Letters a. and b. are True. Letters c. and d. are False. Facilitators had a strong rapport with Alexa who is an AAC user and serve as a functional bridge between her and others. Facilitators can serve as communication partners, but they are to support Alexa's communication with partners. Communication partners have varying degrees of familiarity with AAC users, communication modalities and access methods.

2 Letter c. is the answer. Waiting is not about providing time for a facilitator to program Alexa's message. Answers a., b., and d. validate Alexa's as a communicator who requires additional time and coordination to respond. Preventing her contributions denies her credible place in the conversation and waiting is appropriate for her participation.

○ Section 4 Literacy: What literacy experiences did Alexa have with reading and writing?

When Alexa was a toddler, a woman watched Alexa at a clinic listen with great interest and concentration on each page of a book her mother was reading to her waiting at a clinic. Finally, the woman told Alexa's mother, *I know she can read*. Her mother was inspired by the woman's observation and realized she must continue with pre-reading skills and make sure her daughter did read. Her dad, her mom, or caregiver read books to her every night at bedtime. She heard their voices expressed surprise, excitement, love, and fear presented in each story. She loved this time together. Sometimes they talked about what the characters were thinking, feelings, and reasoning why they acted as they did.

At school, Alexa was assigned to a classroom where a gifted teacher of children with special needs made literacy happen everywhere. Each day the children managed their attendance by turning their written name over. They reached and selected with a pointer the printed names of the day, week and month of the year on charts placed at eye level. They listened to stories, journaled about them, acted them out, looked at, and re-read the books when they had free time. Each day the educator chose one student to write in the journal about an event the child wanted to share. Alexa worked with the class aide to write and share her event. Another child was assigned to guide the class in a review of the written and pictured sequence of events for the day. Her friends and classmates sang songs and recited rhymes. This journal was read aloud at the close of the day. Additionally, the students could choose to look at the collection in the journal in their free time.

The speech-language pathologist focused on Alexa's literacy ability as well. Alexa studied the magnetic letters to associate sounds with letters and blend sounds together to read words and then locate them on her speech generating device. During the book club meeting at school children use speech generating devices to share ideas and text about the illustrations of stories as the speech-language pathologist gave them themes of music, art, myths, and places ahead of each meeting. Written words interpreted by her facilitators became her comments to share. Characters, actions, sequences, and feelings in the books and stories come to life as Alexa shares information through her AAC device. She understands the book club members may have feelings similar to her own and those of her friends. Social closeness was moving into the foreground of her communication. An assistant took exceptional interest in Alexa as she selected software and internet-based programs for reading and math using big key keyboards and switches. Her dad summarized, *Teachers should be willing to be teachable, let the child be the teacher, kinda like sitting at the feet of good teaching, helping the child know how to communicate and what works.* Her friends could not agree more!!!

⊙ Questions for Reflection

Questions for Section 4 Literacy: What literacy experiences did Alexa have with reading and writing?

1 What activities supported Alexa's reading and writing experience (select all that apply)?

- Acting out stories
- Reading books
- Writing about events of the day
- Journaling reactions to reading
- Lining up to go to recess
- Following routines for snack, toileting, and lunch

2 Indicate T=True or F= False to indicate Alexa's reading experiences.

a _____ Alexa engaged with literacy materials such as magnetic letters and accessed tools such as using pointers and computer software, big key keyboards and switches.

b _____ The intervention team incorporated structured literacy during daily routines, journaling, and for communicating through Alexa's speech generating device.

c _____ Writing was not incorporated in group activities.

Answers

1 Acting out stories, writing about events of the day, reading books, and journaling reactions supported Alexa's reading and writing skills. The stories and literacy experiences represented functional tasks and created a demand for participation by all students. Lining up and following routines did not necessarily require literacy.

2 Letters a. and b. are True. Alexa was offered magnetic letters, charts with pointers, and computer software to support literacy development in a structured way that helped her understand her day and communicate with others. Letter c. is False. The teacher incorporated literacy in groups to foster connection and validate the social efficacy of reading and writing.

O Section 5 Vocabulary: What vocabulary does Alexa need for participation?

Alexa's vocabulary is expanding as her friendships and motivations grow. She has more she wants to say across a growing number of topics with her familiar and less familiar communication partners. Alexa communicates social greetings with peers using colloquial quick phrase greetings such as, *Hey what's up?*

Alexa can choose vocabulary to express feelings and emotions. She can share information about precise ideas. *I look out at the red stop sign.* Alexa and her mother smile as they cook and talk about samosas ingredients like *herbs, potatoes,* and *onions* and how to choose to shape them differently. Alexa like to make them into flowers. Therapists asked for more precise vocabulary. *Was the samosa too cold or hot? Did it taste salty or spicy? How did eating it feel ... crunchy, mushy, sticky?* Each conversation begins with a social greeting, then an opportunity to share information, address social closeness with appropriate social etiquette discussing thoughts and feelings of the day, not simply *happy* or *sad,* but *joyful,* and even *awesome.*

Alexa has vocabulary pages representing her unique identity and languages, English and Spanish. She has pictures of herself and family with programmed phrases: *My name is Alexa, My mom and I like ice cream, My dad plays the guitar, I like to swim.* She uses quick phrases and new vocabulary that helps her express her wants and needs. She also has vocabulary that help her manage scary panic attacks at night such as, *I wake up, I am scared, I need help, I call for my mom and dad, they come to me, they tell me I am okay and will feel better, that feels good, I say thank you.* Messages for social closeness allowed Alexa to let others know when she wants people close to her or when she needs some personal space. Since her afterschool caregiver and parents speak Spanish and English vocabulary is programmed in both languages (e.g. *Thank you. Gracias*). Quick phrases such as, *I have something to say,* which got others' attention to her requests and comments, *I'd like a surprise!* or *Could I take a break?* Vocabulary that fulfill the purposes of communication expands her participation in more complex ways across her exposure to English and Spanish, learning both the spoken words, written vocabulary, and visual icons organized on her speech generating device. Expanding her vocabulary leads to more clarity and precision in her communication.

⊙ Questions for Reflection

Questions for Section 5 Vocabulary: What vocabulary does Alexa need for participation?

1   What communication purposes dictated vocabulary that Alexa accessed on her speech generating devices?
    a   Social etiquette with greetings, topic management, and closures
    b   Sharing information about food, friends, wants and needs such as getting help
    c   Social closeness such as keeping people close or needing personal space
    d   All of the above

2 Match the range of vocabulary Alexa uses to build and express her thinking?

a   Core vocabulary   1   _____ Words that represent specific people or things like samosas

b   Quick phrases   2   _____ Words and quick phrases in English and Spanish with visual icons

c   Second language vocabulary   3   _____ Words that are represent common words and actions

d   Fringe words   4   _____ Pre-set phrases and comments for speedier communication on her speech generating device

Answers

1 Letter e. All of the above. Vocabulary was needed to cover all the purposes of communication so that Alexa can be a competent communicator and participate with others. Expanding vocabulary is one way to support her conversations with all of her facilitators and communication partners.

2 Letter a=3, b=4, c=2, d=1. The ease of access provided in quick phrases, core and fringe vocabulary across languages creates timely responses between communication partners.

○ Section 6 Tools and access: One word and the AAC tools that help Alexa communicate?

One Word: Alexa spoke on one occasion. She was inspired by her friends when she was asked to choose a book to be read during an inclusive library program. The children knew she did not speak, yet they encircled and leaned in close to her as she stood in her walker. Two children were programming their voices on the BigMack for Alexa to say, *I want you to read Malala*. Alexa looked intently at them as they insistently repeated, *I know you can. Come on, say 'Malala!' Say Malala, Alexa!* Perhaps they too wanted to hear the story of *Malala, A Hero for All* (Corey, 2016). Malala Yousafzai, the youngest Nobel Peace Prize laureate, was born in Pakistan, and is an advocate for the education of girls. With no response from Alexa, as they turned their attention elsewhere, Alexa let out in a very high voice, a very audible, and very clear speech saying *Malala*. Pandemonium broke out in the reading room of the library. No one could be quiet, not the librarian, other adults, nor any of the children including Alexa who repeated *Malala* twice. The librarian and the children shouted, *I heard her!* The librarian read the story, remembering that this was Alexa's decision, treasuring her unprecedented spoken request.

Each child vied to tell Alexa's teacher they heard Alexa say *Malala*. Alexa's parents were pleased too though she did not repeat it at home. They saw the words in her eyes. They knew the next step was giving her a voice to access the message on her speech generating device.

Single message speech generating device. The children at church recite Bible verses. Alexa and her family ponder the best way for her to access this opportunity. Her speech-language pathologist has an idea. When Alexa turns to speak her verse, Zarah, her weekly volunteer spotter will use a Big Mack© for Alexa to speak the recorded verse, her *voice*.

Dynamic display speech generating device. There is still more communication for Alexa to express. Her parents expect that participation is a given at home, school, and in the community. Her mother investigates how other girls with Rett syndrome communicate. Her parents and intervention team feel that Alexa will benefit from using her eyes to access a dynamic display speech generating device. It turns out that Alexa can do much more than ask for basic wants and needs. Gradually more quick phrases were programmed, some for greeting others, some for telling about Alexa herself, others for sharing information about whom she had seen when she was in the community. Alexa can read and hear a story independently and engage in the narrative questions of *who, did what, where, when, how, and feelings of the character*. Her mother found that while she fixed dinner, Alexa would use her eyes to turn the pages of the illustrated books and hear the text of the story on her device. She is selecting words from eight frames on her *All About Me* page. Alexa can say her name, tell you about her hobbies and jokes and best of all ask others about their favorite books, jokes, and things to do, even say *hello* and *goodbye* in Spanish and English. The speech generating device allows Alexa to understand and share real-life thoughts and events about friends with family.

⊙ Questions for Reflection

Questions for Section 6 Tools and access: How do augmentative and assistive tools support Alexa's communication?

1 How did the implementation of a dynamic display speech generating device support Alexa in expressing the purposes of communication?

    a Linguistic   1 _____ Interaction between communication partners at home, school, and in the community

    b Operational   2 _____ Supporting communication partners in understanding the many ways Alexa communicates (ask for clarification, interpret her messages)

→

c   Social   3   _____ For Alexa, learning, comprehending, and expressing herself in Spanish and English

d   Strategic   4   _____ Using her hands or eyes to activate single message and dynamic displays on her speech generating devices

2   Select the best answer that details the theory behind Alexa's multimodal AAC program?

   a   Now that Alexa spoke one word, AAC tools and devices can be abandoned.
   b   A single message speech generating device and eye gaze support expression of her learning and comprehension.
   c   Non-verbal communication such as her smiles and eye gaze suffice for social interaction in the community.
   d   Non-verbal, single message, quick messages, and dynamic display AAC accessed through eye gaze offer Alexa the opportunity to express all purposes of communication with a modality that is the fastest and most effective for the situation.

Answers

1   Letter a=3, b=4, c=1, d=2. Alexa has access to the four competences of communication that (a) represent her two languages, (b) help her operate her devices, (c) support her social interaction with her communication partners and (d) provide appropriate strategies to support their understanding of her communication.
2   Letter d. is the correct answer. Alexa is using many ways, called multimodal ways, to learn, comprehend, and express messages for many purposes. Multimodal communication modalities give Alexa the flexibility to access the best modality for her at the right time to be understood as an effective and competent communicator.

Case study closing thoughts

For children and communication partners *Making Connections* with AAC is a time in which communication is reciprocally driven from joint motivations. Connections with friends and other communication partners are made and the result is shared information, a social greeting, social closeness and addressing a want or need. Alexa and her parents expect many high-quality interactions. Her rich vocabulary including emotion words recognizes the impact emotion-based vocabulary has on interactions. Alexa's use of language has an effect on others. When Alexa is given time to organize her motor movements, she expresses her unique identity and even demonstrates her ability to follow directions. The gift of time also allows positively impacts developing friendships. Communication is becoming reciprocal. In *Making Connections* we explore how the use of tip cards can aid communication partners in engaging with children that are AAC users like Alexa. We continue to investigate how Alexa uses her body, tools, and devices with access methods to learn that includes literacy, comprehension, and expression with others across environments. Consider the ideas of high-quality reciprocal interaction with shared information and intent in communication activities.

Making Connections with communication activities

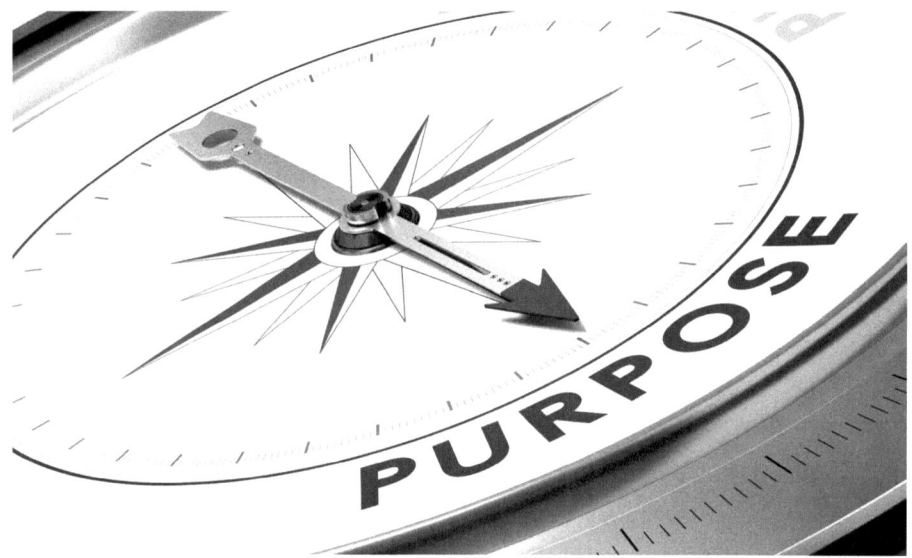

○ Implications of communication on interaction

With our premise now set that children are *Making Connections* between communication skills and the implication communication has on interaction, it is time to add communication rich activities. As you work through the activities we still want to focus on attention within a task and across tasks. Be aware of how multimodal communication can be accessed for effective communication. Watch for language development across communication partners and environments. You will see in the *Making Connections* Activities Pages that vocabulary options are offered rather than communication boards. This is a purposeful change moving from *Making Connections*, to *Bridging Skills*, and finally *Maximizing Communication* because the options of vocabulary can still be relatively small or be quite large depending on *your* child. Use the vocabulary options as a springboard to the best choices of vocabulary for your child, culture, and linguistic needs. Have fun! For each activity ask if vocabulary is represented across the four purposes of communication (i.e. social closeness, sharing information, social etiquette, and wants and needs) even if it is just one or two words or phrases with multimodal way to express messages and access methods to use AAC tools or devices.

○ Activities page – stepping into the purposes of communication

1 Do I Gotta? Daily Routines ... with Implications
2 Circle Time and Other, *Let Me Check My Calendar*, Moments
3 I am the One Asking the Questions Here!
4 A Recipe for Success: Following Directions that Include Transitions!
5 Ah Yes! My Favorite Books: Building Anticipation and Familiarity with Stories, Language, Deeper Learning and Engagement
6 People, Places, and Things – Check Out My Peeps!
7 *No, I Don't Think So* and Other Forms of Negation

Activity: Do I gotta? Daily routines . . . with implications!

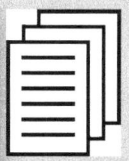

A place to start

We all have our fun and games to develop language and we also have tasks we must do. Focusing on the *must do* tasks is the point of this activity with the built-in idea of not just answering the question of, *Do I gotta?* with, *Yes, you gotta*, but also understanding, *Why*. That leads us to the idea of working on daily routines with the implications of what happens if you DO or if you DO NOT take care of responsibilities associated with daily routines.

Communication partner: what I am doing with my child

You are working on routines with your child anyway so let's make sure there is language support for you and your child. Established routines require less cognitive demand. Establish a consistent way to start a routine. Set a time limit. Establish the steps. Take regard of your child's positive and negative feelings and emotions during the routine. Follow through with a clear ending of the routine so the child knows what finished looks like.

Routines with implications

Talk to your child about the implications, both positively and negatively, of what will happen when a particular routine is followed. Talk to your child about why the steps matter. For example, *You are doing a great job brushing your teeth. Now when we visit the doctor, she will tell you what a good job you are doing.* Use language that resonates with your child. You can take silly pictures or use real pictures of what can happen with each routine. Show your child pictures of a child ready for school and a child not ready for school; a messy face and a clean face; a healthy tooth and a rotten tooth; something that smells nice

Routine Example	Positive Implication of Doing the Routine	Negative Implication of Not Doing the Routine
1 Brushing teeth	• White teeth • Fast dentist visit • Fresh breath	• Yellow or rotten teeth • Long dentist visit to clean or fill cavities • Bad breath
2 Bathing	• Feel better • Smell clean • Fun bathtub time	• Skin may look dirty and/or feel sticky • Smell bad, socially offensive
3 Bedtime routine	• Builds an understanding of what needs to be done and can lead to increased independence • Fun story reading or task • Calm the body down • Sleep helps the body recover and be ready to learn, move, and communicate	• Change in routines or routines completed by another person does not foster an understanding of the tasks and robs the opportunity for learning independence • May impact sleep schedule • May not provide a good environment to calm the body down for sleep

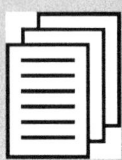

and something that does not smell nice. The images will make you both laugh and serve as a motivational reminder.

What my child is doing

Your child will be in different stages understanding what the implications are of each routine. The idea of implications may be a novel idea. This is why it is a good idea to introduce them in the stage of *Making Connections*. Use pictures to match ideas of routines and positive and negative implications. Use a schedule board so the child can follow routines with you.

My Tool Box Options Depending on the Task You Choose

- Pictures of your child completing steps of a routine
- Icons that represent steps of completing a routine
- Multiple communication options for your child to communicate during routines
  - Nonverbal communication modalities (e.g. eye gaze, head nods, hands, feet, etc.)
  - Communication boards
  - Static or dynamic speech generating devices

Vocabulary by the purposes of communication

Remember that the purposes of communication help us create a framework, an architectural structure, for a complete communication plan.

Do I gotta? Daily routines…with implications!

Social Etiquette	Information Sharing
• *Good morning.*	• *Oh no!*
• *Good night.*	• *I'm helping.*
• *See you in the morning.*	• *I did it myself!*
• *Sleep well!*	• Add sayings and phrases you would expect while playing completing the routine.
• Other family specific sayings	

Wants and Needs	Social Closeness
• *What do I do?*	• *Come here.*
• *What do I do next?*	• *Sit by me.*
• *I want to try/try again.*	• *Sit over there.*
• *I need a second/minute.*	• *You're too close to me.*
• *I am almost done.*	• *I want to do it myself.*
• *I need help.*	• *Do you need help?*
• *Can we read a book, listen to a book on ___ (e.g. tablet, phone, CD).*	• *Can I help you?*
• Core and fringe vocabulary	

Activity: Circle time and other, *Let Me Check My Calendar*, moments

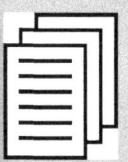

A place to start

In many schools, teachers use circle time to get children oriented to the schedule for the day, discuss the weather, work on concepts such as colors and numbers, and other activities such as students sharing toys or ideas from home. Make a home version. The activities can lead to a new routine and a way to practice skills that your child will use as he or she grows up.

Communication partner: what I am doing with my child

Success with this activity lies in making the activities work for you and your schedule. Decide what concepts and ideas fit best into your home life. Here are a number of options to consider and how they may be adapted at home. These tasks and implementation ideas are just recommendations so feel free to customize away. Choose a few tasks to try. Keep the time you engage in the activities realistic to your schedule.

Circle Time Task	Home Adaptation Options
1 Books	• Reading books is always a great activity. Keep things interesting and listen to books on a tablet or CD. Share ideas and previous experiences related to the text. • Try some phonological awareness tasks: letter to sound association, rhyming, sound segmentation (e.g. *b + a + t makes what word that we are looking at here on this page?*).
2 Concepts (e.g. color, shapes, sizes, quantities, object function, etc.)	• Talk about colors, shapes, sizes, quantities, functions, composition (e.g. wood, metal, paper), or others in activities you typical schedule, • Sort socks, silverware, and supplies. • Give and follow directions to find concept related items.
3 Emotions	• Make, cut out, or buy pictures of feelings and emotions. Match feelings and emotions to characters in books, actors in media forms your child watches, or experiences the child or family members' experience
4 Songs	• Sing or play a few songs you like from your play list. • Sing or play a few songs your child likes from the radio. • Sing or play grade or age appropriate songs.
5 Weather	• Choose a number of weather words appropriate to your climate. • Talk about what the weather will be like during the day, at night, the next day, week, or other. • Think about clothing and outdoor activities that are appropriate to the weather conditions.
6 Calendar	• Use your home calendar and note the day of the week. • Make a calendar for your child and incorporate other ideas on it like the weather of the day, favourite activities for the day or week.
7 Time	• Have a daily schedule that includes a time-based order. • Note the time on a digital vs. an analog clock.
8 Movement and dancing	• Create fun dance moves with songs. • Try a dance move popular with kids. • Sing and dance to nursery rhymes.

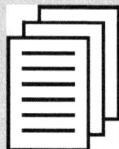

Circle Time Task	Home Adaptation Options
9 Fine motor	• Enlist help with setting the table or picking up items. • Draw a picture menu for a meal. • Draw a picture agenda. • Have a sensory table of dry beans, uncooked pasta or rice for feeling textures.
10 Names and pictures	• Keep a set of pictures of key people in your child's life and have the written name available for matching. • Create a set of pictures or icons of common objects and their labels to work on literacy.

What my child is doing

Your child is actively engaged with you and the operations of what it takes to communicate and participate in the home as well as learning tasks that contribute to literacy and describing items and events in his or her world. Your child is learning so many valuable lessons. Keep the expectation of your child's response reasonable. Have your child use communication boards or speech generating devices to contribute to the success of the activities.

⊙ My Tool Box Options Depending on the Task you Choose

◉ Books, calendar(s), music of all types of genres

◉ Research different types of dance moves to go with popular music

◉ Collect pictures of important people in your child's life for all reasons (e.g. home, school, and community)

◉ Collect pictures and icons of common objects

◉ Card stock for writing names of people and items

◉ Research different weather teaching tasks on Pinterest

◉ Multiple communication options for the child

  ◉ Nonverbal communication modalities (e.g. eye gaze, head nods, hands, feet, etc.)

  ◉ Speech generating device with a single message option

  ◉ Speech generating device with multi-message options

  ◉ Communication board option

Vocabulary by the purposes of communication

Remember that the purposes of communication help us create a framework, an architectural structure, for a complete communication plan.

Circle time and other, *Let Me Check My Calendar,* moments

Social Etiquette

- *Can we play circle time, sing, dance*, etc.
- *Let's do that again.* (Add the words *now, later, next time*, or *tomorrow* as appropriate.)

Information Sharing

- *This is fun!*
- *Oh no!*
- *Yay!*
- *Are you sure?*
- *Look outside.*
- Add sayings and phrases that work for the activity and personal style.

Wants and Needs

- *I want a turn.*
- Questions about the score of the game.
- *Can you help me?*
- *Let me pick.*
- *I want to try/try again.*
- *I need a second/minute to think.*
- *I need a break.*
- *Who is that? What is his/her name?*
- Core and fringe vocabulary

Social Closeness

- *Sing with me.*
- *Dance with me.*
- *Sit over there and I'll sit here.*
- *You're too close to me.*
- *Do you need help?*
- *Can I help you?*
- *You did a good job.*

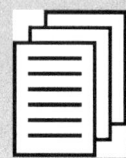

Activity: I am the one asking the questions here!

A place to start

Children are asked questions all of the time. Now we want to get the idea of asking questions into the language repertoire of your child. Let's give your child the opportunity to shape question forms. What types of questions do we ask? Socially we ask, *How are you?* We also ask all types of questions using *who, what, when, where*, and *why*. We also ask other question forms such as *how much* and *which one* but since we are *Making Connections*, start with the question forms that make the most social sense and are most common to your child's experience.

What I am doing with my child and what my child is doing with me

There are two primary questions to ask yourself. 1) Which question forms should I focus on? 2) What level of structure do I need to help my child learn question forms? Talk to a speech-language pathologist to make the best choices for starting to ask questions for your child. Use the list as a general guide. Try a few question forms out that you commonly ask your child.

Making Connections: options with asking questions

Is	Can I/May I/Do you	Where
Are	What	Why

Structured: Select one question form and work with that word and sentence structure with supporting literacy and images on icons. While modeling the production of the sentence using a speech generating device consider placing more emphasis on the target question word for emphasis (e.g. *IS he running? ARE they jumping? WHERE is my book? WHY is the girl sitting?*). Take turns with your child asking different questions. The fun part is that children love to see the impact their language has on others so if your child can ask the question, he or she will enjoy watching and/or listening to respond or find the object of their question.

Less structured: The idea of working on question asking in an unstructured task is not exactly unstructured. The more accurate term would be naturalistic. When you ask your child a question such as, *Are you ready?* have your child ask you the same question in return. Another less structured environment could be asking questions in the park such using the three-tier model from Tyler, Lewis, Haskill and Tolbert (2002).

◉ Forced choice of a specific answer: *Do I push the truck or drop the sand?*
◉ Cloze sentence that requires a specific response: *Are you ready to _____?* The child can answer your question (e.g. play, read, sing, etc.) and then can say the question form independently.
◉ Preparatory set in which a model of the targeted language is offered so the child can produce the sentence form: *Is he swinging? Is she sliding?* Your child may add, *Is he running?*

Ultimately what you are doing is creating experiences whether structured or less structured that introduce and reinforce the opportunity for your child to ask questions. That is a wonderful success! Your child may be asking you questions in the form of a gesture or a facial expression and that is a great thing. Your child may formulate questions that are not in the correct grammatical order. The order of words in sentences for a given language is called syntax. Sometimes intervention is offered to support shaping syntax. Sometimes correct syntax is not the priority and the communicative intent of the question form is the priority. The important thing is to recognize those great questions and foster question forms expressed using communication boards and speech generating devices.

My Tool Box Options Depending on the Task You Choose

- Books, card, pictures, work sheets
- Natural environments such as the park or store
- Multiple communication options for the child
  - Nonverbal communication modalities (e.g. eye gaze, head nods, hands, feet, etc.)
  - Communication boards
  - Static or dynamic speech generating devices

Vocabulary by the purposes of communication

Remember that the purposes of communication help us create a framework, an architectural structure, for a complete communication plan.

I am the one asking the questions here!

Social Etiquette	Information Sharing
• *What's your name?*	• *Is it my turn?*
• *How are you doing?*	• *Are you ready for your turn?*
• *How's your day going?*	• *What's next?*
• *Are you leaving now?*	• *Why are we stopping?*
Wants and Needs	**Social Closeness**
• *Can I do that?*	• *Will you come here?*
• *Can you help me?*	• *Can you sit by me?*
• *When is it my turn?*	• *May we look at this?*
• *Do you need help?*	• *Are you too close?*
• *May I try again?*	• *Who is coming?*
• *May I have a break?*	• *Where can I sit?*

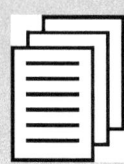

Activity: Ah yes! My favorite books: building anticipation and familiarity with stories, language, deeper learning, and engagement

A place to start

By engaging in shared book reading, your child is *Making Connections* with print, language, interaction, communication, and fun. Bringing to life the richness of text, stories, and interaction opens up a skill base and a positive experience with literacy. Try different shared reading experience tasks. Express enjoyment about language, *I notice the important words in stories, negation and possessive words.* In the book, *Pigeon Finds a Hot Dog* (Willems, 2004), duck asks pigeon, 'Is that a hot dog?' to which pigeon replies, ***Not a*** *hot dog,* ***my*** *hot dog!* Then apply the **not a** and **my** to child's experience (e.g. **Not a** book, **my** book). Share successes with communication partners so they can experience fun with literacy with your child.

What I am doing with my child and what my child is doing with me

The following list has considerations for shared reading experiences with your child. Check out the website Reading Rockets for many tips on reading by developmental stage at www.readingrockets.org/article/key-comprehension-strategies-teach.

Build a relationship between oral language skills and printed language. Build attention skills by moving your finger to show where to look, point out understanding symbols and print, and help your child recognize the difference between background knowledge and new knowledge in the story supporting comprehension.

- *Predict!* Ask your child *What do you think will happen next?* If it is a story you both know, create the anticipation and foster recall with the same question.
- *React*: Ask your child *What do you think about that* (restate details as needed)? *How does he feel? Do you think he is happy or scared? The book said he started to laugh at the silly picture.* Ask other questions like, *How would that make you feel? Would you feel excited or nervous? I would feel nervous. Now you tell me how you would feel.* Give your child time to respond.
- *Comment*: Talk about what you see in the book, the images, the words, the characters, the setting, anything!
- *Relate personal experience*: Relate the events, the images, the story to your child's personal experience. *Remember when we saw a dog at the park? Oh look there is the color red. That is your favorite color. Hey, Pablo the boy in the story looks like your friend Oscar.*
- *Learn sight words*: Kids become excited when they see words they are learning to read in print. Take advantage of that opportunity. See how many words they can find that they know and use those great skills to sound out unknown words.
- *Craft*: Make a project inspired from the book. Or craft your own version of the ending of a story. Craft a new character into the story.

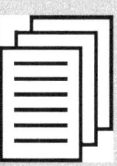

◎ *Pretend*: Pretend to be the characters in the story and tell the story, act out the story, or read parts of the story. Generate scripts of your own.

⊙ My Tool Box Options Depending on the Task You Choose

◉ Physical books, digital books, magazines

◉ Page fluffer or turner

◉ Multiple communication options for the child

   ◎ Nonverbal communication modalities (e.g. eye gaze, head nods, hands, feet, etc.)

   ◎ Communication boards

   ◎ Static or dynamic speech generating devices

Vocabulary by the purposes of communication

Remember that the purposes of communication help us create a framework, an architectural structure, for a complete communication plan. Vocabulary expands beyond nouns and verbs to include articles, prepositions, and adjectives as well as phrases for all purposes of communication. The articles like *a, the, these, those* to go with nouns and conjunctions like *and, or* to tie nouns and actions together.

Ah yes my favorite books: building anticipation and familiarity with stories, language, deeper learning, and engagement

---

Social Etiquette

- *Hi*
- *Let's read a ___ book! (add a describing word)*
- *Come with me!*
- *Let's read again.* (Add the words *now* or *tomorrow, next week* as appropriate.)
- *Bye*
- *See you later alligator!*
- *Thanks, I liked it!*

Information Sharing

- *I see the...*
- *I think...*
- *Look! Wow! Yikes!*
- *What do you see?*
- *What happened?*
- *I don't know.*
- *Do you know?*
- Add sayings and phrases you would expect while reading this book.
- *Yeah, that is like the time when...*

Wants and Needs

- *I want to turn the page?*
- *Can you help me?* (Consider adding: *Move my piece, Pull the board closer, Pick up something,* etc.)
- *I want to try/try again*
- *I need a second/minute to think*
- *I need a break*
- *That is too scary*
- Core and fringe vocabulary

Social Closeness

- *Come here.*
- *Sit by me.*
- *Sit over there.*
- *You're too close to me*
- *You are sweet*
- *Do you need help?*
- *Can I help you?*
- *I don't want you to be like that*
- *I don't want you to do that*

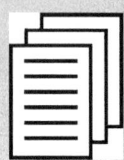

Activity: People, places, and things – check out my peeps!

A place to start

Create a book or smaller individual pages your child and communication partners can use to talk about topics such as family and friends, places the child frequents, activities your child engages in, favorite music, jokes, topics, anything! For your child it can be a wonderful way to not just show his or her unique identity but talk with less familiar communication partners or share new information with familiar friends. The hidden gem of a book or talking photo album with names and brief descriptions is that it is an instant opportunity for a less known or unknown communication partner to have a way to connect with your child. Communication partners come to life and take pride in themselves and in the interaction with your child.

Communication partner: what I am doing with my child

Make some choices about what you think your child would like to share with others. You do not need to make an exhaustive list. On the contrary, a few favorites can be a great way to make a connection with a person that may not have occurred. Some areas to consider for your child's communication book:

People: family, friends, key adults in your child's life
Activities: hobbies, music, books, movies
Fun: jokes, silly stories
Places: school, gym, park, art/music, store
Likes/Don't Like: favorite and least favorite things such as colors, foods, places

What my child is doing

Your child is getting the chance to communicate with others in a unique way that allows others to know a bit about them. The book or card allow for fun and communication. It opens the door to participation. Your child can also have a communication tip card to supplement the book so he or she can communicate more effectively. We have talked about using a communicate tip card. A summary of some ideas is included here:

Communication tip card:

- I will talk to you using my . . . (communication wallet, communication board, speech generating device).
- Give me two choices to answer your question.
- Give me a minute to answer your question.
- Look at my hands/my eyes/my head nod to answer your question.

My Tool Box Options Depending on the Task You Choose

◉ Binder for pages

◉ Card stock thickness of paper

◉ Photos or images

◉ Laminate pages or use laminating sheets (recommended yet optional)

◉ Hole punch and string or a ring clip

◉ Multiple communication options for the child

   ◎ Nonverbal communication modalities (e.g. eye gaze, head nods, hands, feet, etc.)

   ◎ Communication board, wallet, rings, or books

   ◎ Static or dynamic speech generating device

Vocabulary by the purposes of communication

Remember that the purposes of communication help us create a framework, an architectural structure, for a complete communication plan.

People, places, and things – check out my peeps!

Social Etiquette

- *Hi*
- Let's read a ___ book! (add a describing word)
- *Let's talk!*
- *Let's talk again* (Add the words *now* or *tomorrow, next week* as appropriate.)
- *Bye*
- *See you later alligator!*

Information Sharing

- *Look at my book*
- *Look at my communication tips*
- *I like that too*
- *I don't like to*
- *No way!*
- *Me too!*
- Add sayings and phrases you would expect with certain people, in particular places, and with favorite things? while playing this game.
- *Tell me more*
- *What happened then?*

Wants and Needs

- *I have something to say*
- *I want to try/try to say that again*
- *I need a second/minute to think*
- *I need a break*
- Core and fringe vocabulary

Social Closeness

- *Come here*
- *Sit by me*
- *Sit over there*
- *You're too close to me*
- *You are sweet*
- *Do you need help?*
- *Can I help you?*

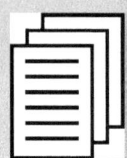

Activity: *No, I Don't Think So, and other forms of negation*

A place to start

You want me to teach my child to say, *No*? Yes. Not only do you want your child to say *no*, you want your child to say *no* in many ways. This is called using forms of *negation*. The ability to say *no* gives your child a way to express a choice. Saying *no* gives your child a way to be safe. The ability to say *no* is a way for your child to express comprehension. Saying *no* is a part of life when we see something that does not belong. We also need to learn to say *no* using the correct linguistic form for a given language. So, yes let's work on ways to say *no*.

Communication partner: what I am doing with my child

There are many ways we can work on saying no. We can say it in funny or different ways depending on our social purpose. We can use different forms of *not* in contractions like *isn't*. We can also use *no* for expressing comprehension of an idea. Each idea is expanded for you in the following list.

1 Social ways to say *No* in English: According to the Oxford online dictionary there are 29 ways to say *no* in the English language. Just for fun check out the link to see all of the variations such as *no way* and *veto* at https://blog. oxforddictionaries.com/2015/10/ways-to-say-no/. Some of these ways to say *no* may be fun to add to your child's communication board or speech generating device such as *thumbs down* and *no way*.

2 Selected forms of saying *no* using grammar: *No, Not, Do not – don't, Did not – didn't, Is not – isn't*. If your child is learning to use negation, starting with choices and answering *no* is a good way to start. As your child begins to use more language structures add appropriate forms. For example, to practice *no* your child can practice items he or she wants and does not want, *I want the yellow crayon*, *I do not want the red crayon*.

3 Express *no* across modalities such as head shakes, hand squeezes, and eyebrow raising. Use pictures with words on communication boards or speech generating devices. Your child can also use a *yes* or *no* response to their understanding of the negation form you are proposing. For example, show the child a picture of a boy and say, *The boy is not running. Do you agree with that?* The child can indicate *yes* or *no*.

What my child is doing

Your child is expanding his or her ability to understand and use negation in language that gives him or her more control over his or her choices, an expression of his or her opinion, and understanding of language. Your child is answering questions and using forms of negation. Your child can make a choice given the following example: *You see a ball and you see a cup. Which one is NOT a toy?* Look at item number three for ideas on bridging your child's ability to say *no* and recognizing forms of negation in sentences. *No* can mean many things. Make sure people learn what your child is saying *no* to in order to avoid communication breakdowns.

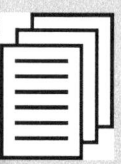

⊙ My Tool Box Options Depending on the Task You Choose

- ◉ Pictures, cards, or books with different items for comparing and contrasting
- ◉ Index cards with the targeted negation word
- ◉ Multiple communication options for the child
  - ◉ Nonverbal communication modalities (e.g. eye gaze, head nods, hands, feet, etc.)
  - ◉ Communication board option with negation word forms
  - ◉ Static or dynamic speech generating device with single message option with programmed negation form

Vocabulary by the purposes of communication

Remember that the purposes of communication help us create a framework, an architectural structure, for a complete communication plan.

No, I Don't Think So, and other forms of negation

Social Etiquette	Information Sharing
• *No thank you*	• *Oh no!*
• *Not right now, thank you*	• *No I don't think so*
• *Maybe next time.*	• *That's not right*
• *No, I will think about it*	• *I can't...*
• *That's not what I mean*	• *No not that one!*
	• *He, she, it isn't...*
	• *Don't even think about it!*

Wants and Needs	Social Closeness
• *I don't want ... (e.g. it, that, to)*	• *Don't go; Please stay*
• *No, I need a second/minute to think*	• *Don't sit so close to me*
• *No, I need a break*	• *That is not necessary*
• *That's not for me*	

Making Connections with facilitator strategies

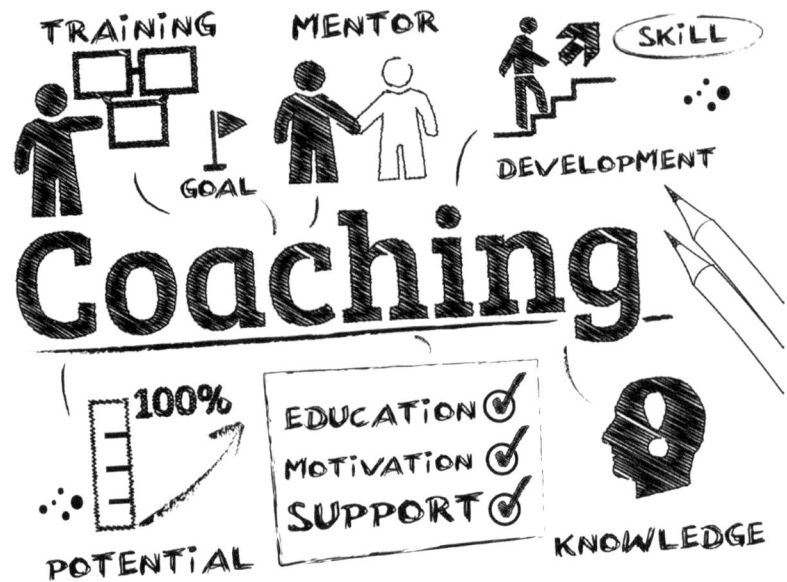

○ Grab and Go Coaches' Corner

Making Connections in communication for a child using AAC is a time when language is budding that shapes messages through words like adjectives, adverbs, forms of negation, and opinions. Core and fringe vocabulary blossom. Vocabulary needs to be on displays that are accessible, available, and attractive. This stage is both exciting and challenging for parents and interventionists. The goal is to make sure your child has the vocabulary and language skills he or she needs to express messages for all purposes of communication. In order for this goal to be met we need to look into a functional multimodal communication program that includes nonverbal, vocal, verbal, low technology, and high technology options. Facilitators need more than just support with technology facilitators need to know how to support language and communication development.

This *Grab and Go* section of *Making Connections* is a collection of ideas to support the language and technology considerations. Just like in the *Building Fundamentals* chapter, facilitator strategies are offered for each activity under the heading *Communication Partner: What I am Doing with My Child*, and *Grab and Go Coaching Tips* are offered by topic in this chapter to help your child's facilitator's help build language and opportunities for participation and interaction. Here are some topics to help you with the consideration process. See each topic for steps to support each tip.

Grab and Go Topics:

1 What is Feature Matching?
2 Tips for Selecting, Teaching, and Learning Vocabulary
3 One Up Environmental Awareness
4 More Word Options or More Phrase Options? What's Best and When?

○ Facilitator tips and steps in Making Connections with communication

1 What is feature matching?

One size does not fit all. When you think about communication devices, whether they are static or dynamic display, the goal is to match your child's skills, capacities, and needs with AAC tools and device. Remember from Chapter 1 that a static communication tool or device is a fixed symbol that does not change and represents one idea found on a communication board or a speech generating device. A dynamic display communication device has symbols that when touched or activated by any access method serve as a link to another symbol or most likely a page of symbols. Think about the size of the device, the number of icons on a page, whether icons can be hidden, whether the number of icons on a page can be changed, the audio capacity, the types of symbols, the weight of the device, and your child's ability to access the device. Then, does the child need switch access, and if so what type? Can the device grow with the child's increasing vocabulary demands (e.g. core and fringe vocabulary across grammar types such as nouns, verbs, adjectives, adverbs,

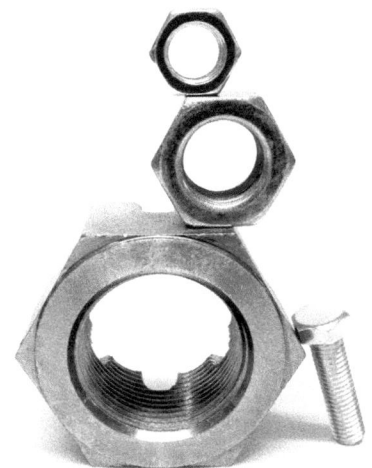

etc.)? Are there options for quick messages, novel message production, and typing? Those features are a good place to start. Rather than scaring you off with feature matching, the point of this *Grab and Go* message is that there are options, many options. Work with a speech-language pathologist or an AAC specialist to help you feature match your child's communication skills with the multimodal communication options. We will talk more about feature matching in *Bridging Skills*.

2 Tips for selecting, teaching, and learning vocabulary

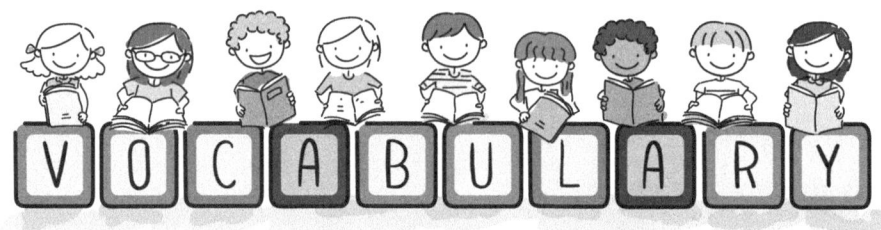

Your number one priority for selecting vocabulary is having a way to meet the four purposes of communication: social greetings, social etiquette, sharing information, and wants and needs. Refer to the *Making Connections* communication activities for tips towards selecting vocabulary. Ways for teaching and learning vocabulary include repeated modeling to the child verbally, modeling the use of the child's device, and opportunities for the child to work together to co-construct messages, and ways to increase independence with vocabulary expression. Implement Tyler, Lewis, Haskill, and Tolbert's (2002) strategy of using a choice of two vocabulary options to answer a cloze sentence. Cloze sentences have a specific answer (e.g. *Is the ball round or square?*) compared to an open-ended question that may have many potential answers (e.g. *What is your favorite color*?). Program core vocabulary in the speech generating device that includes nouns, verbs, adjectives, adverbs, and conjunctions. Emphasize how the child can use articles, adjectives, and adverbs. Show the child how to navigate a dynamic display speech generating device so your child is aware of the variety of choices on different levels for nouns, verbs, adjectives, adverbs, and etc. Make connections and tell how the child's experiences are similar to and different from others' experiences and perspectives. Try these options for working on language that also support vocabulary and word retrieval by Pindzola, Plexico and Haynes (2016):

a   Cloze set sentence completion: You put on your socks and then your _____.
b   Modeling sounds of words: Put your finger to your lips *to say 'mom.'* I see your m___.
c   Describe by object function: I can throw it. You can catch it. You can bounce it. It is a _____.
d   Carrier phase: I need a _____.

e   Gesture: Provide a gesture of the intended word that can be sign language or modeling object functioning (e.g. signing the intent for a ball to be thrown)

f   Request the object function: Tell me what you do with this?

3 One up environmental awareness

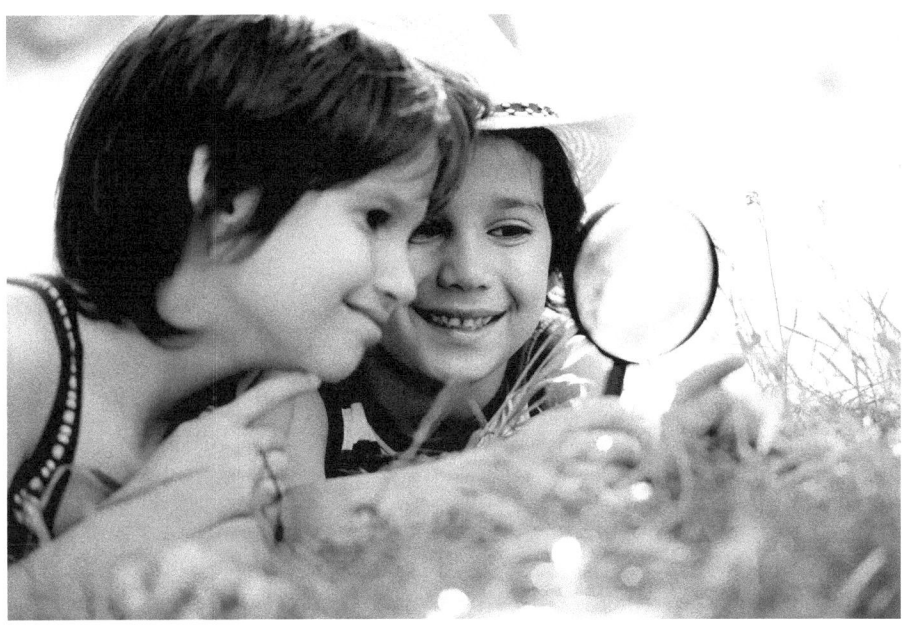

There is a strategy that is used in teaching functional math skills called, *One Up*. The basic idea is for the person to round up the cost of a purchase to the next higher dollar amount. Let's take that same concept to *One Up Environmental Awareness*. Get your child outside with you in one more way than he or she is used to presently. Talk about where you are going. Talk about how long it will take to get to the location. Then, let your child make the connections between language and experience. Let your child experience the atmosphere of a massive home improvement store, the smell and chill of a flower shop, or the bustle of a grocery store. As your child experiences the novel environment watch your child's nonverbal reactions and comment adding descriptive vocabulary to enrich and validate the child's experience and motivations. These ideas are reflective of the Pivotal Response Theory, originated by Koegel and Koegel (2006), in which you are responsive to your child's experience and motivations. Recognize and follow your child's self-initiations and self-management within the situation. Listen to and expand your child's language, providing opportunities to communicate throughout the day across environments and share information with all communication partners.

4 More word options or more phrase options? What's best and when?

You might be asking *How am I supposed to know when to add words, when to add phrases or sentences to my child's communication board or device?* The best answer to answer this question is, what does my child need to say, and

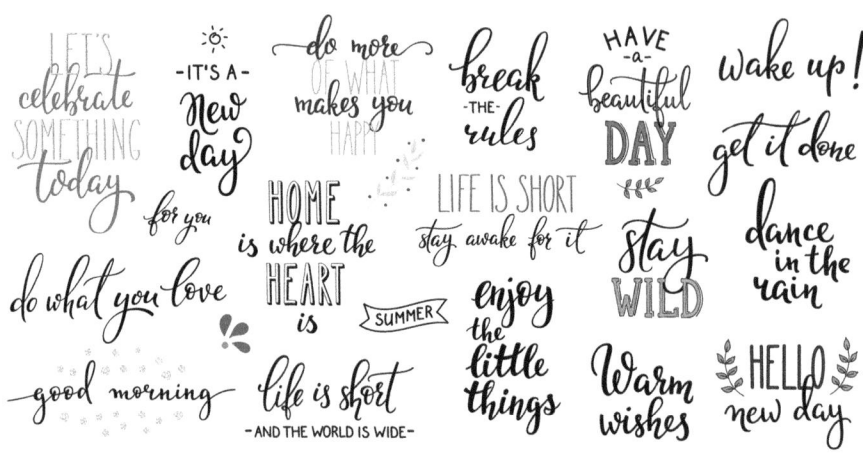

how often will he or she say the same message? While your child is in the stage of *Making Connections* it is still okay to have quick messages for the fastest communication possible. We want an AAC user to communicate as quickly and effectively as possible so having quick messages are great. Equally as great is to have individual words to make novel utterances to express unique ideas. Can you bridge the two? Yes! Consider looking at the words in the quick message. For example, let's look at the following sentence. *I need to go now.* If you think about the words individually, there is a high probability your child can use these words individually to create a new message. Go ahead and add the individual words to the child's communication board or device for novel utterance production. Then use the teach-and-learn methods for your child to produce quick message. *I see you. You **need** the book. I want **to** see you. Make the car **go. Now** is the time! I want that!*

5 How long do I focus on an interaction?

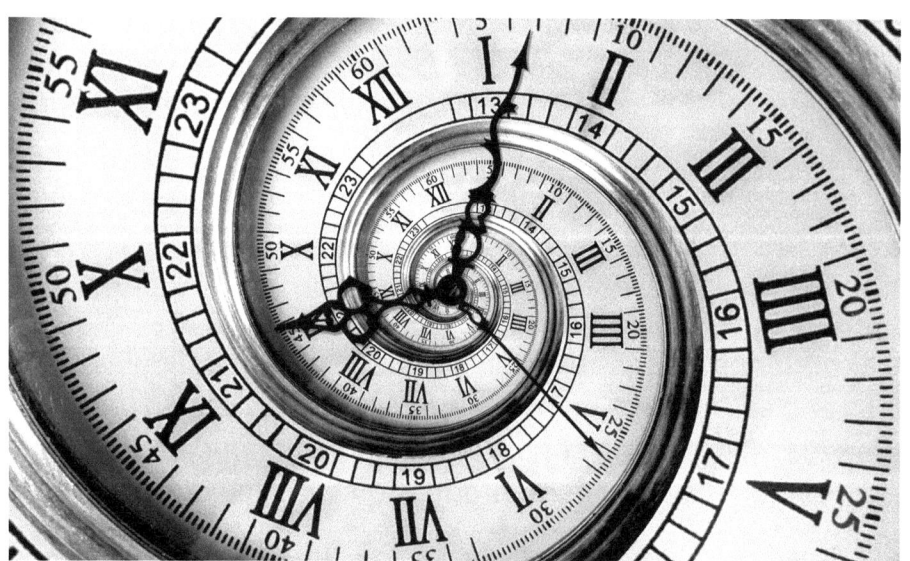

Once you start playing it is hard to stop! That's a sign of good fun. Just make sure your play includes time for your child to use language to communicate. AAC takes time and practice. Make communication an explicit goal. Choose an appropriate number of voice output messages within a 15–20 minute time period or longer. What is appropriate? It's like a great recipe. Make sure you have a large dollop of fun, you are modeling a handful of messages, and your child is mixing it all up with messages of his or her own! You and your child can work together to decide how long to focus on interaction now that you are *Making Connections*, remembering that communication is a two-way street. Be careful though, children with the diagnosis of autism or other disorders may not be able to recognize when they need a break and push themselves to a point of a dysregulation. In this case, chart the length of time a child is regulated across types of interactions and share that information with team members.

6 Literacy skills: a focus on comprehension

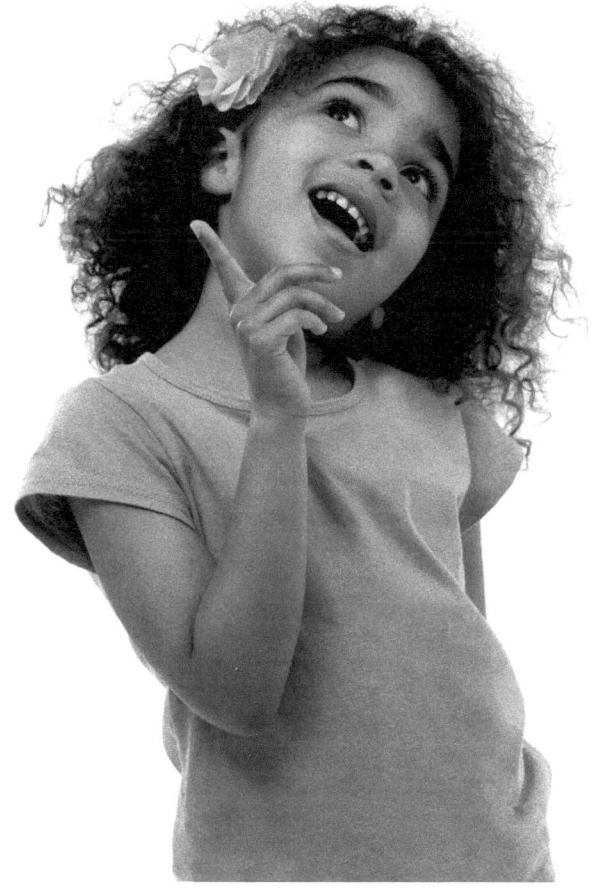

What did (add character) say? What did he do? How does she feel? How do you know that? These are all great questions that can focus on comprehension. Add in a question or two during reading tasks to maximize your child's attention skills and cognitive interaction with the text. Even if you are pointing and answering the questions with your child you are still showing your child what to attend to in the book (e.g. *Do you agree with what she did? Why or why not?*). You are showing them key visual information to attend to in the book or environment. You are showing the child the key details to listen to when reading or hearing a book on tape or an auditory message in the environment. Choose a few questions each time you want to focus on comprehension. Feel free to mix up comprehension and expression of ideas (e.g. *Why didn't she say she was sorry?*) while moving the child along with a good push for language expression and comprehension development.

7 It's time to practice processing

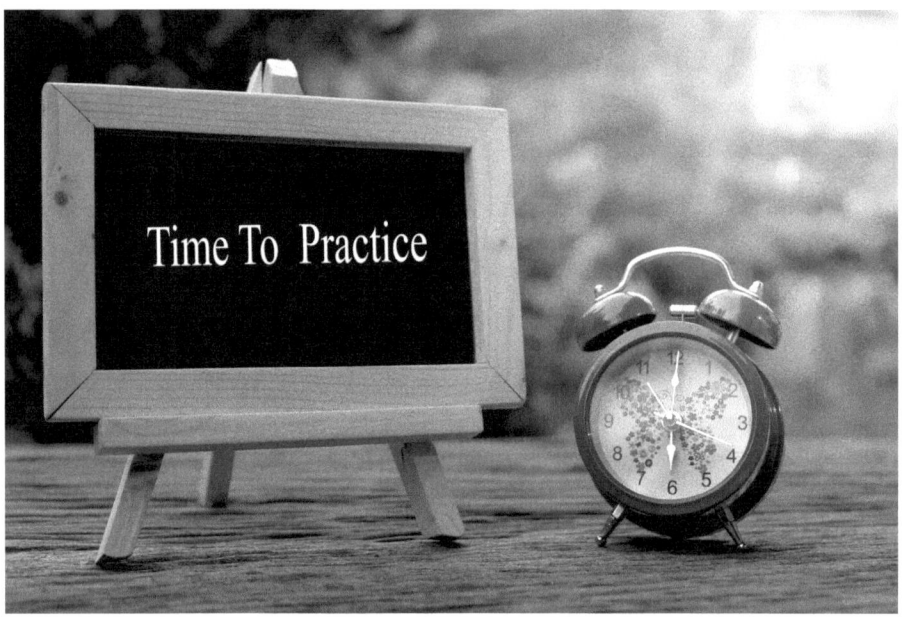

Be careful with rapid fire question asking and even repeating questions. Allow your child to process information whether it is auditory information from speaking or reading to the child, visual information from a text or the greater environment, or a novel setting for example. Teach others to give your child time to process as well. Take some data of how long it takes for your child to process information and write it down for others to know. Then, consider how long it takes for the child to generate a message. Having time to respond and be a part of the conversation is wonderful. Include timing needs on the child's tip card.

8 Give me time to respond: putting data to work

What data can we take? Take a survey of the types of messages your child communicates. See how long it takes for the child to communicate. Take data on the difference between the length of time it takes to generate a message with novel versus known communication partners or if time of day or environment changes the time. The difference in timing may be because of the child's confidence or could be a function of other distractions in the environment. Take a look at what is happening and be aware of the variables. Then put that data to work in letting communication partners know how long it will take for the child to answer different messages under different contexts

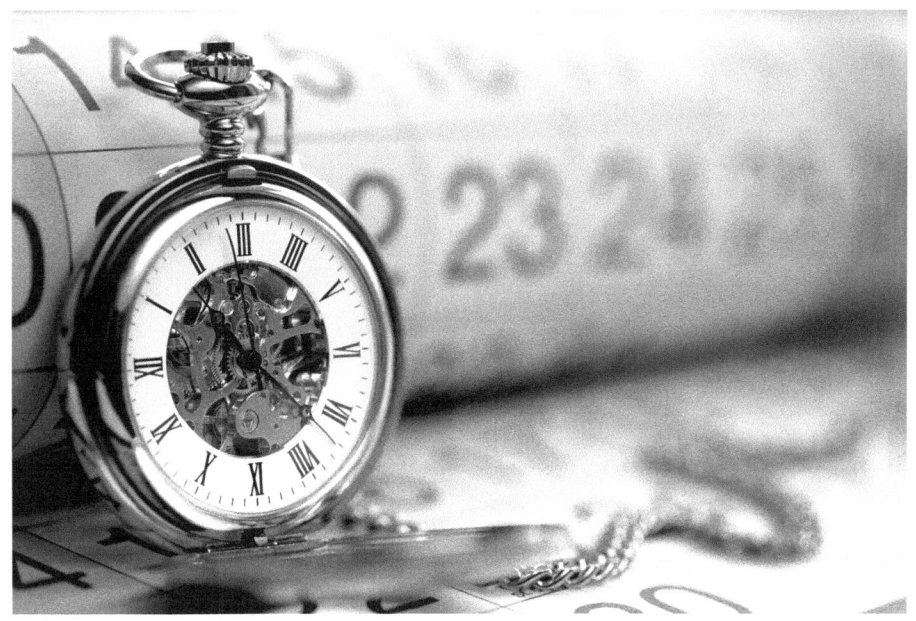

as appropriate. Even a general idea on response time will validate your child in the time and effort it takes to generate and say a message as well as informing communication partners to maximize the interaction.

9 *Language expansion: practice makes a motor plan!*

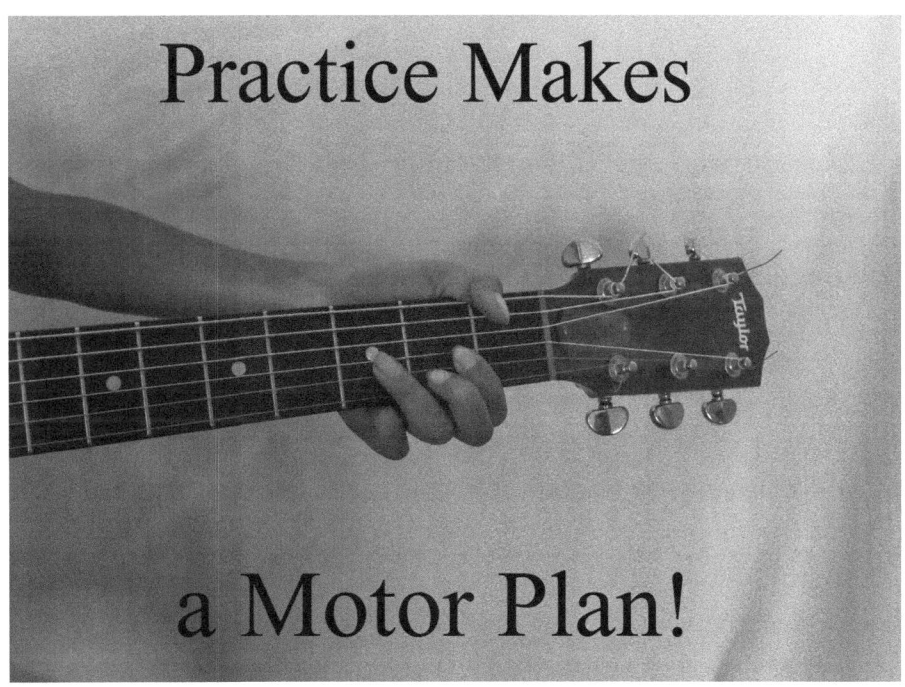

We are *Making Connections* with language. In order to continue in our stage quest we want to expand or scaffold your child's language. To expand a child's language repeat what the child said modeling one more words and pointing to icons representing the language to make your child's language flourish. Scaffold your child's language by using a word or idea the child is expressing, even nonverbally, and support them with the words and structure. Then have your child model the expansion back. However, learning to communicate using a communication board and device is a different form of communication and practice allows the motor plan involved in using an AAC tool or device to be learned. Many say that practice makes perfect. In AAC we can say practice makes a motor plan. Rev those engines. Scaffold more complex sentences, model use of, *and, because, if . . . then*, etc.

10 A second look at vocabulary: what's new to you?

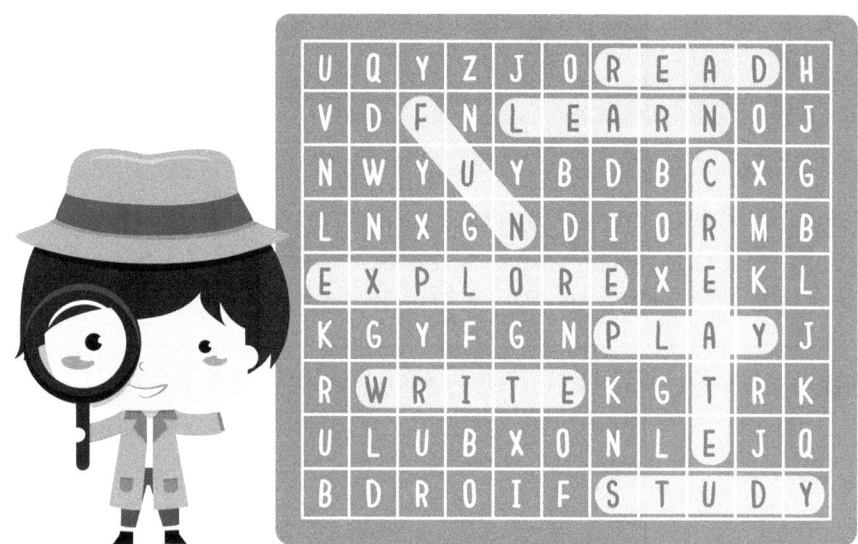

While we expand language, remember to take a grand vocabulary sweep. What language is new to your child in grand ways? For example, did the child start a new extracurricular activity? Did your child change teachers and thus a classroom that may focus on different teaching and learning themes? Did your child start with different interventionists? Did your child get interested in new games and hobbies or would you like to introduce new games and hobbies? Take a look and make sure your child's communication options meet the capacity needs of your child as he or she gets older. Prepare messages on communication displays for the child to interact in novel and typical settings (e.g. field trip, vacation, novel outing, even Dungeons and Dragons!). Include necessary vocabulary and opportunity for practice.

11 Fostering independence in the operational use of an AAC system

Begin to foster your child's independence through the operational use of an AAC system. Teach your child to utilize as many tools as possible and appropriate. *How do I turn my speech generating device on and off, adjust the volume, and brightness?* Teach your child to monitor the environment and alter the AAC device loudness to accommodate for the noise level in any setting. As you start

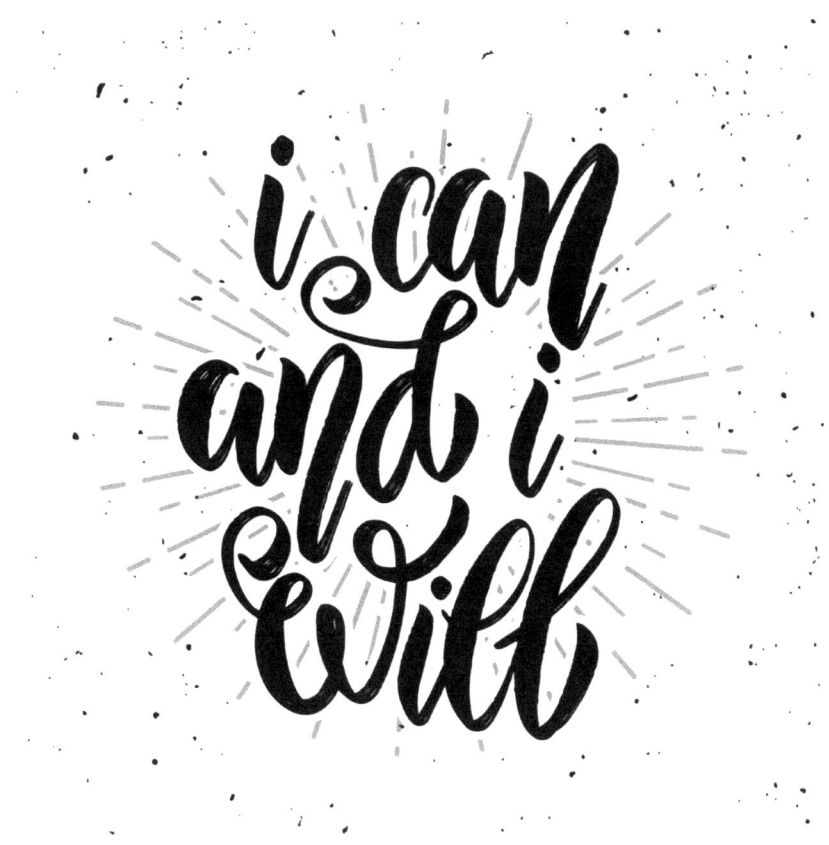

to foster independence consider the level of structure required for your child to be successful. Sometimes a child may require greater support in a more structured environment before that same skill is used in a natural context. For a great resource of types of skills or potential goals across the purposes of communication that includes operational skills, complete an internet search using the keywords Dynamic AAC Goals Grid 2 (DAGG-2) by TobiiDynavox.

12 Tips for teaching visual memory of icons

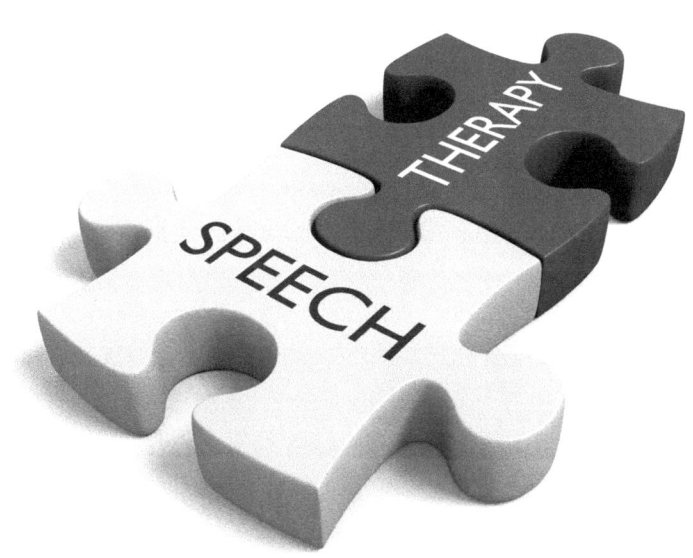

Flashcards! Teach the visual memory of icons on a communication board or dynamic AAC communication display by applying the following three steps.

Step 1: Make a copy of the overlay page that contains the icons.

Step 2: Make individual flashcards out of the copied page by cutting each icon out.

Step 3: Just like learning a new vocabulary word, show the child flashcard with an icon or have the child select an icon and the child can locate the button with the corresponding icon.

Step 4: Celebrate each success with getting the object, acting out a verb, or looking for adjective in the room.

Tip: Monitor the type and number of verbal, visual, and physical prompts you offer and reduce them as appropriate to improve independence and speed of visual memory.

Making Connections with literacy

○ Reading, story telling, and writing

Literacy, literacy, literacy! Does literacy really matter now that my child is *Making Connections* with language? Yes! A solid participation and communication plan includes a balanced learning plan that includes the ability to listen, speak, read, and write.

Listening	Speaking	Reading	Writing

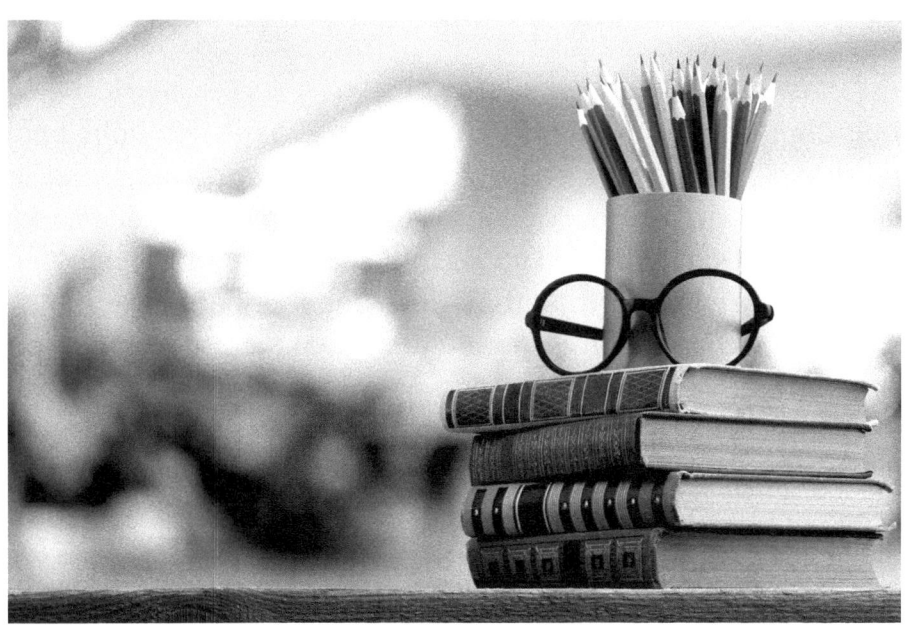

How are we doing so far as we head into the stage of *Making Connections* with literacy? Let's take a look. We are emerging with **listening** to peers through increased perspective taking, some repair strategies, and answering questions across the purposes of communication. Talk about inferences in stories. We are **speaking** using multimodal communication with more complex access to vocabulary on a communication board, in a communication book, using a dynamic display communication device, and low and tech tools too. We are engaged in many **reading** experiences shared through story time, recognizing familiar names, community, and safety signs. Finally, we are **writing** using typing, fun utensils for drawing, copying, and tracing letters and numbers. Listen, read, write, and speak, in any order that works for you and the child, using assistive communication to support communication that is integrated, often simultaneously, into activities.

Now for the *Making Connections* stage with reading and writing: A good question to ask, *What is the difference between my child using symbols on a communication device and my child's ability to read?* Is symbolic understanding of icons different than reading? Yes and no. Yes, letters are symbols of our language and words are included on picture or AAC image icons and they are learned by reading or processing them visually, auditorily, or both. No, a child using image symbols with words does not equal reading. Research is unclear to date on the benefit of learning other forms of symbols on the acquisition of reading (Light & Kent-Walsh, 2003). This means we must be explicit in teaching reading skills. The explicit teaching of letter to sound correspondence in children with autism improved children's literacy skills and resulted in an increase participation at home, school, and society (Benedek-Wood, McNaughton & Light, 2016). Literacy is a bridge to independence (Light & Kent-Walsh, 2003). Therefore, the need for children that use AAC to read is nothing short of mission critical.

Reading

In *Making Connections* the reading goal is to expand symbolic knowledge by learning that objects and ideas are represented in images and letters that represent sounds and words. We do this by targeting two specific reading skills, 1) decoding letters in words so your child can read a word, and 2) developing sight word knowledge so reading words becomes automatic. Erickson and Koppenhaver (2007) note that a child's communication, cognition, physical abilities, senses (primarily vision and hearing), affect, and attention impact the relative success that children experience while participating in literacy experiences. When you prepare icons for AAC tools and devices with pictures and words you have created the opportunity for literacy. Use the words on the icons, vocabulary and images already deemed important for your child to comprehend and express, as your material for teaching reading and writing. The goal is to make literacy fun and meaningful at the child's level of literacy development.

Light and NcNaughton, Accessible Literacy Learning™ (2012)

A fantastic source for children with disabilities that are learning to read comes from Accessible Literacy Learning (ALL)™ by Light and McNaughton (2012; www.mytobiidynavox.com/Store/ALL). The authors also offer steps for teaching reading through the Penn State website called Literacy Instruction for Individuals with Autism, Cerebral Palsy, Down Syndrome, and Other Disabilities at http://aacliteracy.psu.edu/index.php/page/show/id/6/index.html. The step by step reading program with easily digestible instructions with videos is a wonderful starting place that demystifies how to teach a child with a complex communication profile how to read. Consult with your child's educational team on the resources used at school and the goals that are being addressed. Ask about the best practices that you can carryover at home to support the literacy development of your child.

Story telling through development

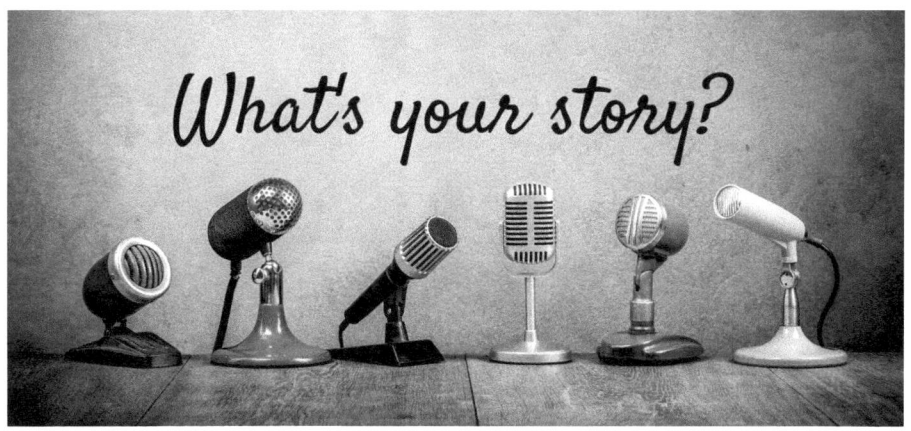

Narrative development. What's that? Narrative development is all about story telling. How fun! Story telling is a wonderful skill to target reading and writing. We can tell stories using spoken language and AAC. We can draw images. We can write words. The best part is your child is at the perfect stage to start working on developing narratives. Let's look at how to do that now. Franke and Durbin (2011), authors of the user-friendly book *Nurturing Narratives*, state that even simple narratives are complex. Now do not let that deter you. In fact, let the following explanation inspire you. When your child is generating a narrative in spoken, written, or visual formats (e.g. video, drawing, model, props), many wonderful skills are demonstrated. First, your child has knowledge of an event or experience that are then put into words and organized into ideas. The authors identify three simple narrative types including comprehending a story, retelling a story, and creating a story. For inspiration, use a video your child loves to watch or listen to and record events of your child's activities (Smith et al., 2018). Videos can be viewed time and again to observe themselves, peers, and friends as characters modeling language that is acted out. Children can incorporate problem solving and solutions, time-based events, and causal events contribute to the story telling. Finally, the child can delve into narratives that include *Theory of Mind*, the idea that the characters in the story can have and take perspectives of others. What should my objective be? Decide what you want the narrative to look like. Start simply. The child can scribble an image. A child can use icons with words that represent parts of a story. For example, the icons including ice cream, a freezer, and a happy face could be used to express a stream of ideas. Parents and interventionists can support the written literacy by working together with the child to create developmentally appropriate sentences.

Simple narrative

Drawing images is a great way to express a story. Encourage the child to trace letters of key words, initial consonants, or each sentence after a story is dictated. Write with formal or invented spelling. Typing a story is an option

First	Next	Last
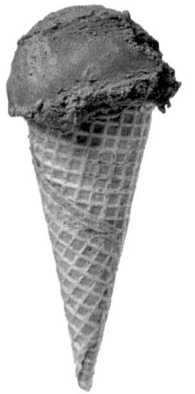	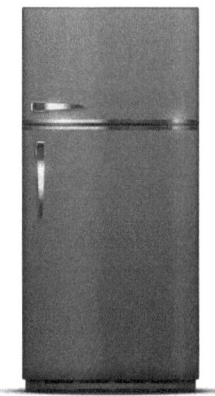	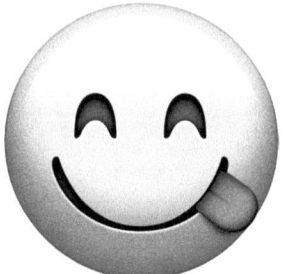

The ice cream felt cold and tasted good.

I like to eat ice cream.

Mom got the ice cream from the freezer in the kitchen.

too. The important part is to focus on idea formulation, story creation, and the connection between the narrative elements. We will discuss more about parts of a story in *Bridging Skills* so feel free to take a peek ahead. For now, let's focus on a few ways to support language including reading and writing with options to support narrative development.

Thinking through narrative development with ice cream

1 Fostering idea formulation: First start with asking great questions: What do you want your story to be about? Answer: ice cream. Who is eating the ice cream? Answer: I am. Who will you get the ice cream? (e.g. Mom is getting the ice cream). Where will you get the ice cream? (e.g. From the freezer). Tell me about the ice cream. (e.g. It felt cold and tasted good.). How do you feel when you eat ice cream? (e.g. Happy).

2 Aided language stimulation: Write and say the story. Have your child imitate each sentence. Use the child's AAC device to model 1) where the icons are 2) how to construct a sentence.

3 Cloze sentence: Start a sentence and have the child fill in the words written on a white board or generated on an AAC device appropriate to the story or sentence contributing to the story. Example: *I like to eat ____ _____. Mom got the ice cream from the _____. The ice cream was _____ and*

_____.

4 Story sort: Print out or write up the story on paper. Cut up the story into strips or sections by images, sentences, or words for each sentence. Match the words to the sentence and then the words or sentences to the pictures. Sort the images into the story sequence talking about what happens *first, next, and last.*

5 Options for publishing My Story

    a   High tech AAC device using icons with words
    b   Low tech AAC device using icons with words

c   Drawing for my child

d   Drawing with my child

e   Drawing (either the child or support person) and dictating my child's story

f   Drawing and supporting my child's writing that may include tracing

g   Use of technology including assistive technology

Writing

Check out the many ways you can start targeting writing skills today. Some of the skills are at the beginning stages of writing while other skills are more advanced. Each skill is helpful in the writing process so regardless of whether a skill is at the *Getting Started* level or *Making Connections*, the skills are fun and help you see 1) where your child is in the writing process and 2) the next steps or options to try in the writing process. For a child accessing only technology, work with assistive technology specialist to maximize your child's access to creative art options and writing applications. If your child scribbles or writes, then note the development levels of fine motor strength and control, elbow and shoulder stability, and head, neck, and torso control during any writing task. Think of the overall benefit of any act of writing is having on your child's mind as a thinker, a doer, a publisher of ideas.

1   Scribble: Drawing lines, circles, and general shapes on paper, chalk or dry erase boards

2   Spell names: Child's, family, friends, pets' names using varying fun writing utensils and AAC device

3   Trace letters: Adult writes a sentence or two using a highlighter that your child writes on

4   Copy words: Copy favorite character names or sight words from books or magazines

5   Word cards or magnets: Have fun with creating sentences using cards or magnets that have words on them to create sentences

6   Word Shape Icons: Use icons or objects to trigger words to be written

7   Invented drawing: Draw representations of shapes and objects

8   Invented spelling: Accept written word approximations

9   Personal word writing dictionary: Use a child spelling dictionary (look for free printable options online)

10 Word walls (Erickson & Koppenhaver, 2007)

11 Carrier phrase writing: I see___. I hear ___. I want a/the ___.

12 Descriptive talking and writing: (color: blue, red) + object; (size: big, small) + object

13 Text to speech of letters, words, sentences, and whole message

14 Word prediction

Are there more? Yes! Try these writing tasks that support literacy development:

1 Match whole words to pictures and vice versa
2 Match whole words to whole words
3 Match letters to spell whole words
4 Match, write, or type consonants in lower case first and then upper case
5 Match, write, or type vowels in lower case and then upper case
6 Choose to select letters in your child's name, preferred toys, and frequently used words
7 Choose to use letters written most frequently. Light and McNaughton's Literacy Instruction (2012) recommends the following order: a, m, t, p, o, n, c, d, u, s, g, h, i, f, b, l, e, r, w, k, x, v, y, z, j, q. See http://aacliteracy.psu.edu/index.php/page/show/id/6/index.html
8 Print rhyming word choices and match them to picture icons or to each other
9 Use multisensory input such as clapping out syllables, tapping syllables in the child's hand,
10 Use Play-Doh, textured material for manipulation, or props to represent word associations or can be used to support narrative development
11 Dictate stories to a communication partner and the child can trace over the writing.
12 Promote sight word recognition by labeling items
13 Have multiple ways of accessing writing using traditional writing tools, keyboards, and craft related drawing options on technology
14 Sing! Singing offers rhythm, increased time of sound production, time to process, a sensory experience, often a shared activity with others, that can be paired with words and pictures

Making Connections with vocabulary

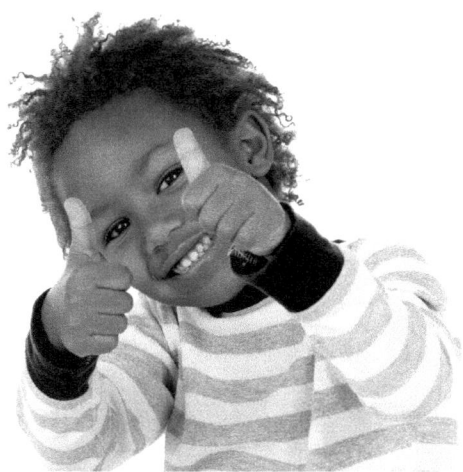

○ Words and word combinations that are important to me!

Making Connections with vocabulary means using words we comprehend and express for an Explicit-Active-Intention. We learn vocabulary by listening and experiencing ideas in action and literacy and solidify that knowledge by applying concepts through self-expression. It can be tricky to accurately measure receptive vocabulary skills of children with complex communication profiles. We can use auditory options for children with degrees of vision abilities. We can apply visual and auditory methods with strategies to support learning differences and disorders. Keep exposing the child to language and literacy. The explosion of vocabulary in the *Making Connections* stage for a child may be on a very broad spectrum between trickling in and significant expansion. You will also most likely see growth spurts, an ebb and flow in vocabulary growth, much like physical growth. This is all natural and as long as progress is being made then that counts as success. How do I choose vocabulary? The key in choosing vocabulary from here on out is to make sure the child has the needed vocabulary to meet the four purposes of communication for social and academic purposes from a quantity and quality perspective. The Prentke-Romich Company's (2018) 100 High Frequency Core Word List is found under free resources at the AAC Language Lab https://aaclanguagelab.com. This compilation of resources serves as a wonderful guide for families and interventionist. Select vocabulary that matters most to your child (Light, McNaughton & Caron, 2019). Not every word on a list is required for communication success. Make relevance to your child the priority.

Prentke-Romich Company 100 high frequency core word list

Social Words	Yes	No	Adverbs	Not/don't	Now
	Hi	Hello		Here	There
	Thank you	Please		Away	Again
	Goodbye	Welcome			
Pronouns	I	Me	Prepositions	On	Off
	My	Mine		In up	Out
	You	It		To	Down
	He	She		Under	Foe
	We	They			With

Question Words	What	When	Determiners	This	That
	Where	Who		Some	All
	Why	How			
Helping Verbs	Be	Is	Conjunctions	And	But
	Am	Are			
	Was	Were			
	Do	Did			
	Can	Have			
	Will				
Verbs	Go	Stop	Adjectives	More	One
	Turn	Make		Big	Little
	Look	See		Fast	Slow
	Find	Put		Same	Different
	Open	Close		Pretty	Red
	Eat	Drink		Blue	Yellow
	Get	Help		Good	Bad
	Want	Need		New	Old
	Say	Tell		Happy	Sad
	Come	Read			
	Like	Feel			
	Color	Let's			
	Work	Play			
	Finished	All done			

Note: Adapted from Prentke-Romich Company AAC Language Lab Resources

Examples of vocabulary across the purposes of communication

Let's talk through some examples of vocabulary across the purposes of communication. Prentke-Romich Company 100 high frequency core word list examples of vocabulary that can be used. Remember to make sure you have examples of vocabulary specific to your culture and family. Family and culture specific vocabulary makes communication more fun and motivating for your child and those that interact with your child, his or her communication partners! Okay so jump in to becoming familiar with the four purposes of communication and think about what would be fun and needed, representative and functional, for your child, family, and community to talk about.

Vocabulary examples using the purposes of communication

Social Greeting		Sharing Information	
1	*Hi what cha' doin'?*	1	*I have something to say.*
2	*Hey what's up?*	2	*Give me a minute to answer your question.*
3	*Hi, how are you?*	3	*Give me three choices to answer your question.*
4	*See you later.*	4	*I know what you mean.*
5	*Catch you later.*	5	*I don't know what you mean.*
6	*I need to go. Talk to you later.*	6	*Can you say that again?*

Social Closeness		Wants and Needs	
1	*Can you sit next to me?*	1	*Can you help me with my _____ (e.g. backpack, lunch, my switch)?*
2	*I need a hug.*		
3	*Go away.*	2	*Hand me my toy/book.*
4	*Not now.*	3	*Can I have milk/water/juice please?*
5	*I want to be alone.*	4	*I need a snack.*
		5	*I need to use the restroom.*
		6	*What's that?*

Now consider the AAC tools and devices that may assist your child in learning, comprehending, and expressing communication.

Making Connections with tools and access

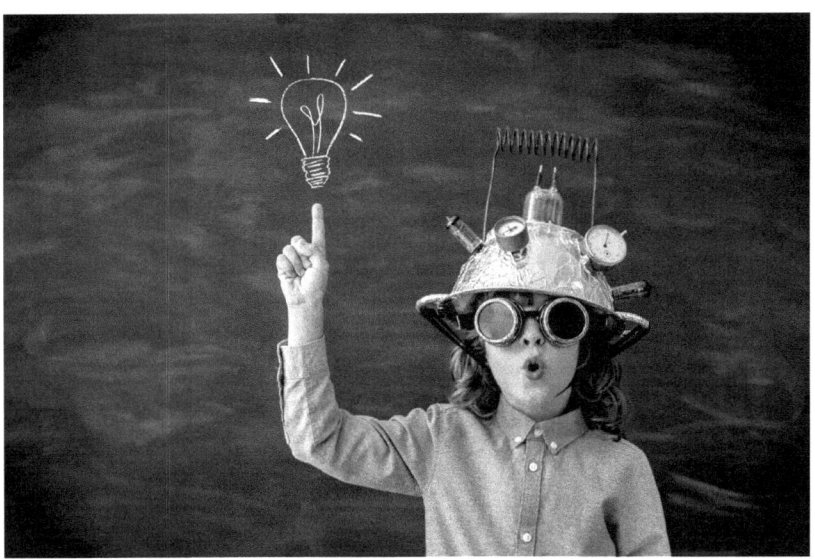

○ I have AAC options!

The purpose of *Making Connections with Tools and Access* is to offer direction in other or additional communication technologies to support communication. Look at examples of high technology AAC devices that use dynamic displays of vocabulary for communication use. Explore options to access communication such as different keyboards, page turners, and book formats to access and improve literacy. Look across all of the chapters for recommended tools and access options for your child. You will see tools and technology repeated across the chapters. Many technologies are applicable across stages and environments to support communication growth.

Static display speech generating device-revisiting Building Fundamentals

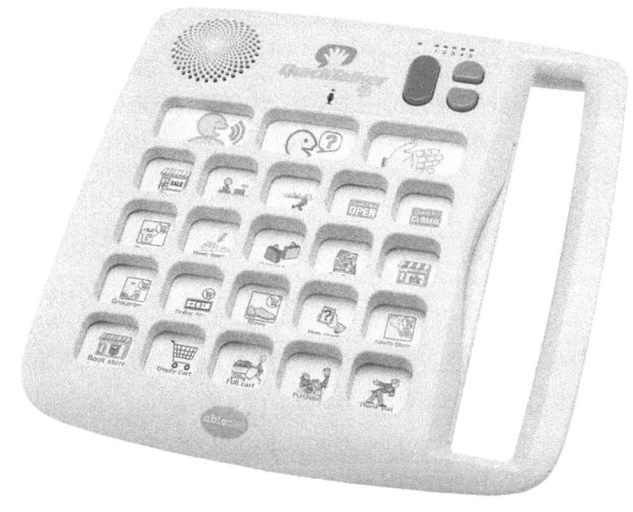

Our static display speech generating device, such as the Quick Talker from Ablenet, allows us to use a mid-level of tech for speech production that can be useful for individuals that 1) are beginning with a limited number of choices, 2) have consistent messages to be spoken during routine events or activities, and 3) are ready to have the option to combine words. A single message static speech generating device can be programmed quickly. Static devices with multiple messages often have accompanying overlays of pictures that match preprogrammed buttons with digitized, or human, voices.

Dynamic speech generating device

Dynamic display speech generating devices allow an individual to express messages across the purposes of communication in forms of commonly used phrases often called quick messages and to produce novel combinations. Children in the *Making Connections* stage of communication are learning how to put words together to express their intent and knowing when it is a good time to use a quick message and when they can put together words to create a message.

Phone or tablet

Hmmm … you may be saying … a phone, a tablet, or a traditional communication device? You want the most efficient communication modality at the time to meet the communication need. Think multimodal. Now, the reality is there is an expense difference between the options but there is also a functional outcome that needs to be considered. If the audio output of a phone or tablet application does not meet the communication need and the audio demands

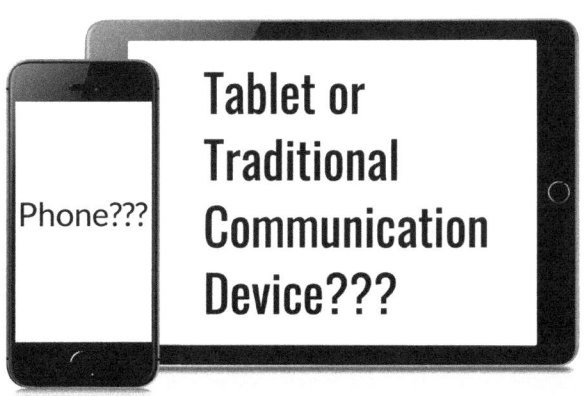

require cumbersome external speakers, then there is your one solid reason to look to a traditional speech generating device. Other considerations are battery life, ease of the device in an environment (e.g. field trip, park, community outing, classroom, home, etc.), the ability to have the same symbol set software across devices. Further considerations include the size and weight of the device for your child and communication partners to interact with participation in activities. A tablet may be the right hardware with applications for your child. Feature match to be sure.

Keyboards

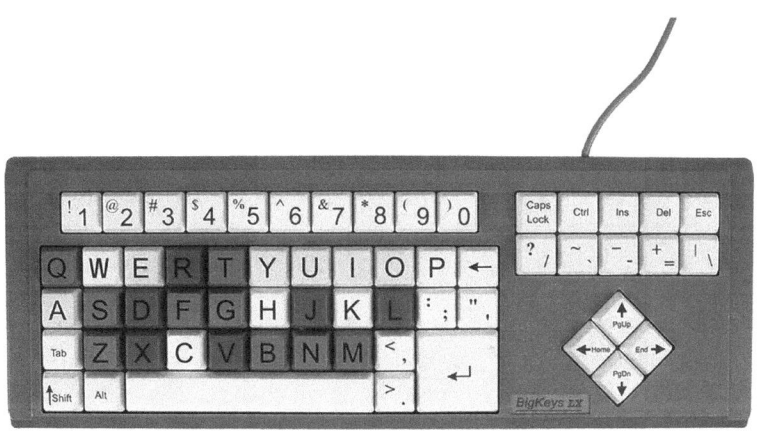

Keyboarding skills. Now? Sure! Start to investigate your child's ability to work with a keyboard. Start with lower case letters rather than upper case letters because most of language is written in lower case letters. There are a variety of keyboards to consider such as a standard keyboard that is wired to a computer or accessed using Bluetooth, ergonomically designed keyboards, on-screen keyboards, laptop keyboards, big key keyboards, and keyboards on devices such as phones and tablets of varying sizes. You may be thinking that your child is not ready for keyboarding but try anyway or set a plan to explore typing that may include degrees of physical support! If at first you do not have success … try in six months, then another six months, and then again for the next few years.

Books in digital format

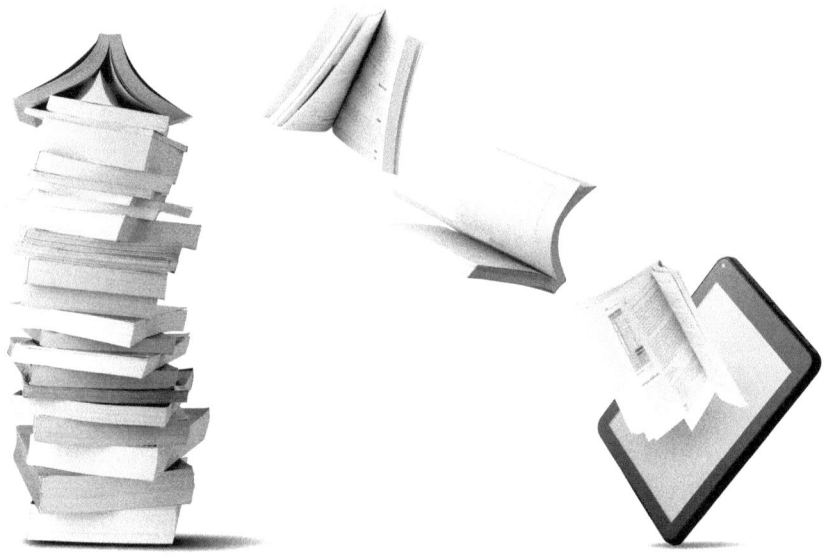

Reading books using a digital format on a computer, tablet, or phone is a novel way for a child to participate in a literary experience and it offers the opportunity for increased independence. It exposes the child to listening to books read by a person or synthesized. Look into the best options for your child. For example, are there images with the book or just audio? When your child is ready then begin to relinquish operational control of books read in digital formats. Consider the operational demands of the digital programs. How will your child turn the page?

Page turners for books: colored electrical tape, pom-poms, and popsicle sticks

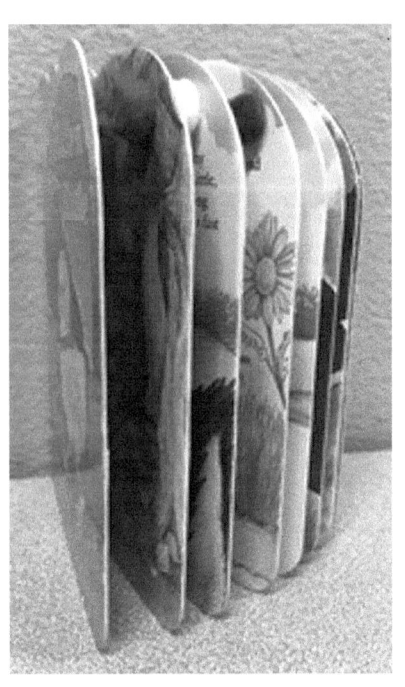 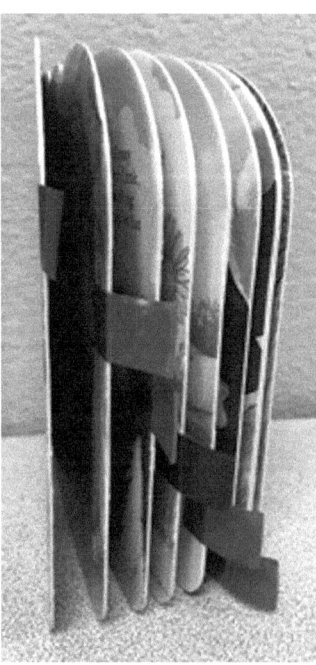 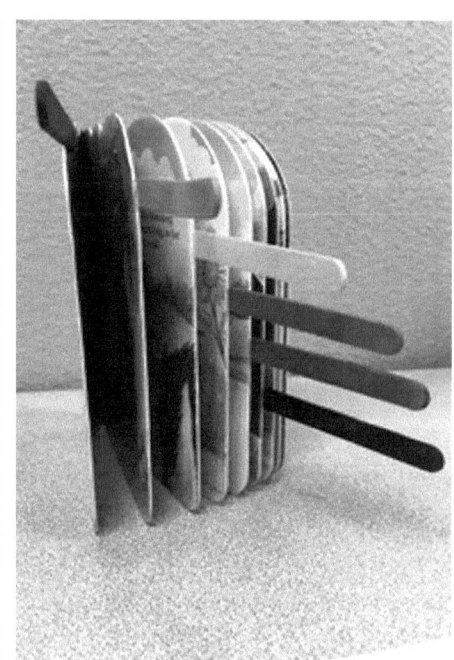

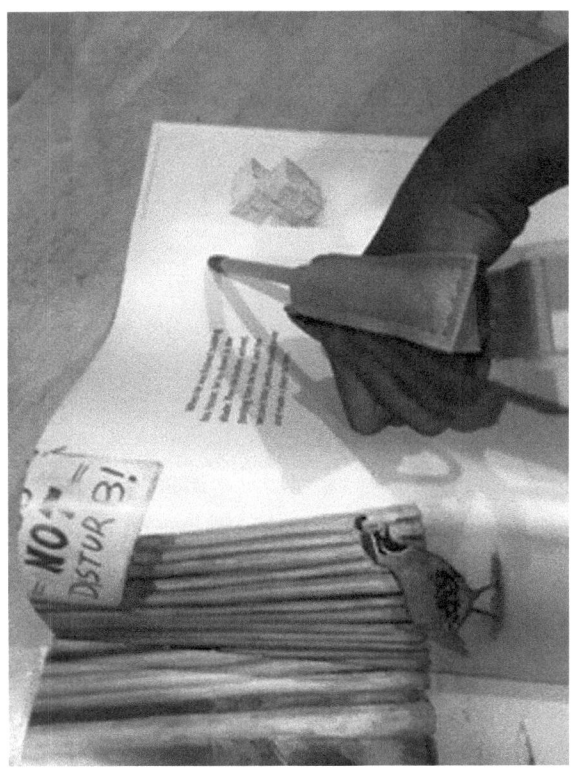

Page turners increase a child's independence in reading. Look into the motor needs of your child and consider the access methods that will allow increased independence for hard copy book reading. Colored electrical tape and Velcro® tabs are nice options for creating space between pages and providing a visual and physical landmark for children to turn pages in a book. A hand cuff with a pencil or stylus is an option for a child to turn thinner pages of a book.

Electronic page turners for hard copy books are an option but be cautious of the significant price range, size, and the functionality of the features the device offers. Some page turners will turn a select number of pages loaded into the device activated by using a switch. Consider the overall impact in improving independence and decide if using electronic books may be a better option. Just as with our communication there may be times you want a manual page turning option for some books and electronic for other book options.

Symbol systems

The discovery and decision making behind the symbol system your child, student, and client accesses is an important device feature. Usually the symbol system is a built in part of the software of a speech generating device. Be sure the symbol system is salient to you and your child. If the icons make sense to you, then you will want to use them with your child. If the symbol system

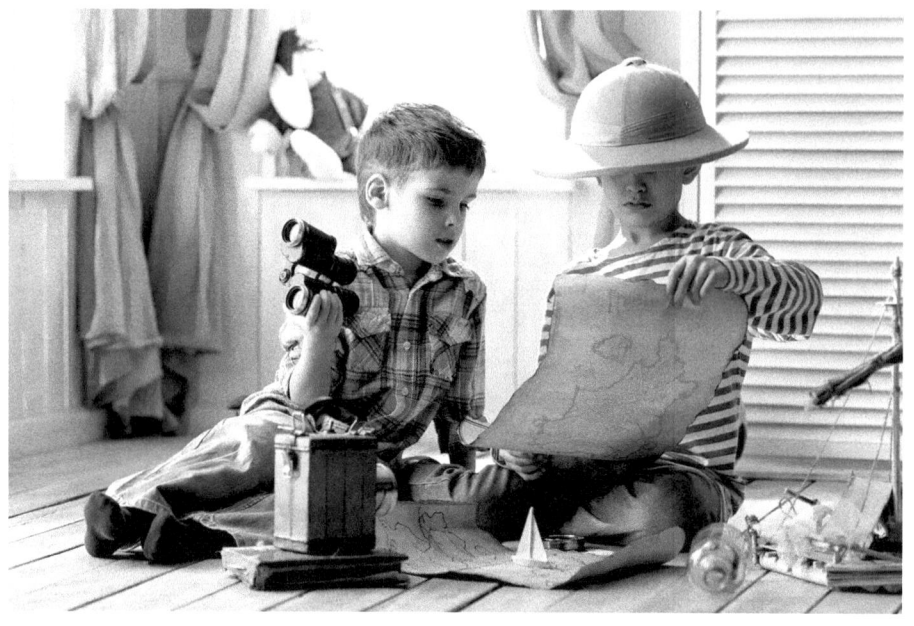

is organized well, you will be able to combine words and so will your child. If there is a quick way for social messages to be programmed, understood, and delivered to a communication partner using salient symbols then you are making a good choice in purchasing that device.

A summary of Making Connections

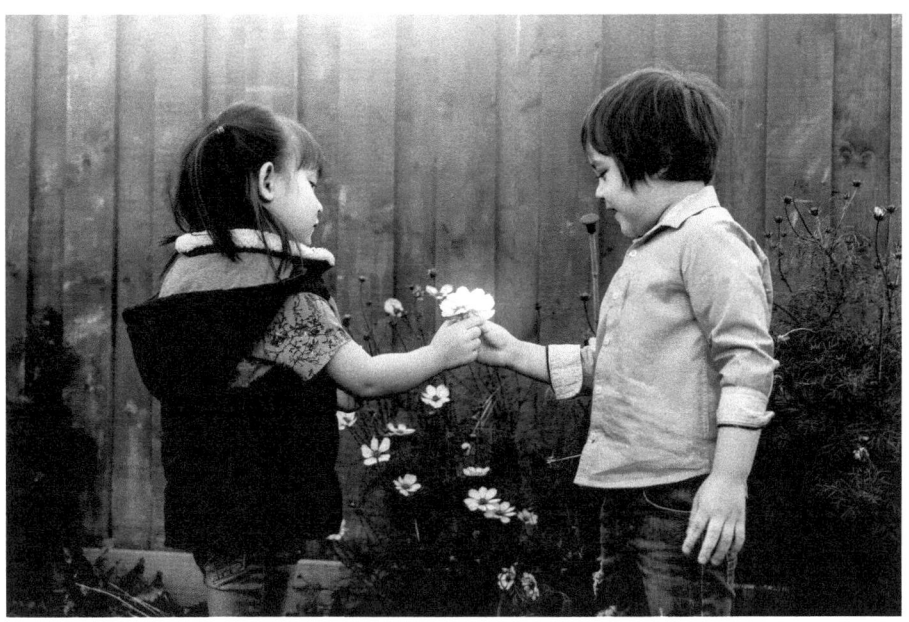

○ Making a difference with others

For children using AAC, *Making Connections* is a time for recognizing their communication is making a difference to someone else that may result in making a new friend. Maybe the result is self-serving and maybe the communication is serving others or both, but connections are being made. This connection will drive motivation to continue *Making Connections* between their communication and interactions with others and the world around them. Fringe and core words can be used to plan activities for the day and to create narratives. High frequency core words and quick phrases can be used for sharing information, making comments, identifying personal wants and needs, and expressing uniqueness. Communication is fun, functional, and engaging. Explore emotion words to check in about each child's feelings. Make a plan to expand your child's understanding and use of emotion words recognizing that the basic emotion words work wonderfully most of the time and to be ready to expand the use of more advanced words when the occasion arises. This goal is accomplished by recognizing the impact emotions have on interactions and that words influence others. Communication, the ability to follow directions, following the social lead, and taking the lead impacts developing our child's friendships.

Before we go: a topic book titled, *The Chronicle of Me*

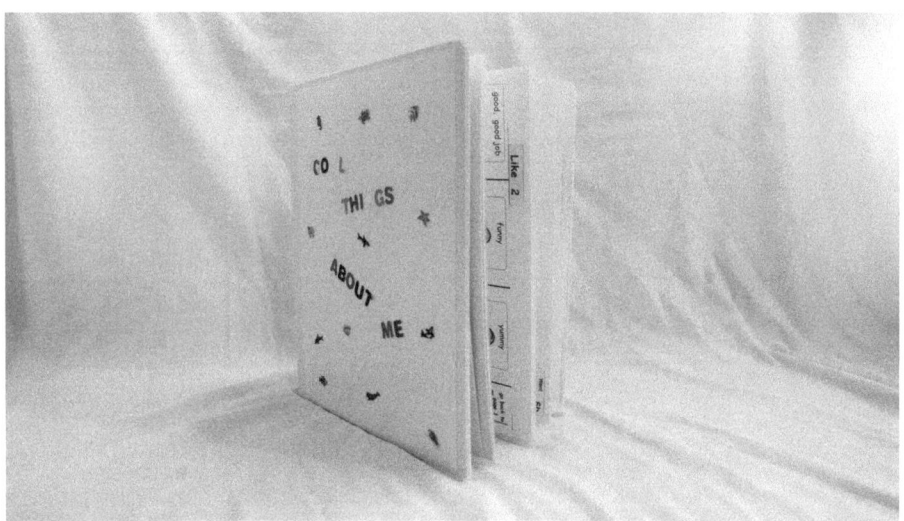

Design a topic notebook with an engaging name that holds tickets, fliers, postcards, pictures, and more. The notebook, binder, or folder is a fun talking point to share information with friends and familiar adults about recent activities. People love to hear about summer trips, that cool new movie, or your visit to your favorite park. Share that information in a tangible way through a binder or folder titled, *Cool Things about Me*, a version of a remnant book, memory book, or scrapbook. Create your own fun title. Consider loading a copy of the book onto the child's speech generating device including photos.

Materials: Binder or a fun folder, page protectors, paper or cardstock, tape or glue

Name your binder: My Notebook, (Name's) Chronicle, My Adventures

Ideas: 1) Include pages for regularly scheduled events, activities, and hobbies. This page may look similar to a choices page but will serve as a list of events the child can easily scan through. 2) Include page protector pages with sheets of paper in them. Tape or glue tickets, pamphlets, brochures, pictures, and maybe even menus from restaurants. Decide which items will remain lose in a page protector so the child or communication partner may select one to take out of the book to read and talk about with your child. 3) Add a note at the end of the page protector or paper that asks the communication partner to tell your child about that person's weekend or what he or she has been up to lately (e.g. *What did you do this weekend? What have you been up to? Tell me about something fun you've done lately!*)

Excellent! Onto Bridging Skills!

References

Benedek-Wood, E., McNaughton, D. & Light, J. (2016). Instruction in letter sound correspondence for children with autism and limited speech. *Topics in Early Childhood Special Education*, *36*(1), 43–54.

Beukelman, D. R. & Mirenda, P. (2013). *Augmentative and alternative communication: Supporting children and adults with complex communication needs*. Baltimore, MD: Paul H. Brookes Publishing.

Corey, S. (2016). *Malala a hero for all*. New York, NY: Random House.

Cowen, A. S. & Keltner, D. (2017). *Self-report captures 27 distinct categories of emotion bridged by continuous gradients*. Proceedings of the National Academy of Sciences of the United States of America. Retrieved from www.pnas.org/content/early/2017/08/30/1702247114

Dynavox. (2019). Accessible literacy learning (ALL™). Retrieved from www.mytobiidynavox.com/Store/ALL

Erickson, K. A. & Koppenhaver, D. A. (2007). *Children with disabilities: Reading and writing the four-blocks way*. Greensboro, NC: Carson-Dellosa Publishing Company, Inc.

Fleischman, A. & Fleischman, C. (2012). *Carly's voice: Breaking through autism*. New York, NY: Simon & Schuster/Touchstone Publishing.

Franke, L. & Durbin, C. (2011). *Nurturing narratives*. Shawnee Mission, KS: AAPC Publishing.

Hasbro. (2019). Hasbro's toy box tools: Making play accessible. Retrieved from https://toyboxtools.hasbro.com/en-us

Koegel, R. L. & Koegel, L. K. (2006). *Pivotal response treatments for autism: Communication, social, & academic development*. Baltimore, MD: Paul H Brookes Publishing.

Lexico. (2019). *No*. In Oxford English Dictionary online (2nd ed). Retrieved from www.lexico.com/en/definition/no

Light, J. & Kent-Walsh, J. (2003, May 27). Fostering emergent literacy for children who require AAC. *ASHA Leader*, *8*, 4–29.

Light, J. & McNaughton, D. (2012). Accessible literacy learning. Retrieved from www.mytobiidynavox.com/#/morestuff/all

Light, J. & McNaughton, D. (2014). Communicative competence for individuals who require augmentative and alternative communication: A new definition for a new era of communication? *Augmentative and Alternative Communication*, *30*(1), 1–18. doi:10.3109/07434618.2014.885080

Light, J. & McNaughton, D. (2019). Literacy instruction. Retrieved from http://aacliteracy.psu.edu/index.php/page/show/id/6/index.html

Light, J., McNaughton, D. & Caron, J. (2019). New and emerging AAC technology supports for children with complex communication needs and their communication partners: State of the science and future research directions. *Augmentative and Alternative Communication, 35*(1), 26–41.

Pindzola, R. H., Plexico, L. W. & Haynes, W. O. (2016). *Diagnosis and evaluation in speech pathology*. New York, NY: Pearson.

Prentke Romich Company. (2018). Language lab. Retrieved from https://aaclanguagelab. com/resources.

Reading Rockets. (2019). Key comprehension strategies. Retrieved from www.readingrockets.org/article/key-comprehension-strategies-teach

Smith, M., Batorowicz, B., Sandberg, A. D., Murray, M., Stadskleiv, K., van Balkom, H., … von Tetzchner, S. (2018). Constructing narratives to describe video events using aided communication. *Augmentative and Alternative Communication, 34*(1), 40–53.

Tyler, A. A., Lewis, K. E., Haskill, A. & Tolbert, L. C. (2002). Efficacy, and cross-domain effects of morphosyntax and a phonological intervention. *Language Speech Hearing Services in Schools, 33*(1), 52–66.

Willems, M. (2004). *The pigeon finds a hot dog*. New York, NY: Hyperion Books for Children.

Bridging Skills with social interaction

Purposeful expression

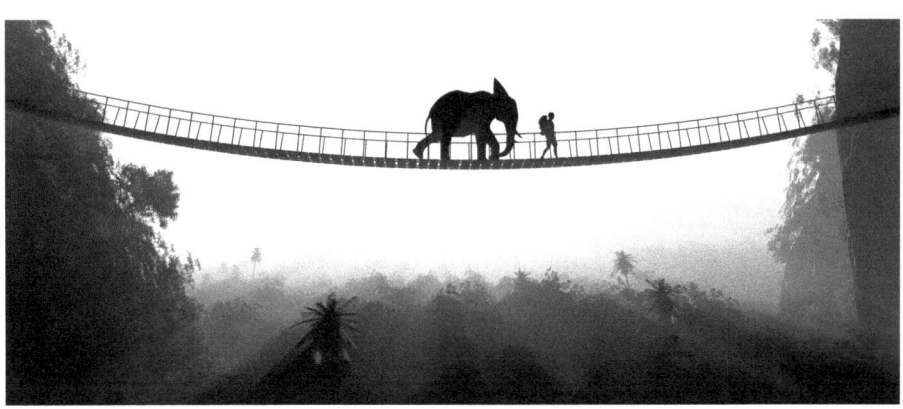

This is our girl and she is teaching me.

—*Parent* (Rogers, 1999)

Welcome to *Bridging Skills*, a time when children, parents, and intervention teams celebrate children's independence in initiating and expressing language using AAC through supported independence. The intervention team endorses children's communicative intent, anticipates their children's meaningful participation, and promotes inclusion across environments. Supported independence occurs within a dynamic communicative environment where your children use a variety of communication tools with various communication partners as prompts are reduced. Children using AAC engage with novel communication partners in new activities across different environments. Your child will practice and implement language more independently, to accomplish tasks your child enjoys and when necessary, have support. Facilitators bridge successful communication and interaction of children using AAC with others to allow growth in problem solving with support to resolve communication breakdowns.

As beautiful and durable bridges are built across waterways, AAC teams look to develop functional communication pathways for children using AAC. Our AAC bridges are built on the foundations of experiences of social interaction (*Why are we building a bridge?*), facilitator strategies (*Who and how will each help us?*), vocabulary (*What words does each child need as a foundation (core words) and words that we need to strength communication (fringe words)?*), literacy (*How can I learn from reading and writing about other bridges?*), and AAC tools (*What tools do we need to access to bridge success?*). As the traffic increases over the bridge, we aim for stability and durability of learning communication that builds over places, times, and opportunities. The purpose of *Bridging Skills* is to generate a meeting of the minds in which the child's communication skills are partnered with new opportunities for exploration and challenge with the level of support required for successful communication using Light and McNaughton's (2014) four competencies (i.e. social, linguistic, strategic, and operational) and purposes of communication (i.e. social closeness, sharing information, wants and needs, social etiquette). Our first then is to organize the thinking that goes into *Bridging Skills.*

Question #1 How do I wrap my mind around providing my child with the *Bridging Skills* necessary to become a more independent communicator using AAC?

The competences a child uses to communicate with AAC are built upon the same principles observed in typically developing children. Start with the pragmatic context such as the social setting, the expectations for social behavior, and a child's social interaction skills. Then add the language skills of children including vocabulary/semantics, phonology or the sound system of a language, and the morpho-syntax or the order of sounds and words for the purpose of meaningful communication between people from a given culture. Investigate the free lesson plans, activities and resources offered by the AAC Language Lab (https://aaclanguagelab.com/) from Prentke-Romich Company to help guide you. Provide facilitators with strategies that enable them to use AAC within their own cultural emphases and patterns important to friends and families. Finally, explore operational skills to access AAC tools and devices. To get you started take a look at the components of bridging social and language skills using the example, *My Friend's Cat*.

Components of bridging social and linguistic/language skills: *My Friend's Cat*

1 Pragmatic/social context: The social interaction skills and expectations of a person in a given circumstance or environment. Developing friendships and sharing information create opportunities for human relations and learning. For example: *When I go to my friend's house, her cat usually jumps on my lap. My friend will expect me to talk about the cat. I can talk about how funny the situation is, how I am a little worried, but the cat is not worried at all.*

2 Semantics/language: Vocabulary of a given language form the basis of verbal, written, and nonverbal interactions. My culture in my experiences day to day has decided how I need to say and think about this animal. For example: *I can describe a cat according to the features of its fur and body, wild or tame, how it purrs, and type. I can talk about the silliness and craziness of the cat. I will need words to share information about the situation, have words to strategize my communication and a way out of the situation, words, for requesting help, and social etiquette words to say good-by to this darn cat!*

3 Phonology/sounds of language/linguistic: The structure of sounds and words spoken, understood, and read. For example: *I hear the word cat and know that c-a-t refers to an animal that jumped onto my l-a-p.* I produce *c* in the word *cat* as a quick stopping sound made in the back of the mouth with no voice. My motor plan to say *cat* on my device requires me to access the *animals* folder button and then access the icon for *cat*, or access my keyboard to spell *c-a-t* and *l-a-p* on my way to produce a full message.

4 Morpho-syntax or grammar/linguistic: Morphology is the smallest unit of language that carries meaning in formation of words and syntax refers to word order and grammar in formation of sentences in the culture that surrounds me. Using the words on an assistive communication device makes me adapt those rules within the access to vocabulary and sentence building on the device. For example: *I know cat is grammatically defined as a singular noun and when I add 's' the word cats becomes a plural. Why <u>does</u> your <u>cat</u> jump on my lap every time I come over! or Why <u>do</u> <u>cats</u> jump on my lap? What do I do when cats jump on me?*

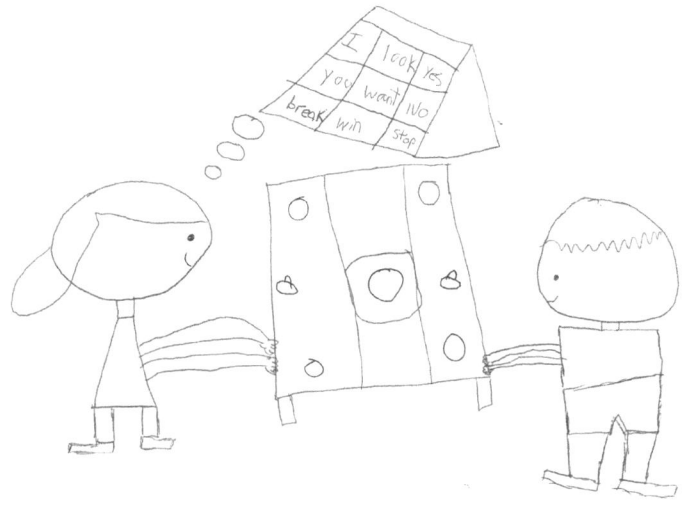

Children who use AAC need the ability to hone their receptive language skills, or comprehension, and their expressive language skills, called producing language. The only difference for children that use AAC is that their voice is expressed verbally through technology. As you recall from *Making Connections*, examples of strategies to support language by Tyler, Lewis, Haskill and Tolbert (2002), such as choice making, sometimes called *forced* choice in which a child can only select from one of two options available as icons on the speech generating device or *open-ended* choice options through spelling out words and sentences. Make sure that these choices suit your child's understood preferences, needs, and emotions. Even with the child making only one of two choices, you can model the language option using aided language stimulation using the child's AAC tools and devices. A child can finish a sentence with a required response, called a *cloze set response*, such as I see the big _____ (fill in the blank with *dog* when looking at the dogs available for adoption). Try expanding sentences adding one or more words to a phrase or sentence, recasting grammatically correct productions, offering a preparatory set such as describing a scene and then offering the child the opportunity to describe a scene (*e.g. Here in this section of the pet store we see dog food, leashes, and water dishes for big, medium, and small dogs. What would you want for your dog here? Tell me about a different section of the store. (Cue the child to look for the cat, fish, birds, and small animals sections).* Model language that talks the child through transitions, offer redirected prompts to allow a child to improve self-monitoring, and scripted play that bridges language with engagement with peers, games, and objects. *Wait a minute. What dog did you think I was talking about when I said 'big' when describing those three animals – a Chihuahua, a Basset Hound, a Rottweiler?* Talk about how the child knows what they know engaging their metalinguistic skill, the ability to talk about what you know. Ask your child, *How did you know that is the tree? The tree is green, has a trunk and branches. Sometimes it has leaves and usually grows in the dirt.* The language learning strategies serve as a solid start, and as often stated in this book, a springboard to other ideas for language development or the spark that leads to a discussion with your speech-language pathologist on recommendations for the implementation of a few of these language strategies or others that best fit the language goals of your child. That leads us to the next question that focuses on participation along with a game plan for success.

Question #2, *What Bridging Skills intellectually, linguistically, emotionally, and physically do I have as a parent or interventionist to support my child to communicate using AAC? How will others and I support my child socially in participation?*

Use the *Bridging Skills Playbook* as a checklist to determine the logical next steps for your child. Assume the competence of your child to communicate using AAC too. Communication depends upon having thoughts and feelings, opinions to express. Now to make sure your child has vocabulary, use of a speech generating devices, as well as physical access and strategies that are effective. Coordinating all of that takes time and sufficient practice. Does the child have access to quality vocabulary? Does my child have comprehension of- and practice with using the speech generating devices? On the device, how does my child locate words, modify them as types of language, categories of nouns, actions, and describing words to arrange these into sentences? If the word is not there, what is the next best alternative? What is the strategy my child prefers when asking a communication partners to wait to hear the message?

Does telling others to say what my child might be thinking work well (e.g. *Your eyes are telling me to wait, Is that correct?*)? Is it possible for communication facilitators and partners to reduce the amount or types of prompting to foster more independence? What is an appropriate wait time for this child's skill level? If you are thinking about the now, the next step, and you are talking with interventionists who can support you in asking the right questions and implementing the next steps, then you are doing everything right!

Bridging Skills playbook

○ **Adding emphases built upon purposes and joint attention**

1 Quick messages: I am working with professionals to determine quick messages my child can use across the purposes of communication using low and high technology options.

2 Combining words to form novel messages: I am encouraging my child to combine words by modeling messages on the speech generating device called aided language stimulation. For example, my model might be to state *milkshake please* on my child's speech generating device and then offer the opportunity for my child to state the same message so she can say her order independently at a restaurant later today. I am working with professionals to determine low and high technology AAC that my child can use to combine words to generate culturally appropriate and novel utterances across communication partners.

3 Language learning strategies: I have strategies that I can use to support the language development of my child. I can expand my child's utterances by stating, *I heard you say 'Time, book?'* Encourage your child to state, *'Time for a book? Is it time to read a book?'* I am working with professionals on the best way to grow my child's language skills. I am using fewer or different hints or cues to speed communication along as success with language increases with unfamiliar communication partners.

4 Self-monitoring: I am increasing my child's awareness of his or her communication skills including positioning when speaking with others, using eye contact and facial expressions, demonstrating attention, and using language across environments (e.g. asking for repetition of question or phrase, requesting time to respond using AAC, stating an opinion in another way, noting when others make a mistake).

5 Feelings and emotions: My child has access to and the use of words that represent a range of feelings and emotions with support by communication partners and facilitators. My child and I are learning to understand and interpret verbal and nonverbal initiations and responses regarding feelings and emotions.

6 Self-correction: I have ways to help my child self-correct such as modeling body posturing, correct word combinations and giving a verbal, vocal, or nonverbal cues.

7 Schedules and routines with flexibility: My child makes transitions best with predictable routines. I have schedules with pictures and words, physical cues, and offer time to support my child's transitions. I will eliminate unnecessary routines and increase or decrease steps to facilitate independence, self-reliance, and reduce uncertainty to promote security, familiarity, and reliability.

8 Motivation: From *Hear Me into Voice*, I identify interests and activities that are usually motivating to my child. I have incorporated driving motivational experiences as incentives, new knowledge, arousal to move around, and build anticipation into my child's day that naturally foster the desire to communicate. Motivation supports my child's sense of control during communication and participation such as initiating, managing, and ending interactions.

The playbook is a sound foundation for working on *Bridging Skills*. Read the following case study and let Jada's experience and the experiences of her family and intervention team provide you with an understanding of her *Bridging Skills*. Consider the ideas of supported independence and language development as you learn from Jada.

A case study in Bridging Skills: meet Jada

Jada is a tall and slender nine-year-old girl who wears her glossy brunette hair in a long attractive braid that cascades down her back. She is a daughter and a sister who is dearly loved and cared for, who began communicating effectively with her father and mother long before she was given the diagnosis of autism and intellectual disability. She misses her brother who is away at college, but she has the company of her grandmother along with three dogs, two cats, two birds, and a few fish that add perfect variety to their home. Her father, a gifted primary school teacher, uses his experiences with Jada to differentiate learning in his classroom. Jada's mother, a geology laboratory technician at the city college, is also an artist. When Jada was three years old, her mother sketched a portrait of herself with her daughter. She titled the drawing *Within Autism*. A mother sits on a nearby rock smiling with a caring look and ready to help. *This is my daughter. How will she participate? Who will come when she calls? What would she like to do?* Separating the mother and daughter is a tall wire mesh fence forming an image of separation/a kind of mutual imprisonment. The daughter's mouth is wide open as if she is begging for someone to interpret her communication, her emotions and thoughts. Her mother wonders, *Is she angry, dismayed, searching, talking, yelling, puzzled? How can I listen to her?* The portrait demonstrates the complex relationship between her daughter with the diagnosis of autism and her mother and the questions they have asked about participation in the world.

For Jada, *Bridging Skills* is a time to expand participation and communication. Her mother recognizes that Jada requires physical and emotional support to be successful and she is okay with that reality. Jada needs help with her uneven gait and awareness for safety in the community. The information her parents and intervention team reported in the protocol *Hear Me into Voice* indicates Jada's unique personality, physical differences, safety needs, and communication partners. Her mother sees communication as a barrier to participation and she wants Jada to have assistive technology that she can access easily wherever she is. The intervention team at school sees her as a capable person who now benefits from increased independence, a person who is a participant in life experiences, a thinker, and a doer. Now, her family and interventionists will use *Bridging Skills* to support Jada's communication with familiar and less familiar communication partners across environments and social dynamics with a variety of topics and interests.

○ Section 1 Social interaction: How does Jada express herself in social interactions?

Even though many shoppers frown or simply stare when Jada reaches out to greet them with a smile and a touch them as they go by in the grocery store, Jada's mother knows this is, *her way of saying hi*. She said, *I am going to make a sign that says I am proud of my autistic daughter. I will wear it when we go shopping together.*

Jada could say *hello* using her communication wallet. She kisses her parents to express *goodnight, I am going to bed.* Other times her parents think her kisses mean, *If I kiss you and I am cute, I get my way and I will not go to bed.* Maybe she is trying to stay up longer or maybe she wants to stay with them just to be socially close. When asked, *What would you like?* Jada sometimes responds with *ju* as in *juice*. *Ju* also mean *different types of food or drinks like Diet Coke*, a clear indication of her wants and needs. She likes to laugh and jump with excitement saying, *yeh, yeh* whenever she sees the favorite part of movie reruns of *Rocky and Bullwinkle*. Jada leans into her communication partner to show her affection and to greet them. Her dad expresses his pleasure in her puzzle skills as she completes puzzles noting, *She was pleased with herself for doing it right*.

Jada's mother especially appreciates caregivers who interact so positively with her daughter such as the caregiver who interacted with her daughter by saying, *This girl has more than what we are led to believe. She is such a warm person. She has her own idiosyncratic meaning to words, gestures, and smiles*. The occupational therapist observed that initiation of a task was difficult for her without a touch cue on her arm. Sometimes her completion of a task is more a *question of her interest than ability*. She also has a counting board with numbers 1–10 that help her regulate care routines like brushing her hair and teeth. In fact, Jada may cry out a joyful 10! to punctuate the point that she finished a routine or task and wants to be done.

Jada expresses herself nonverbally with a limited number of signs, using her body, occasional verbalizations, portable low-tech communication tools like communication boards and a communication wallet. Her preschool teacher taught Jada sign language to say *all done*, *please*, and *more*. Now Jada points to communication board images posted on her mirror at home that allow her to say quick phrases as she dances and watches her reflection. Her intervention team designed a tip card expressing her interests and inviting question asking to expand her low-tech options; but wearing it around her neck bothered her, so it was laminated and added to her communication wallet that she carries in a pocket. With her parents, Jada verbally says a few words consistently, *mine* for *it is mine* and *moogie* means *movie*, but watch out because it can also mean, *Whatever!* Other favorite words include *mookit* for *music* and *open* usually means she needs help *opening* the cupboard where the movies are, and *bees peez* is a polite request for the movie *Beauty and the Beast*. Other times she uses a string of vowels and consonants as she 'reads' a flyer at home. Jada had success with the implementation of low tech tools so the team clearly sees the advantage high tech tools like speech generating devices, tablets, and tools may bring.

Jada struggles with self-regulation such as making transitions during activities during the day and falling asleep at night. Transitions are especially difficult when favorite people leave for the day or if she has to move on from a project, like putting all the pieces in a puzzle before she has to catch the school bus. She often requires medication to help her fall asleep, though her reactions to sedatives actually became sleep avoiding stimulants. Her parents are *vigilant* to monitor her *stuffing* a whole piece of pizza into her mouth before chewing. Communication partners know to offer visual cues to remind her to regulate her actions in making transitions and in chewing her food.

The role of sensory overload for her has been a concern. Jada was uncomfortable carrying the heavier computer-like speech generating device as she asked for different activities. Though she also carries a communication wallet, Jada's speech generating device allows her to participate in activities, sharing information using more complex language. She likes to read and write. She understands how her words impact others that reduce her self-injurious behaviors, such as hitting herself when frustrated. Her speech-language pathologist is working on her metalinguistic skills, meaning she can think about her language in new ways with familiar communication partners and friends using a speech generating device as well to participate with less familiar communication partners. At this time novel communication partners need an efficient way for Jada to express *wait, say it again*, her message using her assistive technology. She watches as others write and is encouraged to write her own responses.

⊙ Questions for Reflection

Section 1 Social Interaction: How does Jada express herself with people across settings?

1   Match how Jada's social interaction skills using AAC tools and devices express her communicative intent?

Jada's Social Interaction using Multimodal AAC	Communication Intent
a Speech generating device to talk to friends	1 _____ Ask for a movie, snack, or book
b Nonverbally leaning into people	2 _____ 'All done,' 'please,' *and* 'more'
c Communication wallet in the community	3 _____ Jada's spoken and written words
d Verbalizing at home	4 _____ I like you and I am saying 'hello'
e Sign language	5 _____ Say 'hello' and quick messages

2 Jada has verbal and vocal productions that carry different meanings. Indicate T=True or F=False for the statements that represent different ways her verbal and vocal skills represent communicative intent?

a _____ An unintelligible string of sounds represents a protest

b _____ A word approximation represents a word or phrase 10! = I am finished!

c _____ Jada uses AAC so she must not be able to produce oral speech

Answers

1 a.=3, b.=4, c.=5, d.=1, e.=2. Jada's multimodal AAC plan allows her to communicate many different types of messages across people and environments. For Jada and her team there is no right or wrong AAC tool or device just the right tool or device in the moment she needs to share information, greet someone, share social closeness, or make a request for wants and needs.

2 Letters a. and b. are True. Jada has a variety of verbal productions with different meanings. Letter c. is False. There is a tendency for people to label AAC users as nonverbal when in reality many children have degrees of oral verbal skills, nonverbal skills, and low and high tech voices.

○ Section 2 Communication activities: What communication activities does Jada participate in?

At home, Jada's favorite activities are watching movies and looking at flyers that come in the mail. She looks through school supply catalogs and magazines. Her mother teaches Jada to use a highlighter to mark items she wants on the grocery flyer. In its own way, creating this shopping list is a communication activity. At the market, Jada smiles as she holds the flyer, takes command of the shopping cart and pushes it through the store, taking a box of her favorite cereal and salty crackers along the way. She and her mother mark each item off the list. Her mother also supports Jada by practicing aided language stimulation to ask motivating questions using her speech generating device to say, *When, can, I buy, marker, pencils, book, Angels*? Her father will be taking her to Angels School Supplies Mart soon. Participating in activities gives Jada opportunities to communicate using including oral speech, verbal approximations, a communication wallet, visual schedules, and speech generating devices. She reads some sight words, uses movement of her body and eyes, vocalizations, and gestures to enter into these activities. Her dad follows through by taking her to the school supply store where an entire wall holds bins with every type of markers and pencils from classic #2 yellow pencils, to birthday wishes, animals, aliens, stripes, and dots. Jada's eyes light up when she sees the display and heads over to choose one before heading home. Success.

Jada benefits from having physical therapy as she walks with an uneven gait. When an accompanying adult walks with her, Jada seems to gain stability and follow safety rules as they navigate at school and in the community. Occupational therapy and a play center have focused on social inclusion where she uses communication boards to select activities and to state, *This is fun*, and, *I need a break*. Attentive adults monitor the centers where Jada enjoys the balance beams, swings, and pitching areas. Jada joins other children with disabilities on the weekends where teams learn the rules of playing baseball. Jada, however, soon protests that she really, *needs a break* using her communication board because she does not like playing baseball after all. Swings are much preferred and make up for any inconvenience baseball caused her.

Jada's parents learned through their experience to adopt the view that failure, even repeated failure, is a gateway to opportunity. They follow both that sentiment and the motto coined by Seth Godin (2014), *If I fail more than you, I win*. Jada had been 'failing' in segregated special day classes with limited communication models, activities, and low expectations for social interaction and literacy. Her inappropriate behavior was a warning sign. Her parents sought a winning educational plan in the full inclusion general education program in which Jada has a day-to-day gateway to literacy with more opportunities for social communication and accommodations to support learning. Jada's peers and educators learn that when they ask her about characters and actions in illustrations in a book, she will respond by purposefully taking the person's hand and firmly directed it toward the image. Jada leans into her friend who is writing a biography and indicates she wants to follow suit. The educator at school reports that Jada still *demonstrates frustration with tantrum behaviors at times, but she can be redirected with verbal directions now*. The visual schedule helps her direct her attention to take more appropriate actions to self-regulate physically and emotionally. She is energized and follows her classmates who are reading and writing throughout the day. Jada complies with school rules much more effectively now in a more stimulating inclusive learning environment. She feels the support and in turn the support drives her to continue to monitor and regulate herself. She learns with and through her peers and instructors as role models with supported independence, the marker of a person who is *Bridging Skills* with AAC.

Questions for reflection

Section 2 Communication Activities: How is Jada's communication influenced by her participation in activities?

1 How does participation influence Jada's multimodal communication?
   a Jada is motivated by the opportunity to buy pencils using her speech generating device
   b Jada indicates playing baseball is not her favorite activity with her communication board
   c Jada engages with books, writing, and friends through AAC tools, devices, and her body
   d All of the above

2 Indicate T=True or F=False for the statements representing how and who Jada communicates during activities across environments.
   a _____ Jada's communication is limited to immediate family due to her disability
   b _____ Jada shops with her parents for food and fun from lists she makes and reads
   c _____ Jada plays baseball enthusiastically with her peers using her device to say so
   d _____ Jada's tantrum behaviors increase in an inclusive educational setting

Answers

1 Letter d. All of the above is the correct answer. Jada communicates in multimodal ways because she is motivated by the participation in shopping, baseball … okay less-so, literacy activities, friends and family.

2 Letter a. is False. Jada has familiar and less familiar communication partners! Letter b. is True. Jada reads the shopping list to find the food items at the store. Letter c. is False. Jada plays baseball but will request for a break to swing on her AAC device. Letter d. is False. Jada's inclusion class setting increased her literacy motivation and appropriate physical and emotional behaviors with fewer self-injurious and tantrum behaviors.

○ Section 3 Facilitator strategies: What strategies do facilitators and communication partners use to support her communication and participation?

Jada's strongest facilitators, her parents and caregivers, are willing to try new strategies to bridge her increased communication and participation. When Jada is overly distracted or excited, her mother notes, *Her latest way of getting comfort is going out on the back porch with a pile of blankets and lying in them quietly for up to half an hour paging and looking through a book.*

Jada's other communication partners include educators, therapists, bus drivers, school personnel, classmates, and others in the community. They may have to repeat an instruction so she can focus more accurately as they wait patiently while she accesses one of her communication tools. Their responses with relevance and feeling help Jada to know she is being heard and understood. They interpret her responses as having a *real, deep empathy for people*, an empathy that not only extends to others her age but helps her communicate with others. They too have learned how to support Jada's opportunities for participation confirming with Delpit (1995): *Our task is to ensure that voices of children become embodied in the way in which we teach [and interact with] them.* Instead of pressing Jada to play baseball, for example, they offer she watch and cheer. At school a touch cue helps Jada initiate her jumping on the trampoline, getting off the bus, and writing with a pencil. A touch cue did not work every time for every situation. A touch cue does not help her to follow the 'Pick Up Your Jacket Rule' at school but a visual schedule met that need. The occupational therapist along with saying, *You can do it!* knew to touch Jada's hand as she clipped paper clips together to form a chain. The afterschool caregiver talks to Jada. She does not dismiss Jada's comprehension, and clarifies requests or commands Jada makes of others. Jada's team at school helps her locate and repair messages on her speech generating device and/ or use her communication wallet.

For Jada, who is *Bridging Skills*, her voice through a speech generating device conveys her more complete thoughts by her accessing icons with quick phrases or novel utterances. Her facilitators know their goal is to support her personal, social, and academic communication growth for social closeness, social etiquette, wants and needs, sharing information (Light & McNaughton, 2014). This does not mean that each communication partner will always accurately interpret Jada's every communication intent, however facilitators can support other people in understanding and practicing the best strategies for Jada, modeling more complex language, providing prompting as needed, and satisfying Jada's unique interests. Facilitators expect Jada to have increased independence to comment, ask questions, take turns, tell jokes with multiple communication partners, and express her unique requests in important multi-dimensional ways.

Questions for Reflection

Section 3 Facilitator strategies: What strategies do facilitators and communication partners use to support her communication and participation? *Circle preferred response:* I agree, I Disagree

1   The role of a facilitator is to support independence for personal, social, and academic purposes which does not mean the person knows every intent of the child but does mean the person understands optimal strategies to identify the child's intent.

I agree.   I disagree.

2   The role of the communication partner is not to use AAC or to listen to the child's productions but rely on facilitators to interpret communication.

I agree.   I disagree.

Answers

1   The correct answer is *I agree*. Facilitators do not always have the answer but strong familiarity, connection with the child, careful observation of behaviors, successes, and failures create potential for success.
2   The correct answer is *I disagree*. Many communication partners require training to communicate with children using AAC including aided language stimulation (an adult or peer modeling a message on the child's device), prompting, modeling and turn taking.

Section 4 Literacy: How does Jada's access to technology change her communication participation with reading and writing?

Literacy is a priority as expressed by Jada and her parents. Jada loves it when her parents read books, catalogs, and movie covers to her. Her favorite, of course, is a school supply catalog where she sees books and finds pencils and markers. By school age, Jada's mother had created a *Golden Alphabet* book on a tablet with words and illustrations. She scanned pictures from the *Peter Pan* book Jada loves. She typed simplified text of the story to pair with the images. Now Jada seeks access to her mother's tablet each morning to independently read her favorite books. They begin locating live webcams of zoos and aquariums around the world, pausing the footage, and naming what the animals are doing, unless they are sleeping; but then they talk about where the exhibit is, other animals like birds they can see, or zookeepers maintaining the habitat.

In a classroom when Jada was first in school, books were put away since Jada tore several books by several leafing through them repeatedly. Without her own classroom books to look at, Jada bolted to other classrooms to see their book displays or headed to the library as soon as her teacher was not watching. Her mother laughingly notes that Jada's grandmother was a librarian who like Jada too may have been described, as being *obsessive* about books. The assistive technology specialist who supports Jada matches her interest level with her reading skill and chooses the most successful level on applications and books on her tablet and speech generating device. She gave Jada a purple gripped pencil and paper to draw or write letters on a dry erase board. With a touch cue she began making swirls with the pencil. They talked about who Jada is to motivate her and connect words to the pictures they created together.

For some time, Dr. Seuss's books and videos have been Jada's story time favorites, and often a good fall back for free time at school. Her parents had read about Schuyler, another girl about Jada's age, who found phone and tablet technology 'so cool' (Rummel-Hudson, 2011). They proceeded to add technology to Jada's daily use of communication devices. She expands her vocabulary and she is learning to read and write across multiple electronic formats, tablet, speech generating devices including phones. Jada's interest and ability to work with computer technology prompted the use of worldwide accessible book programs like *Bookshare* (www.bookshare.org/cms/) and *Tar Heel Reader* (https://tarheelreader.org/) developed by the researchers and educational innovators at University of North Carolina at Chapel Hill Center for Literacy and Disability Studies. Literacy is accessible at home and at school now throughout the day and enables and rewards her participation academically and socially.

Along with her educator, Jada associates letters with sounds and blends sounds and letters into words. She sees how words became sentences that bridge to stories that she loves. Together Jada, her parents, and her interventionists begin identifying the story elements in the stories they hear and read. They read the names of the characters (e.g. the King, the Queen, Court Jester), discuss the setting (e.g. village, castle, forest), outline the plot, spell out the conflict or action to be resolved, and even articulate the feelings that prompt the characters to act the way that leads them toward the solution, and sometimes even describe the consequences of their actions. Jada now is supported through her speech generating device as she writes, types, and/or draws the words and illustrations as she forms sentences about what she is reading. Each skill reinforces the other. Her parents and educators see how much Jada's behavior improves with the rich literacy opportunities in seeing peers read and having her accessible books to read. Interestingly, as if in tandem, her interests and complexity of the language of her book selections has grown. She now consistently seeks two particular books to read: her father's physical education teaching text book and another text in Spanish. She swipes through the illustrated pages of the physical education book whose edges have become dog eared and worn. Her parents believe that since Jada hears her peers speaking Spanish, this may drive her to read the Spanish text.

Jada's parents and intervention team value Jada's use of assistive technology in building literacy and using communication tools. Their learning is reinforced by reading themselves and attending conferences with nationally known speakers who advocate for teaching reading and writing to all children, including Jada. Assistive technology expands her communication participation across communication partners and environments.

⊙ Questions for Reflection

Section 4 Literacy: How does Jada's access to technology change her communication participation with reading and writing?

1. What are indications that Jada enjoyed reading and writing?
   a She likes reading her father's physical education and Spanish textbooks.
   b She leafs through books and magazines.
   c She reads stories on different forms of technology.
   d She expands her vocabulary from reading and writing using technology.
   e All of the above

2. What materials and technologies are used to teach Jada reading and writing? Indicate T=True or F=False. Watch out for a tricky statement!
   a _____ Visual schedules in printed words and illustrations.
   b _____ Books with high interest content are matched to Jada's reading level and paired with writing activities.
   c _____ Use of Bookshare and Tar Heel Reader support accessible reading.
   d _____ Books for reading and writing are avoided so Jada does not become obsessive.

→

> **Answers**
>
> 1   Letter e. All of the above is the correct answer. Building upon Jada's interest in textbooks, movie covers, leafing through books and magazines as well as reading stories at home and school in traditional print and electronic formats sets the stage for developing literacy skills.
> 2   Letters a. and d. are False. Letter a. is the tricky statement. The primary function of a visual schedule is to support transitions and not to formally teach reading. While Jada is highly motivated by books, confining access to literacy is not used as a form of rewards or punishment. Letters b. and c. are True. Pairing interest level with reading level motivates Jada to read more.

○ Section 5 Vocabulary: What vocabulary did Jada need for participation?

As Jada is becoming an adolescent, she requires new vocabulary to develop and foster friendships and learn. Her parents decided to move to a state that promoted more communication and scheduled more inclusive activities of children with the diagnosis of autism. At the same time, her parents had to find a home and learn about a new environment. Jada would have a different school with unfamiliar communication partners, named with new names *Sondra, Miguel*, and *Carmelo*. Hopefully, her parents, new facilitator and aide would quickly catch onto Jada's unique communication and interests. The administration at the new middle school was open to including more complex assistive technology so childrem could access the curriculum even though the educators and aides had to master additional skills.

Jada often participates in social interaction with access to written and spoken vocabulary. She greets people less frequently now by touching them and adds quick phrases at school and in the community with phrases for social greetings like, *Hi, What's up!* or *Adios amigo, Hasta la vista.* Yes, she has her distinctive hand wave gestures that familiar people understand but Jada wants to talk to new communication partners too. She wants to relate to others by moving closer and showing empathy and now needs vocabulary that shares, *I want to do that with you. Leave me alone now. How can I make you understand?*

She wishes to express her wants and needs. She needs to ask for help pouring her juice or milk into the glass. Jada interacts by naming her educator, her therapists, and favorite classmates on her speech generating device. For class activities, Jada communicates *all done* in her words that matches her interests and attention but needs the more age appropriate phrases with the vocabulary of, *I am done with the puzzle, Didn't I do a good job?* as she works with familiar and unfamiliar communication partners.

She would like to use quick phrases to order in a restaurant or ask for food in the cafeteria, *I'd like a hamburger, please. How much is that? Thank you very much, See you later!* From her dad's physical education book, she learns new vocabulary that she could relate to like, *balance, walk forward and backward.* As part of her routine, she needs a simple, *Here!* to answer when her name is called. From the science book, Jada's vocabulary highlights measurements in *sizes* and *weights*. A must in this curriculum had become vocabulary about *earth, space* and *life sciences* from *climate change* to *eco systems*.

Jada shares information with her peers as communication partners as she points to her communication wallet with her name, street address, and phone numbers. She compares her information with theirs. How would she share her novel experiences and unique perspectives? Her mother wants Jada to tell her who she walked to class with her and who sat with her for lunch. Jada sees that the words in her books are words she has ownership of and now needs vocabulary that access these messages. She smiles and points at printed words *exit, women's restroom, enter*, to say, *I know that word!*

She expresses her emotions as she expresses her *fear* that she sees in some movies. From her sustained interest in movies, she watches scenes with complex emotions such as *scary, threatening, mean, distressing, evil, angry, destructive*, and yet overcoming with acts of *love*. However, sharing more precise feelings with her communication partners as they read and hear stories now require her to have access to other feeling words like *mad, sorry, sad, excited, loved*, and *surprised*. Then, she can begin to explain *She looks happy now*, *that made me happy*, or, *I have watched that too long, I want a different movie*, or *I am bored*.

Jada welcomes vocabulary in quick phrases that express negation of choices and contractions in everyday activities such as, *no like, don't, not, didn't, can't, won't* and more. She reads and already hears negation in her world, *No, that is not what I meant*, to share information, *That was not a good idea for him to jump*, or to serve as a strategy, *No, I want to write*. Her parents asked themselves what words would might help Jada regulate her own actions, such as *not now, but later*.

Jada requires vocabulary that includes prepositions for telling stories, creating novel utterances and describing events to request activities at home (e.g. *in the swing, by the dog, on the couch*). Dr. Seuss's book *Green Eggs and Ham* (Geisel, 1960) had taught her her prepositions and phrases *in the house, not with a mouse, not in a box, not with a fox*. Now vocabulary included everyday life such the tortoise *in the box, in the garage* and in fictional movies such as *into the castle, through the forest*. Jada likes the repetition and the fun that show how words are related to each other.

Jada needs help to anticipate the steps of an activity. At school she is learning *first, then, next*, and *last. First, I walk to class with ____. Then I change my clothes. Next I go outside to the playing field and watch. Last I change back into my clothes and walk back to class*. This sequence helps her understand her daily routines and routines in her environment and use effectively on visual schedules. Waiting…waiting … was probably the hardest thing for Jada to do. Counting from 1 to 10 helps her to wait when her mom was brushing her hair works but there is a lot of waiting in the world. She needs a way to talk herself through *waiting*. Her parents wrote a Social Story they learned from a framework by Carol Gray (2015) as a great way to support Jada and to help others understand how to help Jada with waiting.

Waiting

Sometimes I have to wait for help.
Lots of people wait for help at stores, at work, and at school.
I get bored and frustrated and other people do too.
While I wait, I can ask for a timer, ask to draw, or count to 10.
I will be helped soon, and my wait will be over.

Vocabulary supports Jada as she sequences the day, meets new people, waits for responses, and learns with peers what is expected as a new middle school person!

⊙ Questions for Reflection

Section 5 Vocabulary: What vocabulary does Jada need for participation?

1   All EXCEPT which vocabulary words were motivating and needed for Jada?
   a   Prepositions and describing words
   b   First words and toddler vocabulary due to Jada's dual diagnosis of autism and intellectual disability
   c   Words and phrases for jokes, shopping, movies, and names of important people
   d   Words for expressing feelings and emotions, negation, and approval

2   What vocabulary would support Jada's information sharing and her curriculum?
   a   Fringe words: people's names, specific books, activities, and places
   b   Core vocabulary: feelings, colors, preposition words
   c   Sequence words: first, next, last
   d   Negation words: not, no, didn't
   e   All of the above

Answers

1 Letter b. is the correct answer. Jada requires vocabulary that meets her social-emotional and academic needs that include all grammatical forms such as negation, preposition, and words for feelings and emotions. First words and toddler vocabulary does not represent her receptive language knowledge.

2 Letter e all of the above. Assignments and daily communication at her age level require fringe words, action words, prepositions, sequences, and negation at her age appropriate level and are included on her communication boards and speech generating devices.

○ Section 6 Tools and access: What were Jada's important multimodal communication tools?

Jada has been introduced to assistive communication tools such as communication boards, tablet technology, and speech generating devices that allow her to express herself. Many times, she wants to interact socially with peers in and outside her classroom, yet she faces difficulty socializing because most children do not understand her nonverbal communication and have limited or no experience with assistive tools. How could Jada tell new and unfamiliar communication partners about who she is and what she is interested in? Training and sharing!

Colorful and inviting cards are made for Jada to let people know who she is and offer quick social greetings. People engaging with her can read her tip cards or communication wallet to hear about her interests and read questions that ask them to talk about themselves. A facilitator listens to Jada and then works with her peers to teach them how to use a touch cue at her elbow to get her started with expressing her message. They learn about she uses physical proximity and eye gaze to express her intent. With the speech generating devices, Jada and her peers are seeing how to put together sentences through well-organized vocabulary to share new information at school, home, and participate in community activities she likes. Her communication experiences are broadening to new communication partners and environments thus enabling her to develop her own thinking skills. As she asks questions, her own thinking is brought forward into the discussion and eases some of her frustration in social closeness and sharing information.

Her parents want Jada to express her thoughts and feelings in as efficient and effective way using AAC like her friends do. The communication wallet and tip cards have limited vocabulary. The only problem with the six-pound speech generating device is that Jada finds it physically too heavy and awkward when she walks unevenly to the library, cafeteria, and home again. Through teamwork with the vendor they find a protective and functional carrying case that allows her to position the device at her waist so she can carry the device and access it wherever she goes and wants to communicate. The device is made more age appropriate by accessorizing it with pins, key chains, stickers, and rings. Her school team also agrees to try a lighter tablet with AAC with complimentary applications and feature matching to her dynamic display speech generating device vocabulary and organization. She can decide which device to use to talk about her feelings and emotions, even complain about loud sounds, but also access stories and text. Jada has a choice in selecting the best device for her to meet her physical and communication needs in the moment. Communication makes sense in a new way to Jada. Her path to *Bridging Skills* with multimodal communication walks hand in hand with her team who interpret a range of unaided forms of communication through her voice, gestures, and facial expressions. They now want to add phones as an aided form of technology from pencils, tablets, computers, single message and dynamic display speech generating devices (in a carrying case, that is!).

⊙ Questions for Reflection

Section 6 Tools and access: What are Jada's multimodal forms of communication?

1 What considerations by the team bridge Jada's communication skills for improved participation?
   a Determine appropriate tools and devices to improve speed of communication
   b Develop communication pages that meet her academic and social needs
   c Provide education, experience, and tools like tip cards for communication partners
   d All of the above

2 Match the form of communication to the types of messages Jada expressed.

Form of Communication	Type of Message Expressed
a Nonverbal gestures, facial expressions, manual signs	1 _____ On the spot, easily programmable phrases to express an idea or make a choice
b Communication board, book, wallet, ring	2 _____ Most limited form of expression for Jada, communication partners had to infer meaning

c   Single or multi-message
    message (static display)
    speech generating device

d   High technology (dynamic
    display) speech generating

e   Verbalizations, vocalizations,
    word approximations

3   _____ Jada's quickest form
    of expression with no voice,
    communication partners infer
    meaning

4   _____ Easy to transport, quick
    visual form of communication
    with picture icons and words

5   _____ Quick messages and novel
    utterances are spoken with a
    digitized or synthesized voice

Answers

1   Letter d. All of the above is the correct answer. There are many
    considerations the team needs to make. Included in those decisions
    are determining appropriate tools and devices to improve Jada's
    speed of communication, developing communication pages that meet
    her personal, academic, and social needs, training for the team and
    communication partners, and providing guiding tools for communication
    partners.

2   1=c 2=e 3=a 4=b 5=d. The forms of communication that make up Jada's
    multimodal communication plan allow her quick access, vocal access, and
    verbal access across types of devices and her natural voice. Opportunities
    for Bridging Skills support the use of all forms of communication including
    reading and writing that are available to the child.

Summary

Jada, her family, and intervention team embrace multimodal communication that allows her to expand her language, participate in social interactions with new communication partners around valued activities that match her own preferences, interests, and learning style. The educator with other students surrounds Jada with models for literacy and encourage her more appropriate behavior. Her communication technology that includes single and multi-message speech generating devices allows her to learn and express herself especially with adapting to a carrying case for her portable devices. Yes, Jada needs supports in terms of initiating her physical movement with touch cues, motivation to communicate and use speech generating devices, and teaching about language use but she now has a way to generate more complex messages and interact with less familiar communication partners.

In reflection, her dad suggests that the protocol title, *Hear Me into Voice*, should be, *If a tree falls in a forest and no one is around to hear it, does it make a sound?* (Rogers, 1999). He believes that if there is no one to hear his daughter because no one observes her and accurately and sensitively interprets her communication, no one knows her for the amazing person she is today. The bridge to communication focuses on Jada's skills and experiences with learning and using new vocabulary with new yet supportive communication partners. Together they match her uniqueness, affirm her interests and strengths, program the vocabulary and quick phrases into her speech generating device, and support her as a successful communicator as she participates more effectively in everyday activities using assistive technology. Now we need others to engage with Jada's communication because she is saying to us using my own body, voice and the speech generating device, *Hear Me into Voice*.

Bridging Skills with communication activities

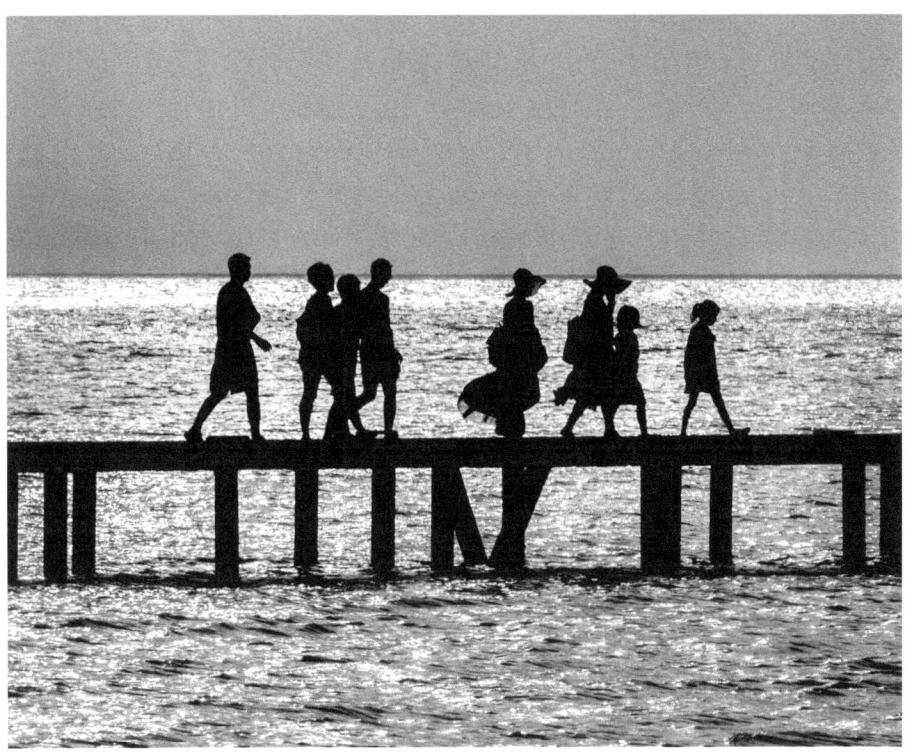

○ Supporting independence

Communication activities in *Bridging Skills* is our next stop. Here we offer facilitators and communication partners ways to support a child's independence communicating with AAC. As you investigate activities remember to consider the social interaction groundwork reviewed in *Bridging Skills.* The communication activities introduced in this section simply look at where your child is successful both socially and academically with others and consider the next steps. What are the good questions to ask during *Bridging Skills*? We consider the child as a part of a social dynamic and the needs of this particular child as an individual by listening and engaging each child in social interaction so that relationships are developed (Klein, 2017), information is shared, and the child's contributions are made. Communication partners continue to advocate for increased use of AAC in inclusive activities so the children can say anything they want to say. Most of these questions extend from our initial questions in *Getting Started*, *Building Fundamentals*, and *Making Connections*. Now we want to frame the competencies into functional questions.

1 Social: *Who does my child like to play and be with? What do they like to play? Where do they like to play? What is my child's social role in the making of friendship with peers and adults?*
2 Linguistic: *Does my child have access to vocabulary and breadth of language skills? Does my child need additional practice with novel people in familiar environments, familiar people in novel environments, and novel people in novel environments?*

3 Strategic conversational and device management: *Does my child have the tools, strategies, and time to engage, ask, respond, maintain, and manage transitions within and between topics and activities? Does my child use words and positioning to cue others in participation?*

4 Operational: *What is my child's AAC device and tool inventory? What AAC devices and tools are used in my child's environments? Are they successful or do the AAC devices and tools need modifications (e.g. Does my child need more practice with no modifications to the devices or tools, or does my child need different AAC devices or tool to meet the social and/or linguistic participation goals including academic needs?).*

These questions take your child to a new level of interaction, participation, relationships, and independence, which is exciting. With increased independence your child may fatigue more, blossom more, need time to adjust, or need a creative environment in which to be independent. Now that we are equipped with social communication strategies and good questions for supporting independence let's jump into *Bridging Skills with Communication Activities.*

Bridging Skills

Activities Page – Purposeful inclusion for initiation and expression

1 Yes, I Talk on the Phone!
2 Email Me!
3 Talking Points and TV
4 Let's Go Out! Community Fun
5 Let's Go to the Game!
6 Let Me Ask You Something: Questions for Peers
7 What's Your Strategy? Taking Responsibility to Get Your Point Across
8 Webcams Bring the Zoo to You: Orangutans! Pandas! Penguins! and More!

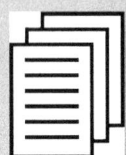

Activity: Yes, I Talk on the Phone!

A place to start

Children work on expanding their communication skills by talking on the phone, even to answer the phone at home. This includes children who use AAC! AAC users can take advantage of free Speech-to-Text or Speech-to-Speech, forms of the Telecommunications Relay Service (TRS) in the United States and Canada (Federal Communications Commission, n.d.). A person can quickly access their TRS call center from any working phone. Web-based text relay services are available in Europe. The National Relay Service in available in Australia. Communication assistants are trained to speak and relay messages between people with communication disabilities especially speech intelligibility issues and their communication partners. Check with phone plan carriers regarding relay service options via text, speech, and video.

Facilitator plan

If you are feeling like jumping straight to communications through a communication assistant may be too big of a leap, then take a look at a blog called PrAACtical AAC authored by Carol Zangari (2012). She discusses five phone tips at http://praacticalaac.org/praactical/call-me-later-5-supports-for-phone-communication-by-people-who-use-aac/ that include having pre-programmed phone numbers, practicing phone skills, using free speech-to-speech relay systems, Voice Over Internet Protocol (VOIP), and phone or tablet applications. Phone conversations are a perfect time to sketch out dialogue across the four purposes of communication including words for social closeness, social etiquette, wants and needs, and sharing information.

My child's action plan

My child will gain valuable skills in learning that he or she can talk, text, or both on the phone to relay a message. How fun. My child can practice even using FaceTime with one friend using a social greeting to say, *Hello*, share information about his or her day, use strategies such as using a quick message to state, *Wait a minute for me to respond*, and a give a closing message, *It was great to talk to you. Let's talk again soon. Bye!* After some successful practice at home, try a message from school to home.

My Multimodal Toolkit

- Two phone sources, one for the child and one for the communication partner
- A script for my child to follow to generate messages

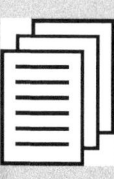

- ◉ Optional: external speakers
- ◉ Optional: toy phones for introductory practice
- ◉ Multiple communication options for the child
    - ◉ Speech generating device with a single message option
    - ◉ Speech generating device with multi-message options

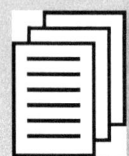

Activity: Email Me!

A place to start

Email me! Kids see and or hear you on your phone all the time, talking away, clicking keys, reading and sending messages. Regardless of the stage of literacy your child is at, take advantage of the fun, of the message, of the anticipation of a return message, and the connection that is made through email. Co-construct a message. Send photos and artwork. Send images of a message from your child's AAC device. Get inspired. Email grandparents, a cousin, a friend.

Facilitator plan

Make a list of people to email. Make a list of fun things to email like images and photos. Lists are for offering inspiration when the creative juices are low. Let's face it, you are busy. Making lists will help. Here is a good one. Take a picture of your child writing a message on his or her AAC device and send the photo in email. Better yet, make a video of the message being constructed and send the video so the receiver has the benefit of hearing the message as well as seeing it and expressing appreciation for the child's communication.

My child's action plan

Your child will be motivated to send a message and anticipate a message in return. Make sure the writing includes a message to the receiver to write a response with their opinions and ideas. Investigate the twelve action plan ideas for emailing:

1   Select and scan image your child likes, dislike, or thinks is crazy! Write three things about the image.
2   Send a drawing created by your child.
3   Take a photo of the child drawing the image.
4   Send a photo of the child doing something fun.
5   Co-construct, which means write a message together. You can generate ideas together or you can write a sentence and have the child write a sentence, type in keywords, or fill in the blanks to the story.
6   Type a message for a social greetings and closures unique to your child and your family.
7   Type a message demonstrating social closeness such as, *I miss you. I love you. See you soon!*
8   Type a message that shares a story about what's happening now.
9   Tell a joke.
10   Make a plan to get together.
11   Send an image of the child creating a message on his or her AAC device.
12   Send a video of the child stating a message using his or her AAC device.

Keep the message as simple or as complex as meets the inspiration and motivation of your child. Sometimes a short and sweet message does the

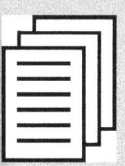

trick. As your child heads through *Bridging Skills*, add a touch of expectation to complete an unfinished task so the child learns follow through. Sometimes a simple, *finish this idea and we will send the email off*, is all it takes!

My Multimodal Toolkit

- Emailing technology
- Optional: A source to take a picture of a drawing or message
- Optional: A video source to record the child generating and speaking the message through a speech generating device
- Optional: A script for the child to follow to generate email messages
- Multiple communication options for the child to generate a message

  - Speech generating device with a single message option
  - Speech generating device with multi-message options
  - Communication board narrated by a facilitator

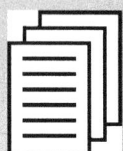

Activity: Talking Points and Media!

A place to start

Television, computers, phones, tablets, gaming consoles and more! We all have our screen time moments. Whether you are surfing channels, the internet, or streaming, use screen time as talking time. Comment on what you like or don't like, what is funny, or quite dramatic. Talk about alternative endings and feelings with expanded sentences and rich vocabulary.

Facilitator plan

Use TV time as an opportunity for your child to learn valuable social interaction and language tools. Consider the possibilities:

1 Make a choice of shows to watch
2 State preferences through likes and dislikes of genres, characters, and actions
3 Talk about ideas such as humor and levels of drama with feelings and emotions
4 Predict what will happen next in a scene or the next episode
5 Ask communication partners how they feel and think about aspects of the show
6 Discuss alternative endings
7 Expand commenting and other sentence forms
8 Respond to comments to keep a conversation going
9 Work on other language targets
10 Set a future plan for another *Talking Points and Media* opportunity

When it comes to *Talking Points and Media* consider the role of the facilitator, the person who is setting the stage for your child to communicate with others. Also consider communication partners who will be an active contributor to the interaction. Make sure your child has multimodal access to communication. Practice the communication options including nonverbal, verbal, vocal, and low- and high tech speech generating device options as applicable. You will make sure siblings and peers have their needs met regarding their comfort with the media, the environment, and understand how your child communicates with AAC. Then, as the interaction ensues, facilitators bridge communication either in the form of encouraging your child to use an AAC method, supporting independence to have a communication need met, helping repair communication breakdowns, and providing any physical or social support needed.

My child's action plan

Your child will watch a show and share information, make requests, and participate with peers and siblings. Inform your child that you will facilitate, if necessary. Working on self-implementation of communication modalities, with support as needed is the goal.

My Multimodal Toolkit

⊚ Let the kids decide on the form of media and show.

⊚ Suggest multiple communication options for the child.

  ◉ Nonverbal communication modalities (e.g. eye gaze, head nods, hands, feet, etc.)

  ◉ Speech generating device with a single message option

  ◉ Speech generating device with multi-message options

  ◉ Communication board options

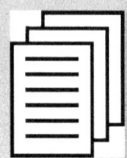

Activity: Let's Go Out! Community fun

A place to start

Community fun. Let's go outside and do . . . anything! Generate opportunities to go to a park, a movie, a restaurant, a mall, the bookstore, the free museum day, theme park etc. Errands! Is there one errand you can run and include your child and the opportunity for communication engagement, even a social greeting that was not occurring before? Remember to be aware of the child acquiring social etiquette, information sharing, as well as the wants and needs.

Is going to the movie a regular event or a special treat? Ask your child to watch you and then purchase his/her own admission ticket using a communication board or speech generating device. Go to the bookstore and have your child select a book and pay the clerk. How about following the routine of going to the swimming pool, taking towel and suit, changing clothes, getting in and out of the water, swimming, drying off, changing back into street clothes, getting back in the car with a laminated visual schedule? How about ordering a pizza, selecting crust and toppings, asking for price, thanking the clerk on a four-message communication board or speech generating device?

We all tend to do the same activities and that is not a bad thing. It either functionally works, it's fun, or it's required. Every once in a while, it is a good idea to entertain new activities to broaden the mind and experience in the world. Where better than now, in *Bridging Skills*, to do a quick check on community engagement with your child using AAC. Ask yourself *Is there a place we can go in the community that we haven't tried, that we haven't been to in a while, that we were waiting to try, that didn't work last time but we can try again?* If the answer is *yes* then you have your place and now move right on to your facilitator plan. If the answer is *no*, then make a list of community options to try and then move right into your facilitator plan. Either way, go for it.

Facilitator plan

You have your list of community options. How can you support your child in using a social greeting, commenting, asking questions, stating an opinion, etc.? How can you support your child in expanding the use of a language form, the number of times your child responds to a person or in the setting, or using a complete grammatical form, etc.? Think about what success with communication in the environment you choose looks like. Use the following chart as an example to spark ideas for your plan. You do not have to write a dissertation for an action plan. Think ahead. Collect some ideas. Write them down so you can look back and gauge success.

Jamie's communication plan: Disneyland February 14

Purpose + Look for Augmentative and Assistive Communication	The Communication Plan	Successes and Next Steps
Social Greetings and Engagement Nonverbal: wave, smile, point to messages on a communication board Verbal: Use a *SGD single message, quick message, novel message	• Jamie will use any modality to say *hi or bye* five times to a Disneyland cast member. • Jamie will make brief eye contact with Disneyland cast members when they talk to her.	Successes: Jamie said *hi* to ten people today. It was great. Next Step: Jamie didn't say *goodbye* and eye contact was a bit tough when cast members talked to her but she tried when I reminded her to use her eyes to say *goodbye*.
Sharing Information-Commenting Nonverbal: eye gaze, face/body gesture Communication board SGD quick message SGD novel message	Jamie will comment three times today something like: • *I liked that.* • *Can we do that again?* • *Fun!* • *Look!* • *Wow!* • *What is he eating?* • *Let's go there.*	Success: It kinda worked. Jamie commented with her communication board when we reminded her. She used *fun and I liked that* messages. Next Step: Initiation is still tough so I am going to make sure her quick phrases are easy to get to and prepare her by saying, *Okay, after the ride tell me what you think!*
Social Closeness Nonverbal: eye gaze, face/body gesture Communication board SGD quick message SGD novel message	Jamie will comment two times on social closeness: • *I'm scared.* • *Can you pick me up?* • *Put me down.* • *I can do that myself.* • *I'm fine.*	Success: Jamie responded to us when we asked her how she was doing so that was great. Next Step: We need to try to cue Jamie to use her feelings and emotion vocabulary.
Wants and Needs Nonverbal: eye gaze, face/body gesture Communication board SGD quick message SGD novel message	Jamie will comment on her wants and needs three times during the day: • *Can you pick me up? I want to see!* • *I'm hungry.* • *I need a break.* • *Can we cross now?* • *When will we go?*	Success: Jamie let us know what she wanted nonverbally so we cued her to use her boards and SGD. We praised her. Next Step: We want her to keep using her boards and SGD. We want her to learn she can speak with anyone at any time to participate fully.

*SGD = speech generating device

My child's action

I see my facilitator has gone over a purposeful communication plan with me so I know my role and what will happen next. I want to keep the focus on the fun of participation first. I will independently sprinkle in some extra messages. I see how successful I am and know what I will work on next.

⊙ My Multimodal Toolkit

◎ Decide on a place to go and complete a communication action plan.

◎ Optional: Checklist for things you need such as sunscreen, a hat, etc.

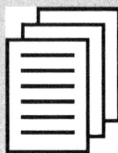

◉ Bring along multiple communication options for my child.

    ◉ Nonverbal communication modalities (e.g. eye gaze, head nods, hands, feet, etc.)

    ◉ Speech generating device with a single message option

    ◉ Speech generating device with quick messages

    ◉ Speech generating device with multi-message options

    ◉ Communication board options

Activity: Let's Go to the Game!

A place to start

It's Super Bowl Sunday! The Olympics are in full swing. World Cup soccer is on! Okay maybe you're not going to the game, stadium, or pitch for a major sporting event but maybe you are! Watch the sport on TV, listen to the sport broadcast through media sources, or read about the competition events on the Internet. You have multimodal options to go to a game so let's create multimodal options for your child to enjoy the game and cheer on your team! What about a game close to home? Check out your local high school, middle school, and children's sports leagues. Then tell your family and friends, *Let's Go to the Game!*

Facilitator plan

Check out the variety of sporting options you and your child have interest in that work with your time, and budget. Select and create a communication plan. Consider the audio requirements. Take an external speaker to boost the output of your child's AAC device. If environmental noise is overwhelming, keep earplugs or headphones handy. Make a poster. Decorate the wheelchair. Dress up for the game. Go have a blast. If you need to leave at half time, do it. If you need to show up at half time, do it.

My child's action plan

Think of the fun of attending a sporting event where you get to cheer on your team. There is fun in the planning, fun in the anticipation, fun in the dressing up, fun in decorating, and fun in having so much to say. Make sure your communication tools are packed ready to go with words such as, *YES! YAY! DE-FENCE, OH NO!* Have phrases such as, *Way to go! Are you kidding me! Nice call!* Program quick phrases specific to the team name and mascot. Your child will be in the community, socially engaged, and communicating. Even if the audio isn't perfect, who understands anyone's exact words when they are cheering at a sporting event any way. You are trying. You are out there. You're expressing yourself along with a collective group of peers.

My Multimodal Toolkit

- Dress up for the game.
- Decorate the wheelchair.
- Make a poster for your team or favorite player.
- Bring external speakers for voice output with AAC.

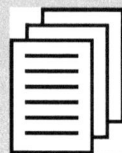

◉ Take multiple communication options for the child

    ◉ Nonverbal communication modalities (e.g. eye gaze, head nods, hands, feet, etc.)

    ◉ Speech generating device with a single message option

    ◉ Speech generating device with multi-message options

    ◉ Communication board options

Activity: Let Me Ask You Something: Questions for Peers

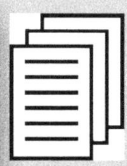

A place to start

It is time in our path to *Bridging Skills* to purposefully practice your child's ability to ask questions with peers . . . and of course adults. In the speech therapy world, we call this *Wh questions – who, what, when, where, why, which*. Yes, *how* can join in the fun too. We also ask questions starting with a verb (e.g. *is, are, do, was, and were*). Many times, interaction with a child that uses AAC is based on a peer or adult asking question and response. Using AAC, we prefer that the children ask their important questions. Let's work on that. This is language building.

Facilitator plan

Teach your child to ask questions asking using the purposes of communication. *Why* ask questions across purposes? *Because*, when we teach someone to ask questions, you are not just teaching the *Wh* or other question form, but you are teaching the reason, the motivation, to ask a question in the first place. Facilitators bring social closeness and social etiquette the next stage. Children gain information and express themselves. Step one, however, is to make sure your child understands question forms. The choice of the question word (e.g. what, where, why) may be a matter of personal preference. Work with your speech-language pathologist on making a progress monitoring tool to measure how well your child comprehends and generates *Wh* questions and other forms such as, *When can we play? Where do you want to go?* Do you need to focus on all of the question forms? No, you do not. In *Bridging Skills* it is a good idea to select forms your child can work with now that represent a good push and save harder question forms for *Maximizing Participation*.

My child's action plan

I am gaining the opportunity to explicitly practice asking questions across the purposes of communication. I like that I am learning that I can use quick messages to ask a question. I will start off asking one question and enjoy what happens with my communication partner. Sometimes that one question serves as a springboard to more questions, more comments, more communication. Look at these question forms to get your own ideas.

Examples: Purpose of communication question forms

Social greetings: *How are you? How are you doing? What are you up to?*
Sharing information: *Who is this about? What did you do? How did you do that? When did that happen? Where are you going? Why did you do that?*
Social closeness: *What do you think? Do you want to sit by me?*
Wants and needs: *What do you like? What would you like to play? Is that fun? Are you ready? Was your friend there? Were you cool?*

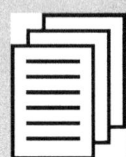

Asking questions through a language development task: From the list of recommended questions set a goal, use your newly developed progress monitoring tool, and plan an activity. *Bravo!* Use the following chart as an example. First you set a goal of one question form. Program it onto a communication board or speech generating device. Work with your speech-language pathologist on a selecting a measurable goal for asking questions. Sample Goal: Nathan will ask three questions with peers given AAC tools and devices in a structured social setting in 2/3 opportunities as measured by charted data. Celebrate your child's success in asking questions!

Activity	Examples by Question Forms
1 Structured Book Lesson	*Which book should we read? Why do you like that one? Whose turn is it? When do we need to stop reading?*
2 School Group Assignment	*Who is in our group? What part will I/he/she take? When is it due? Where will we meet?*
3 Setting Plans	*What are we doing? Where are we going? Who else is going? When will we go? What time will we finish?*
4 New Friend	*What is your name? What is your favorite _____? Where do you like to go? Why do you like it?*
5 Catching Up with a Friend	*How are you? What's up? What did you do this weekend/ yesterday? When can we get together? Did you see (add in a show) last night?*

The beauty of question forms is that many can be written as quick phrases on a communication board or programmed on a speech generating device. The faster the question can be generated the sooner social reciprocity begins.

⊙ My Multimodal Toolkit

- ◉ Work with a speech-language pathologist to determine appropriate *Wh* or other question forms.

- ◉ Add quick phrases in questions forms gradually so that the child is able more easily to accomplish each purpose of communication.

- ◉ Include multiple communication options for your child.

  - ◉ Nonverbal communication modalities (e.g. eye gaze, head nods, hands, feet, etc.)

  - ◉ Speech generating device with a single message option

  - ◉ Speech generating device with multi-message options

  - ◉ Communication board options

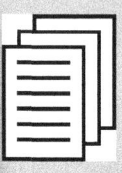

A place to start

Now that we are asking questions (see, *Let Me Ask You Something: Questions for Peers*), let's take on another explicit task, repair strategies. Communication breakdowns are inevitable in all conversations. In *Bridging Skills*, we want your child to start to recognize when the breakdowns occur and employ a strategy to repair their message, or intent, for successful communication.

Facilitator plan

Help your child learn to take more responsibility in communicating with familiar family and friends, less familiar peers, and people in the community when a familiar adult is present. Start with explicit practice with familiar people. Practice using a quick phrase programmed on a speech generating device or pointing to a quick phrase on a communication board, in a communication wallet, communication ring, or a tip card for communication partners. The tip card can state messages to communication partners such as, *Give me a minute to answer your question, Can you say that again? That is not what I meant to say. Hold on, let me fix my message.* Choose a quick phrase that would works more often than others. Tell your child you will practice using repair strategies for pretend. Start a conversation with your child. Cue them to point or speak a quick phrase repair message. A possible script could be the following.

Mom: *I had a great day at work today. Oh, I picked up some Valentine's Day supplies for us to make cards this weekend for your friends. What did you do today?*
Child: *I went to the park.*
Mom: *You did?*
Child: *Hold on, let me fix my message.*
Child: *I went to school today. I read a book. I played with Emma.*
Mom: *Fantastic!*

Next try it on shopping trip (preferably not a rush hour and with patient clerk).

Child: *Where is the apple?*
Clerk: *Aisle 10 by the fruits.*
Child: *Hold on, let me fix my message.*
Child: *Where is the applesauce?*
Clerk: *Aisle 12, canned goods. Left side.*
Child: *Got it, Thank you.*

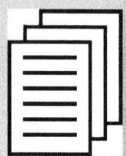

My child's action plan

I am going to learn a new sense of control. I am learning to be an active participant in expressing a message and taking charge to fix the communication situation. My plan is to be successful with familiar people in a practice environment using or combining a number of repair phrases. Then I will practice a repair strategy in new environment. I can call it ping pong, zig-zag, or piggy back, or whatever phrase I choose with repair strategy between 1) familiar, less familiar and novel people with supervision and 2) familiar, less familiar, or novel environments. Repair strategy quick phrase options: *Wait I need a minute to change that. That's not what I meant to say. What did you say? Did you say _____? I didn't hear you. Say that again, please. You can use my AAC device so I can read your message! Please write your message down so I can read it. Hold on. Let me fix that. Oopsie! Let me try again.*

My Multimodal Toolkit

◎ Quick phrases for repairing communication

- ◎ Communication wallet or board

- ◎ Speech generating device with a single message option

- ◎ Speech generating device with multi-message options

Bridging Skills with facilitator strategies

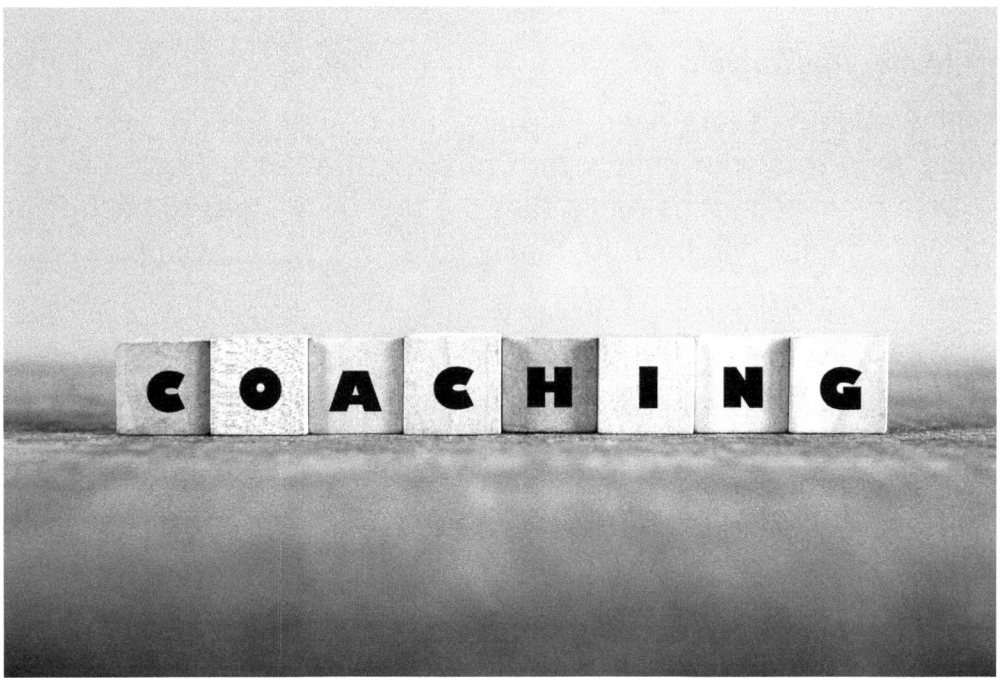

○ Grab and Go Coaches' Corner

The *Grab and Go* section of *Bridging Skills* is a collection of ideas that guide facilitators with options for supporting a child who is ready for increasing responsibility for expressing communicative intent. Just like in the *Making Connections* chapter, facilitator strategies are offered to help your child build language and have opportunities for participation and interaction. Review the topics and steps to support each tip. Provide the child with opportunities at home, school, and community daily to increase the child's independence with social interactions and communication.

Grab and Go Topics:

1 Talk to Me! Tips for You!
2 Code Switching
3 Fading Prompts
4 Eliciting Opinions
5 Asking Leading Questions
6 Joke Time
7 Compare and Contrast
8 Writing for Communicative Intent
9 Honoring Multimodal Communication Preferences
10 Answering a Question, Comment, Ask a Question

○ Facilitator tips and steps for Bridging Skills with communication

1 Talk to me! Tips for you!

Communication partners need help too! Interventionists structure therapy sessions. Now it is your child's turn to structure communication partners. How? Give them some tips too! Adapt the following ideas to best meet your child's word choice and how the family holds a typical social conversation.

- *Hello! Yes, say hello to me any way you want to. I say hello with my eyes and my speech generating device. We named my device Fred.*
- *What have you been up to? I'd love to hear about it. Look at my communication book or my binder and you can see what I like to talk about.*
- *Okay I gotta go! Great talking to you! Catch 'ya later!*

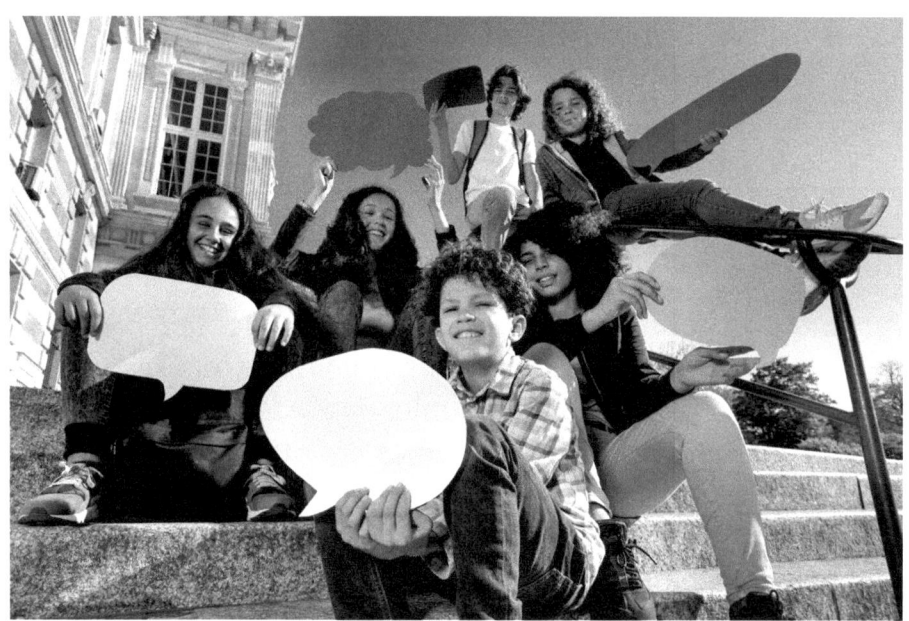

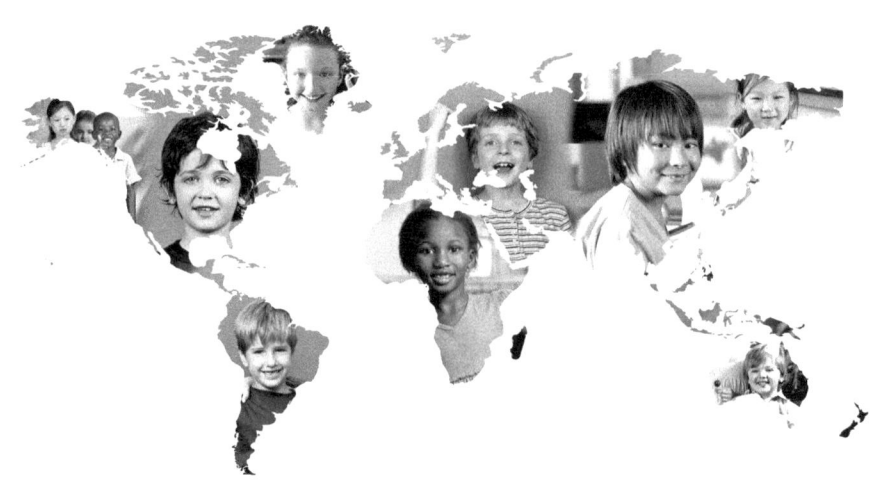

2 Code switching

Ray says, *Hello Dr. Ness*, to his teacher and, *Hey Bryan, What's up?* to his friend. Code switching is the ability to use the right words, cultural, or linguistic practices with a person in an environment at the right time. Practice culturally appropriate social interaction and language with your child. Generate communication tools that allow a child to interact across their cultures, environments, peers, and adults. Include social language. Include formal language. Then, enjoy the moment when your young child uses slang with the school principal. It is all a learning process. Priceless.

3 Fading prompts

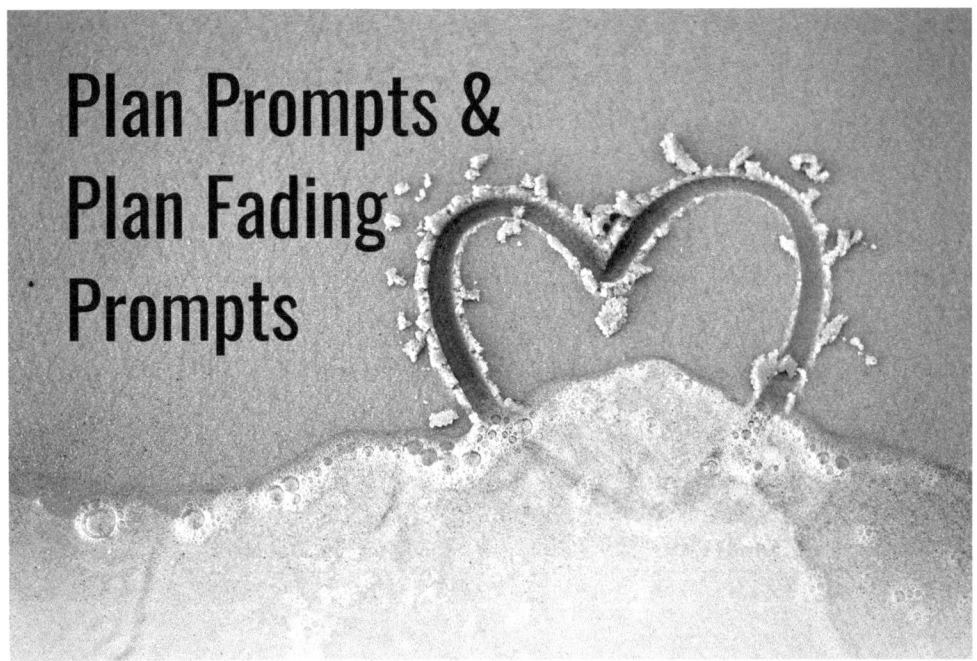

Verbal, physical, and motor prompts as talked about in *Getting Started* and *Building Fundamentals*, are great because they help us be more successful with many types of tasks. However, sometimes children become prompt dependent for communication and other tasks. For example, a child waits for someone to give a prompt to get started and will not start until the prompt is given. Sometimes, facilitators do not realize how many and what types of prompts are used. Take note of the types and amount of prompting you use with children that use AAC. Begin to fade the amount or type of prompting with your child to improve independence. Use a partial physical prompt such as touch cue rather than a full physical motor prompt to initiate a point. Instead of navigating between pages on a speech generating device, point to show where the child can take control and change the page. Provide a model of the communication on an AAC device (aided language stimulation) rather than a verbal command to imitate. Move from a verbal prompt, the hardest prompt to stop using perhaps because the easiest for us to offer, to a gestural prompt to a more natural cue such as clearing your throat to cue attention.

4 Eliciting opinions

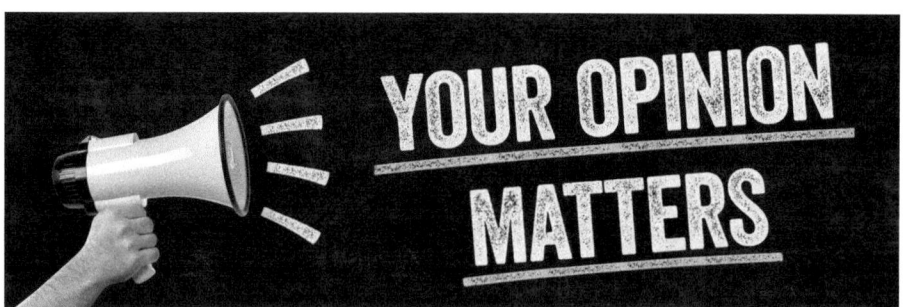

Elicit your child's opinions on topics about communication or environmental activities such as, *How did you like that game? How did you like that book?* Make sure you are willing to hear the opinion your child offers. An opinion is not necessarily a choice. There is a time and place for most opinions, however there are times when a choice or an opinion is not an option and a set course of action must take place. Elicit opinions when the information can be appropriately heard, acknowledged, and acted upon.

5 Asking leading questions

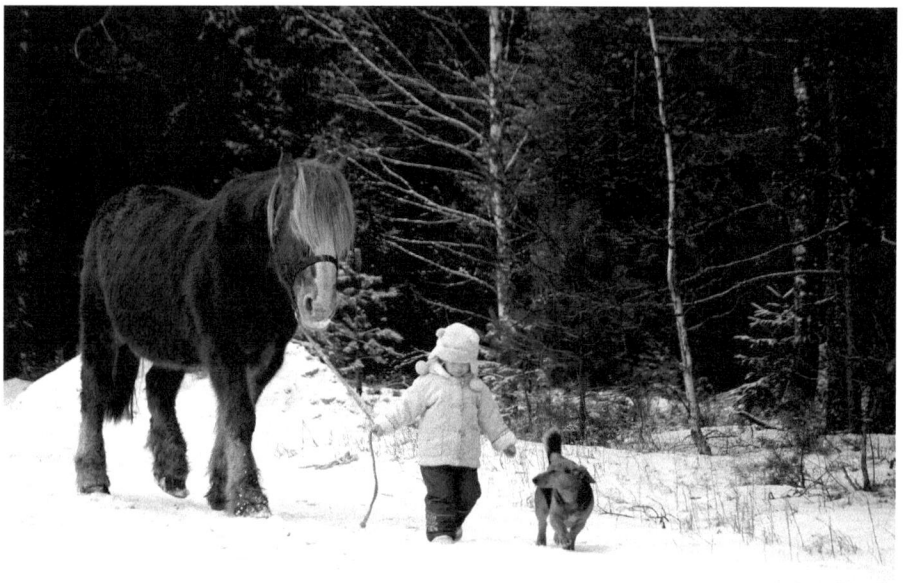

There are many ways to ask a leading question, perhaps suggesting your child answer in a particular way. Ask leading questions about a topic to get to a specific answer, to engage in prediction, to yield an interpretation, or check for comprehension of words, context, events or behavior. Feel free to ask a *yes* or *no* question to springboard towards a deeper meaning, intent, or information. You can also expand on your child's responses because now you want to strive for increasing novel communication and independence. For example, *Did you read Stephen Hawking's book for kids called George and the Big Bang? You did? Me too. What was your favorite part? Tell me about it.*

6 Joke time

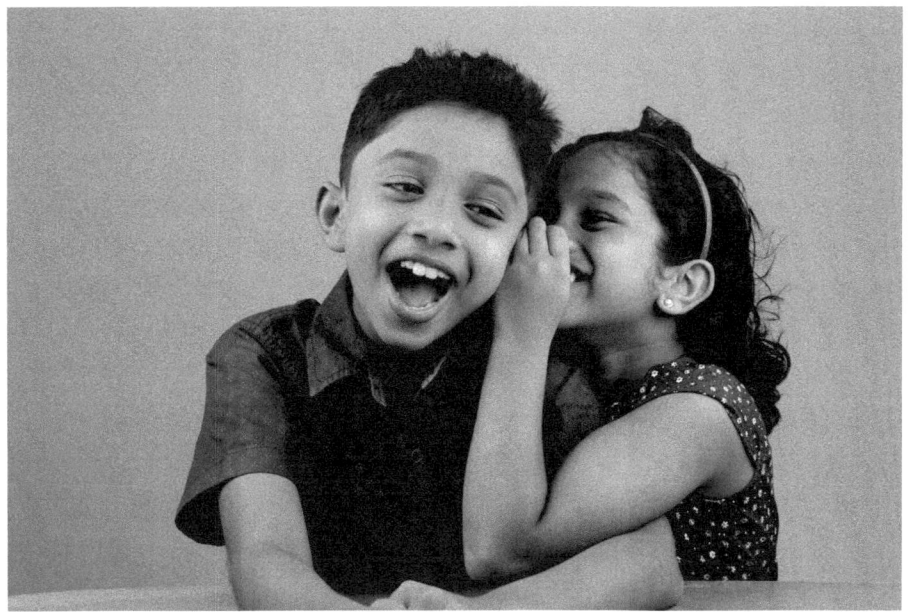

Program your child's communication device with age appropriate jokes. Telling and responding to jokes is a great way to generate fun in social interaction. Try a joke of the day. Your child will have fun as will your child's peers and other communication partners. If you want to use a communication board or tool option you can create one icon that says, *Do you want to hear a joke?* Then create two more icons, one with the joke set-up and one icon with the punch line. *What do you call an alligator in a vest? Give up? An investi-gator!* Jokes are often a play on words. For extra fun, program a laugh after the punch line, *Hee-hee-hee.*

7 Compare and contrast

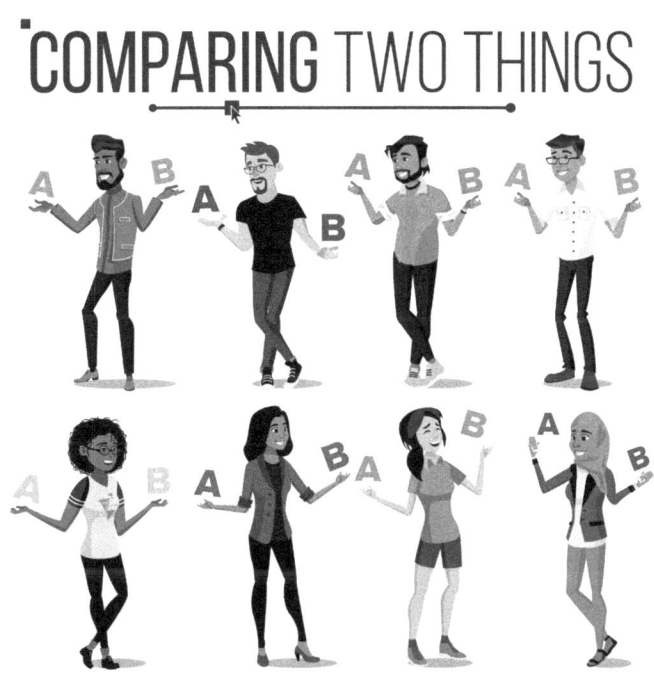

COMPARING TWO THINGS

Teach comparing and contrasting. Talking about silly pictures and actions is the most fun way to compare and contrast. Talk about how categories or two items are the same and different. Comparing and contrasting is a great way to generate the use of adjectives and adverbs in phrases or sentences. Use words that describe color, shape, size, quantity, composition, function, preferences, and locations. Check out the company Super Duper (2019a; www.superduperinc.com/) for many product options for purchase to build language skills. A particularly fun product is called That's Silly Fun Deck Flashcards (2019c; https://superduperinc.com/products/view.aspx?pid=FD29&s=thats-silly-fun-deck&lid=41E46A95&view=read_reviews) that provides a fun way to work on contrasts or their Compare and Contrast Cards (2019b; www.superduperinc.com/products/view.aspx?pid=FD45&s=compare-and-contrast#.XYfprJNKh0s) are great fun too.

8 Writing for communicative intent

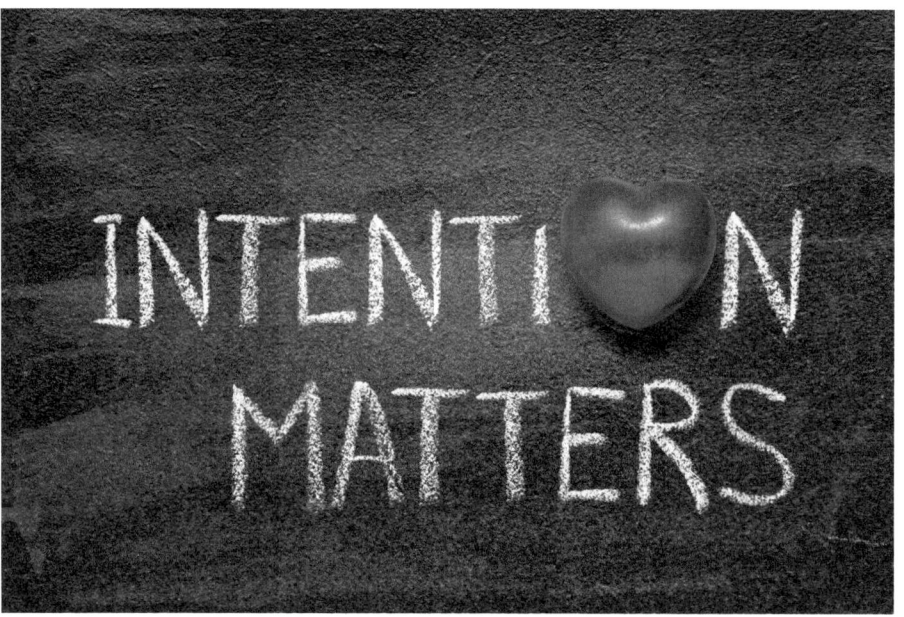

Did you understand your child's written communication even if the words were not in the right order or some of the function words like articles (e.g. a, an, the) were missing or verb tenses or irregular plurals were not correct? If the answer is 'yes' then you have a great example of writing for communicative intent. The goal in this stage does not necessarily require the child to write with perfect grammar, or written competency. Keep the focus on message, the communicative intent. The act of writing, referred to as orthography when grammar, spelling, punctuation, and other formal written aspects are required of a given language, is generally considered the most formal expression of a language. A change in grammar may or may not change the intent of the message (e.g. He is here. He was here). Sometimes we may want to look past the grammar and focus on intent.

9 Honoring multimodal communication preferences

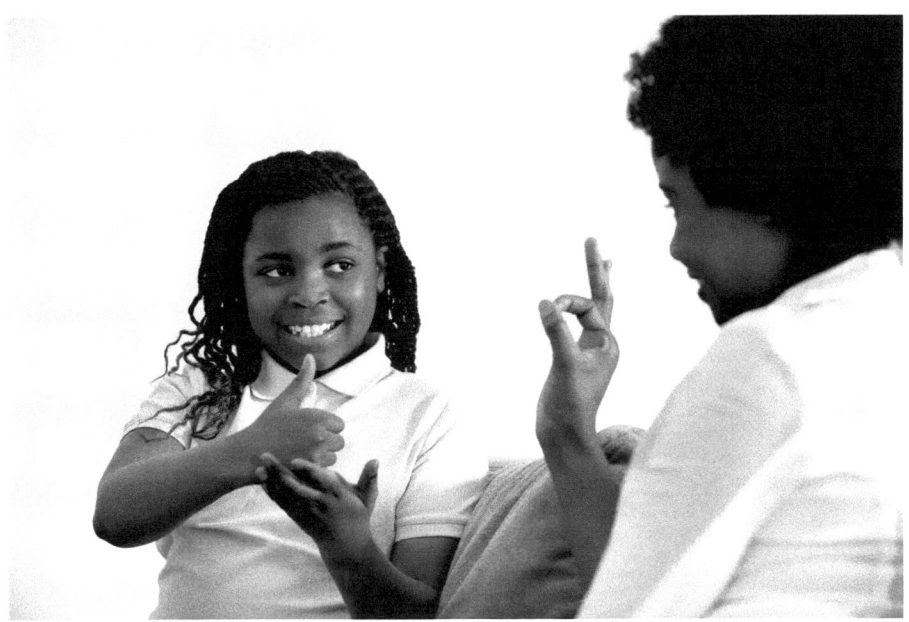

Honor your child's preferences for the types of symbols, speech generating devices, aided communication, and nonverbal choices for communicating across the purposes of communication and topics your child may prefer. We have spent a lot of time talking about using multimodal communication. Now keep in mind to honor your child's preference for communication modalities. It is great to allow your child to choose to how he or she wants to express the message. We all have our preferred methods!

10 Answering a question, commenting, asking a question

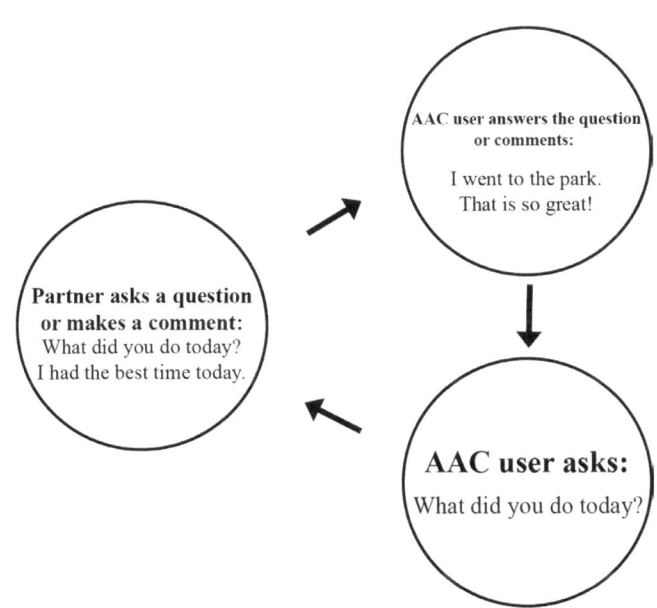

Follow a three-step model to keep a conversation going. Use the following questions, comments, and options for answering questions. Write down questions, comments, and ways you commonly answer questions in your home as the best set of ideas to work with. Establish a set of three to five questions, comments, and answers for your child to work on and add more to expand your child's skills when he or she is comfortable with the format. Program quick phrases on AAC device or make communication board icons for routine questions, comments, and statements.

Question Asked by a Peer or Adult	Child Answers a Question	Peer or Adult Comments on a Topic	Child Asks a Reciprocal Question
What are you reading?	I am reading my new book.	That sounds like fun.	What are you reading?
Where are you going?	I am off to the park.	See you soon then.	Where are you going?
What do you want to do?	I want to help mom.	That's interesting.	What do you want to do?
What is on your schedule?	I am going to the store.	Thanks for letting me know.	What is happening next?
What time are we going?	After 3:00 p.m.	Okay I got it.	When will we be done?

Bridging Skills with literacy

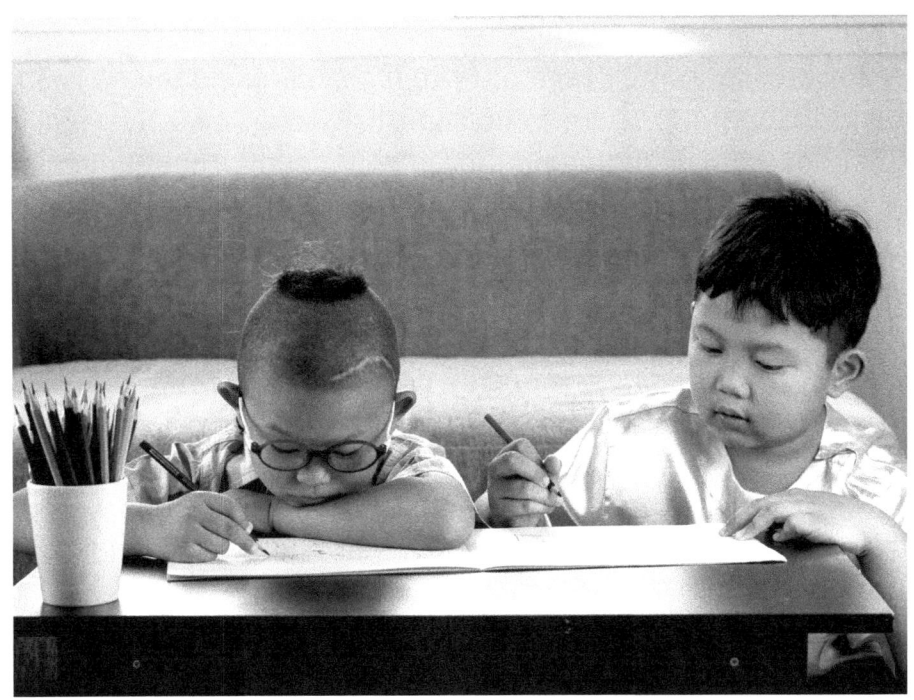

○ The power of words

The power of words! Words make a difference. We speak them, hear them, read them, and at every turn, interpret them. Our voice, whether spoken using any modality, or written makes an impact on others and ourselves. As we discuss *Bridging Skills with Literacy* see your child as entering into a world of expanding possibilities with literacy. Make word choices explode imagination. Make word choices create rich images. Make word choices change the mood and in turn change how your child sees his or her day. Read the following story of a young girl who is not having her best day. See how the power of literacy turned isolation into participation.

The power of words: from frustration to happiness

A young girl, frustrated with her day, sat on the couch. She was not interested in engaging with anyone and demonstrated no aspiration what-so-ever to communicate with her AAC device. However, it was time for her speech therapy. Her somewhat desperate yet keen speech-language pathologist went to her on the couch and began to read. It was a story with rich language that talked about fascinating interactions, vibrant colors, and exciting actions. The young girl became rapt in the story. The girl with no motivation or inclination to communicate, not only began to communicate, she flourished. She looked at her therapist as if to say,

'You're not going to test me?' Her therapist brought over her AAC device and the girl used the device to say, 'Keep reading.' Then she navigated to the emotions page and stated that she was happy.

Literacy for a child in the stage of *Bridging Skills* includes a broad spectrum of reading and writing. There is no right or wrong level for your child to be on. Instead focus on including literacy in your child's communication plan and moving your child forward. Now let's take a look at some options to consider for reading and writing at the *Bridging Skills* stage.

Reading

1 *An Inventory of Decoding and Sight Word Knowledge Mastery: Revisit the stages of Accessing Literacy Learning (ALL)* by Janice Light and David McNaughton (2012) http://aacliteracy.psu.edu/index.php/page/show/id/15/index.html. Your child may be ready for a new level or work across levels in the *Bridging Skills* stage of development. Determine your child's reading skills. Meet your child where he or she is across the stages of development and continue to move your child forward.

2 Reading fluency for comprehension: Reading fluency is the act of increasing the speed in which a person can read text silently. The increase in speed allows the reader to read more text thus allowing the opportunity to connect ideas in sentences that lead to a greater understanding of a paragraph and ultimately a story. Reading fluency is different from decoding and sight word knowledge. Remember that decoding is the skill of reading a word by processing sounds to letters and seeing the patterns of letters; sight word reading is knowing a word by sight without having to think through the sounds that make up the word. Children that use AAC as their primary mode of verbal communication can use decoding and sight words to increase their reading fluency. Facilitators offer children the opportunity to read the answers before they read a text, a strategy for increasing comprehension. Then read text. When the child is finished, offer comprehension questions for your child to answer to demonstrate their understanding of the text by giving them 3–4 choices of answers, use a word bank to complete a sentence (see cloze sentences in *Making Connections*), or elicit a short open-ended response. Reflect on the emotions of the stories. Recall the time order and spatial sequences that tell the story. Relate to child's own life experiences and those of others. Remember to provide your child with rich language in which to answer questions. Of course, ask engaging, meaningful questions, sometimes ones that you do not already know the answers.

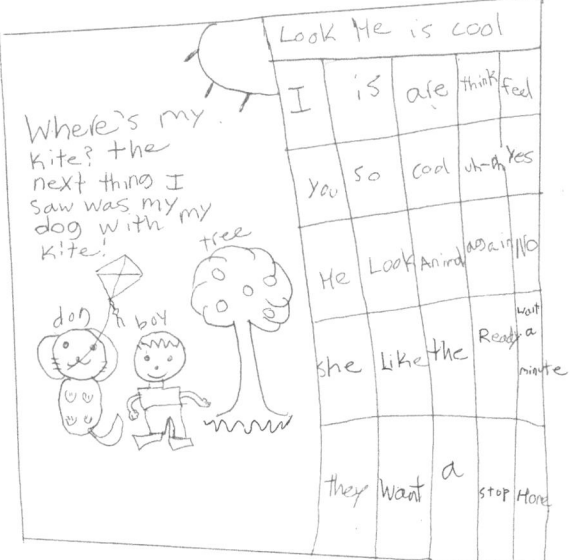

Construct stories focusing on a sequence of connected events. In earlier stages of story telling the events in a story may be unrelated or may look more like a list of events such as what your child played with at recess or what activities happened during the day (Westby, 2019). Later help your child see that events may be connected as you discuss the timing of events or the location of what happened in the story. Then use the ideas to help your child build stories of their own whether they are telling or writing narratives. Check out the website Tar Heel Reader (https://tarheelreader.org/) for free, easy-to-read accessible books and add your child's story to the growing list of titles!

Ways to building an understanding of how narratives are constructed

1 Recognize a temporal sequence of a story for *first, then, next, last.*
2 Create a logical order of a story with a beginning, a middle, and an end.
3 Talk about time as it relates to the story whether the events occurred within hours or less, a day or longer. Look for how time- and location-related details in the story predict future events.
4 Label parts of a story that you read with your child to improve reading comprehension. Identify the setting, the characters, and the plot. Then advance to recognizing problems, making inferences, solving problems, making decision, determining consequences, seeking resolutions, and deciding on final results.

5 Reflect on your child's and your own experience as it relates to the story. The child is able to generate a sentence description, supply past experience, and begin to add components of social thinking such as perspective taking and projections, making inferences about actions and people.

Investigate *The Story Grammar Marker* (Moreau, 1994; https://mindwingconcepts.com/), a physical tool used to build story and language skills. Children can say or recall story elements as their hands feel the different textures associated with characters, action, emotions, and resolution to improve story telling.

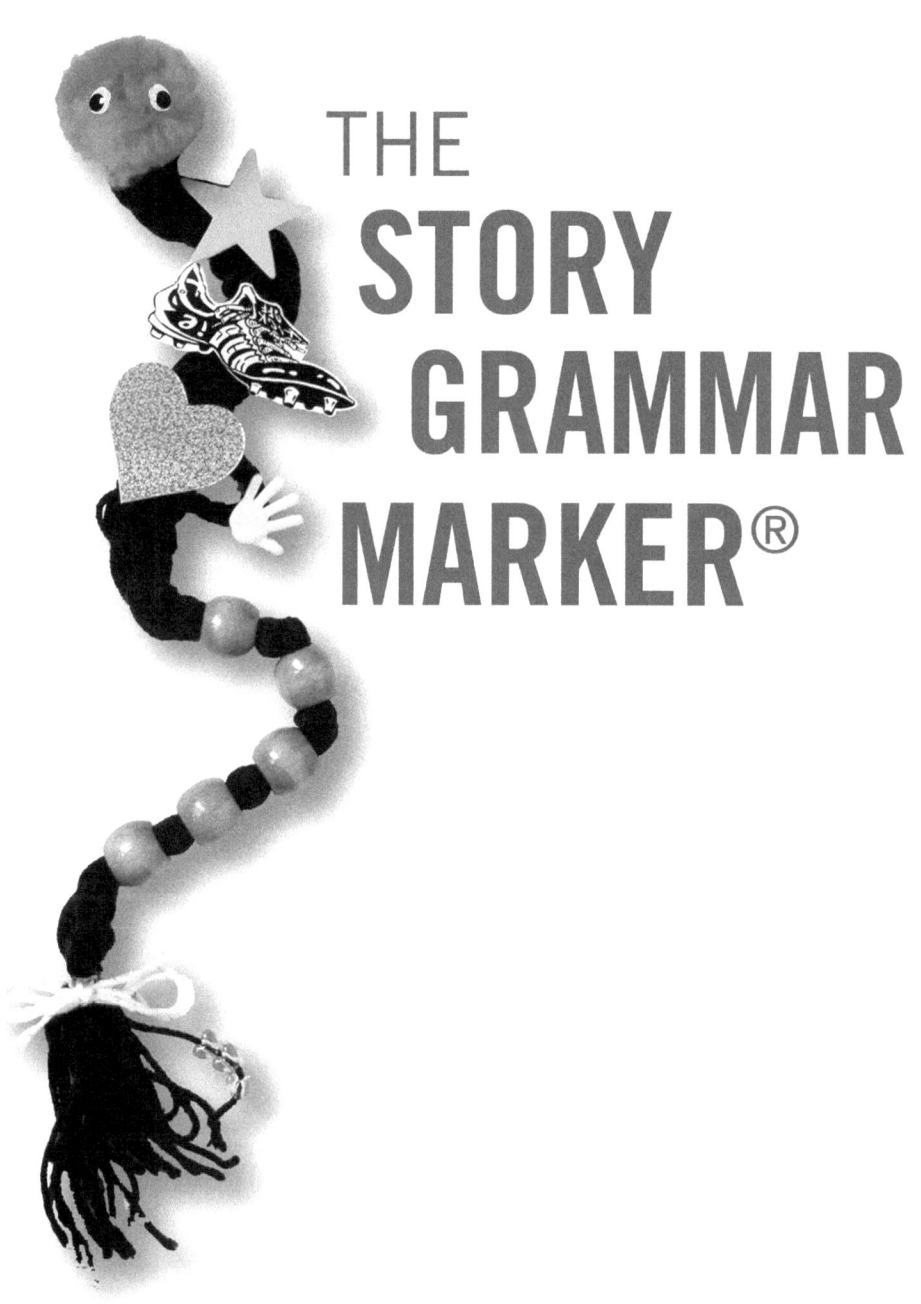

THE
**STORY
GRAMMAR
MARKER**®

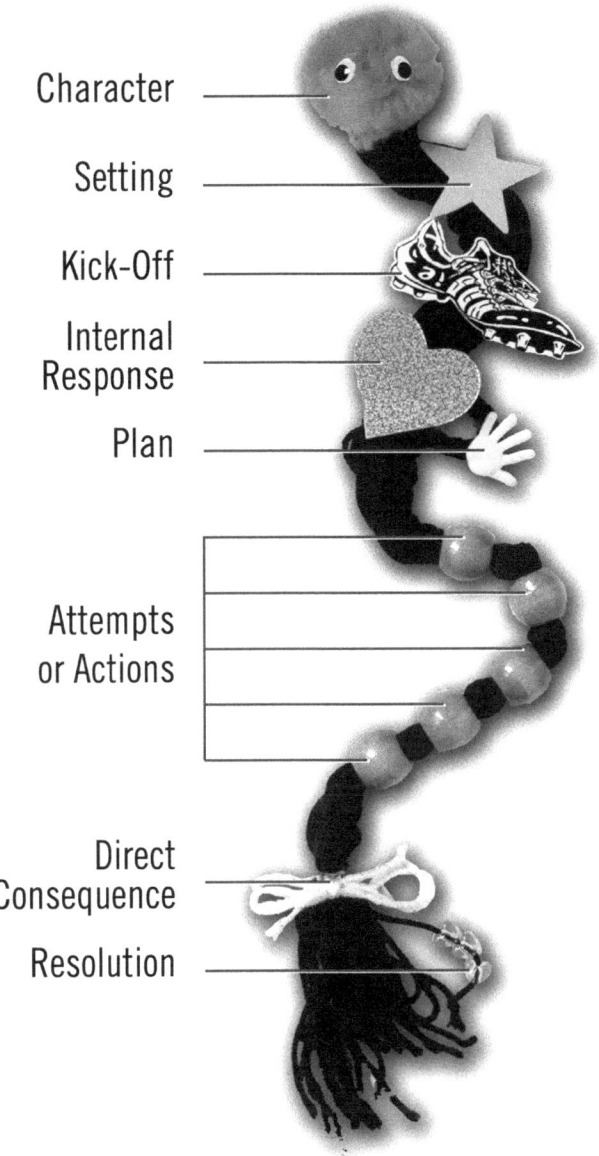

Character ——————

Setting ——————

Kick-Off ——————

Internal
Response ——————

Plan ——————

Attempts
or Actions

Direct
Consequence ——————

Resolution ——————

Writing

AAC users publish their ideas. Sometimes ideas are handwritten or drawn, emailed, texted, or generated on a speech generating device. Consider the best way for your child to demonstrate and share written output. Focus on the different number and type of words the child can use to write. Focus on the sentence types that are being produced such as simple sentences, sentences that ask questions, sentences that have negation in them, sentences that have compound words, lists of ideas, and phrases. Listen for clauses that explain using *since, however*, and *but that change the direction of the sentences*. Build on the child's quality and complexity of output.

Your child does not have to master each type but considering each type is a worthy task. As you see your child develop, consider adding new sentence formations that then makes sure these words as included on the communication tool.

Sentence types

1 Simple sentence: *That cloud looks like a fish.*
2 Compound sentence: *That cloud looks like a fish and that one looks like a whale!*
3 Complex sentence: *Because you are imaginative, you can see fish shapes in the clouds.*
4 Compound-complex sentence: *Because you are imaginative, you can see shapes in the clouds; and I get to enjoy your company.*

Bridging Skills with expository writing

Bridging Skills into expository writing explains, describes, and/or informs facts and opinions in for science, history, and problem solving in mathematics, and more. This type of writing does not assume the reader having prior knowledge but provides support for making inferences and predictions with specific vocabulary. Since reading and writing is to be learner led, allow students to ask questions as they read and experience vocabulary embedded in sentences and then write the facts and opinions themselves.

Creating a supportive literacy environment

The following tips are a compilation of known strategies wrapped up in a new package for you and your child to create a supportive literacy environment so that reading and writing become socially and functionally dynamic. In *Bridging Skills*, you and your child are seeking the balance between the known and unknown in learning to read, write, speak, and listen. Create a list of two to three ideas you can help your child connect with literacy given the following ten ideas.

Ways I support literacy development

1 Motivation through shared interests and stories: Think about how the interests you have. Think about your child's interests. Talk about them. Discuss stories about your interest of other stories that connects interests in books, magazines, and other forms of printed or electronic material.
2 Structure literacy: Where are you going to start on the Accessible Literacy Learning (ALL, Light & McNaughton, 2012) stages of development and where you are going based on your child's skills? Is your child beginning with sound blending and decoding? How is your child building comprehension skills?
3 Social interaction and participation: Literacy provides a solid foundation for the quality interaction children that are AAC users need with adults, siblings, and peers. Seeing other children reading, writing, and talking about what they are reading opens the door to access for social interaction in a rich and engaging way that supports children's responsivity and increases their responses with communication partners and the child using AAC.

4   Access, independence, and ownership: How does your child access literacy? What modes of access work and work best? Under what conditions is your child dependent on others to access literacy? Under what conditions does your child access literacy independently? These are all great questions to ask and answer yourself, or with the support of others that may have additional knowledge that supports literacy through about assistive and instructional technology (Light & Kelford-Smith, 1993). Relinquish degrees of the literacy independence by having the child choose a favorite writing utensil such as markers, colored pencils, pens, paints, and others. You can provide a variety of texts ranging by topics and complexity to make each child's reading more accessible. Take a few notes on books that are motivating to your child, accessible modes of writing, motivating utensils for writing, ways your child is dependent on others for writing, and ways your child reads independently.

5   Share original ideas and stories: Generate opportunities to share your child's literacy skills by showing books of interest to others such as interventionists and peers, writing and sending messages and stories to others, talking about books and other written forms or media using AAC. Create different endings for stories and events of the day. Reflect on perspectives from other cultures. Begin to write your own stories of events the child has experienced.

6   Time, time, and more time: Make the time, give the gift of time, time, time to read and write at home, in the car/bus/train using books, magazines, environmental signs, computers, tablet applications, phones, and more! Marvel at the mystery of discovery with reading and writing.

7   Publish and post: Have books, student work, posted and available (e.g. places at home or school). Children love to see their work acknowledged.

8   Generate access: Locate forms of access to books and libraries that may be online or electronic sources and print sources (e.g. home library, school library, public libraries, literacy programs, literacy intervention programs, internet-based libraries on the computer or tablet technology).

9   Support comprehension: Ask questions that help your child understand a word or concept. Check for understanding of specific words and ideas. Pause to allow for processing time. Ask cloze questions that require a specific answer and make use of open-ended questions that elicit a variety of responses or opinions.

10 Writing: Giving children opportunities for writing are important because they give your child that uses AAC another voice, another visual form of expression, that represents a quantitative and qualitative experience with a tangible outcome. Some options include tools (e.g. writing utensils, keyboards), technology (e.g. paper, writing utensils, tablet, computer). Look at the purposes for writing such as for homework, quick social message, sharing information, expressing opinions. Introduce your child to self-editing, peer-editing, adult-editing for the purpose of capitalization, periods, organization, grammar, clarity! See how others send written messages such as mail, email, post, text, or handing in homework?

Remember we want to make sure of two things. First, does your child understand the symbol on the icon and that it represents vocabulary on the communication tools or speech generating devices? Secondly, can your child read the word associated with the symbol? Sometimes learning the symbol and reading the word will occur simultaneously and sometimes the symbol will be learned before the written word. Focus on both symbolic understanding and reading the vocabulary word text to maximize your child's understanding and ability to produce novel utterances with vocabulary that represents quality and quantity. These supports only increase delight in reading and writing messages. Remember to check out the Center for Literacy and Disabilities Studies at www.med.unc. edu/ahs/clds/ for reading and writing resources. Visit the website Literacy for Children with Combined Vision and Hearing Loss at http://literacy.nationaldb. org/ for emergent literacy, writing, and vocabulary development.

Bridging Skills with vocabulary

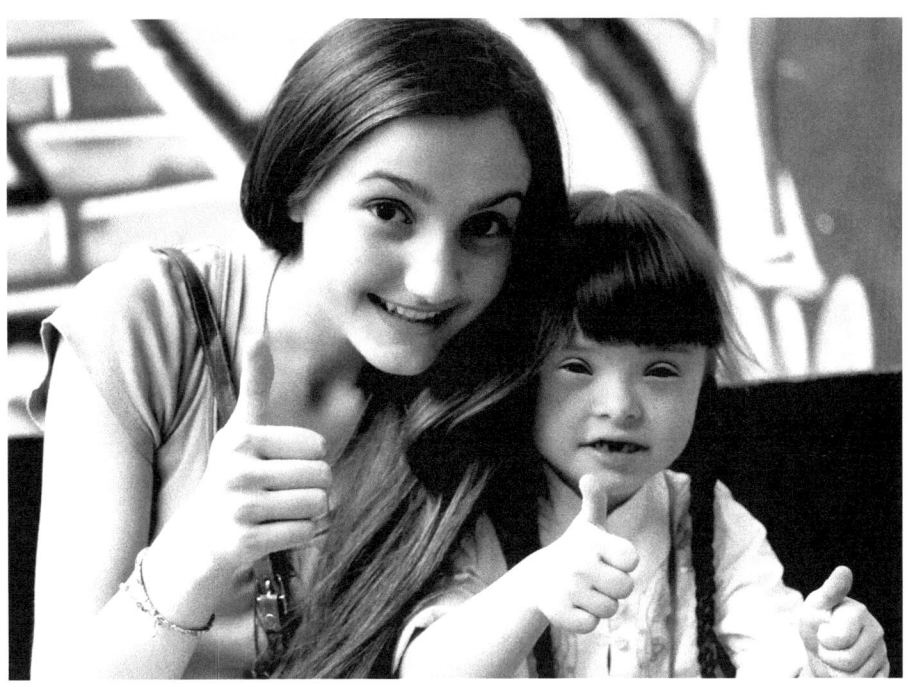

○ Quality vocabulary with meaningful quantity

In *Bridging Skills* place the focus of vocabulary on your child producing quality vocabulary with the quantity desired to meet the intent. How can we do that? We want to take a look back, take a look around, and then take a look forward at vocabulary. First, look back at the previous vocabulary stages in *Getting Started, Building Fundamentals*, and *Making Connections*. Note your child's vocabulary development. It is very possible your child is learning vocabulary across stages. Light, McNaughton and Caron (2019) state that it is important to focus on meaningful words that are developmentally appropriate. Use word lists and core vocabulary tool as guides to making choices yet maintain the focus on the child's communicative intent and the message. Now let's discuss a way to address vocabulary called Tiered Vocabulary by Beck, McKeown and Kucan (2013). The authors designate vocabulary according to three tiers including Tier 1 for basic vocabulary, Tier 2 for more specific vocabulary, and Tier 3 for domain specific vocabulary like words for science, technology, engineering, and math or other industry specific terms. Is your child learning beginning Tier 1 vocabulary such as *hot, cold, big, little, car, house*? Is your child learning Tier 2 vocabulary such as *boiling, frigid, enormous (gi-normous ... for fun), tiny, vehicle, domicile*? Reading simple descriptors to progressive descriptors: The following chart provides an example of simple and progressive descriptor words that would be found in Tier 1 and Tier 2 words. As your child grasps descriptive language begin to offer more complex synonyms and antonyms. When your child has a broader use of language, he or she increases his or her 'file cabinet' of language possibilities to be used for literacy and communication purposes. Add Tier 3 vocabulary that is academically specific to your child's grade by course.

Simple Descriptor	Progressive Descriptor
Small	Miniscule
Yes	Agree
Happy	Gleeful
Red	Scarlet
Round	Sphere

Is the vocabulary on your child's AAC tools and devices meaningful to him or her? If so, great. Next, take a look <u>around</u> at your child's vocabulary. You may feel like your child has more vocabulary than is often expressed. This gap between children's vocabulary knowledge and use was Sara Smith's motivation to create the Expanding Expression Tool (EET; www.expandingexpression.com/). Smith (2020), a speech-language pathologist and lecturer, states that it can be a challenge for children to talk about even common objects. The EET provides children with a tangible multi-sensory approach to organize thinking to express vocabulary for descriptive tasks such as oral expression, written expression, vocabulary, defining and describing, making associations, stating object functions, categorization, and similarities and differences. Children and interventionists apply her tool to promote expression across all verbal modalities including AAC through speech generating devices. With the EET you can start at a single word level or advance to phrases, sentences, paragraphs, and even reports which makes it an ideal tool for students of all ages and abilities who use core vocabulary based AAC systems (Smith & Browning, n.d.).

Next, we want to look forward and see how we can expand vocabulary. EET supports the learning of new vocabulary in addition to the use of existing vocabulary. Review the following tips to support your child's vocabulary and other language development skills. Your child may know some of these vocabulary concepts and some may need to be learned or polished. Take a look at the concepts, address them, and even categorize them to help you understand how your child's language and vocabulary is growing across domains.

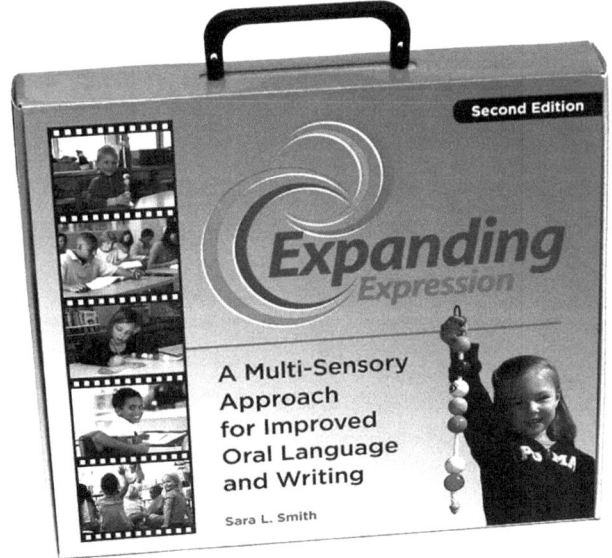

○ **Tips for building sentences: add words, phrases, and clauses…**

1 Vocabulary for opinions: Include language for opinions including negation: I think…, I don't think…, I feel…, I don't feel…, I agree…, I don't agree…

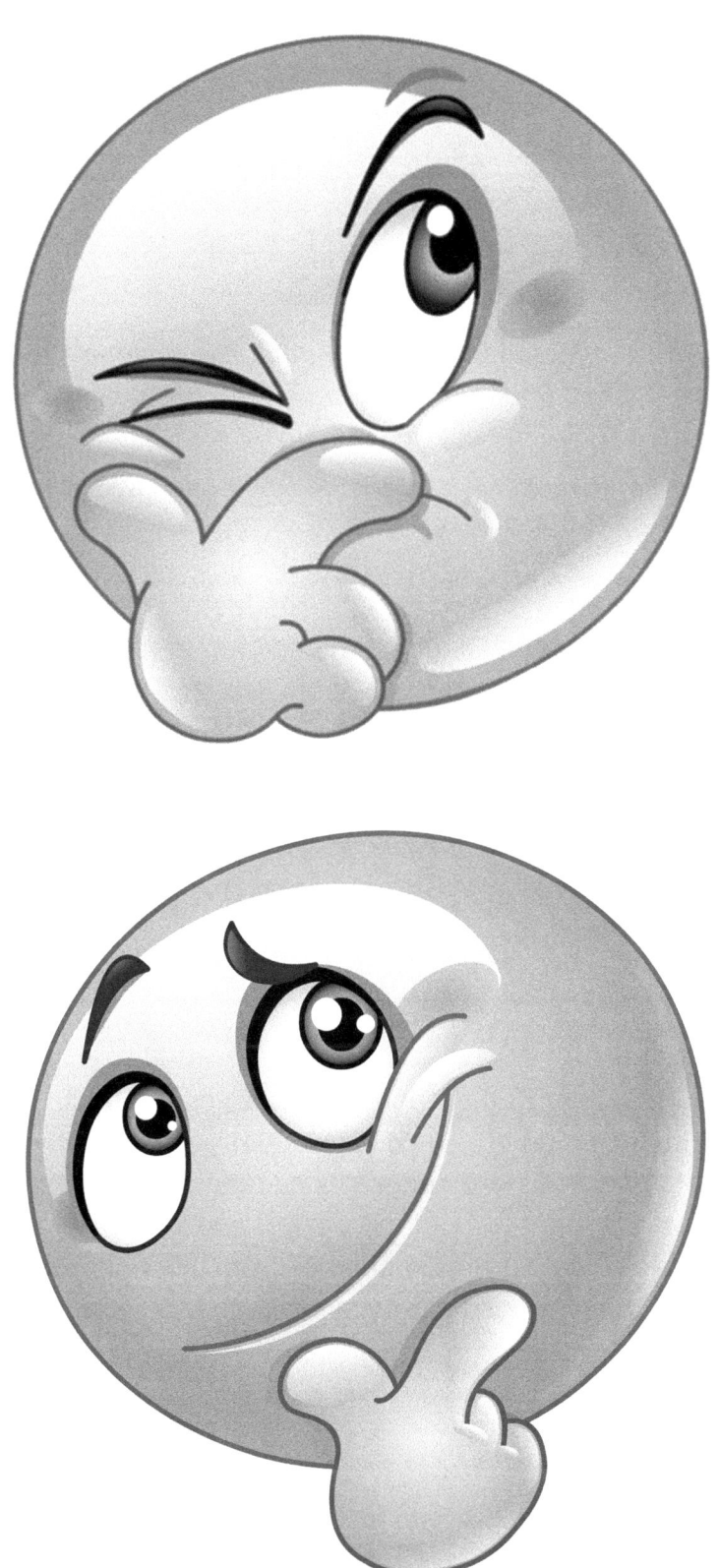

2 Vocabulary for complex ideas: Use more complex concept words such as adjectives, comparison words, and superlatives that help us compare and describe differences. Words to expand language like conjunctions (e.g. and, but, or), and phrases called adverbial phrases to expand your child's use and comprehension of language.

Adjectives, Comparisons, Superlatives	Conjunctions	Adverbial Clauses or Phrases
Big, bigger, biggest	And, but, for, or, if, yet, because, although, since, unless	…carefully across the street.
Small, smaller, smallest	Then, when, such as still, too, in particular, after	…quickly to the playground.
Cool, cooler, coolest	But, therefore, also	…slowly to the desk.

3 Vocabulary with prepositions: Sensory-language anyone? Prepositions tell us to GO *in, on, over, under, next to, between, through* and more. Practice sentence expansion while your child follows your aided language stimulation model of, *Go through the door.* Then your child can give a command for peers, a whole, class, parents, or interventionists to follow!

4 Vocabulary for *If, Then* conditional statements: Adding conditional statements allow a child to state a dependence of one factor on another. Conditional statements allow the child and communication partners to understand the relationship between two objects, events, feelings, and others. Look at the following examples.

Objects:	*If I push the car, then it will roll across the floor.*
Events:	*If I go to the birthday party, then I can play with Sam.*
Feelings:	*If I show that I am happy to Jill, then she may be happy too.*
Combination:	*If you learn to swim, then next summer you can have fun in the pool with Sonia and Grace.*

5 Vocabulary for safety: Comprehend safety signs in and around the child's community focusing on stop signs, walking signs, train tracks, and lines on streets that show where pedestrians should walk to be safe. It is one thing to recognize the symbol for *stop, go*, and *wait*. It is another thing to read the words. Make sure your child has the symbolic knowledge and the ability to read the words on safety signs such as *entrance, exit, danger*, and *caution*.

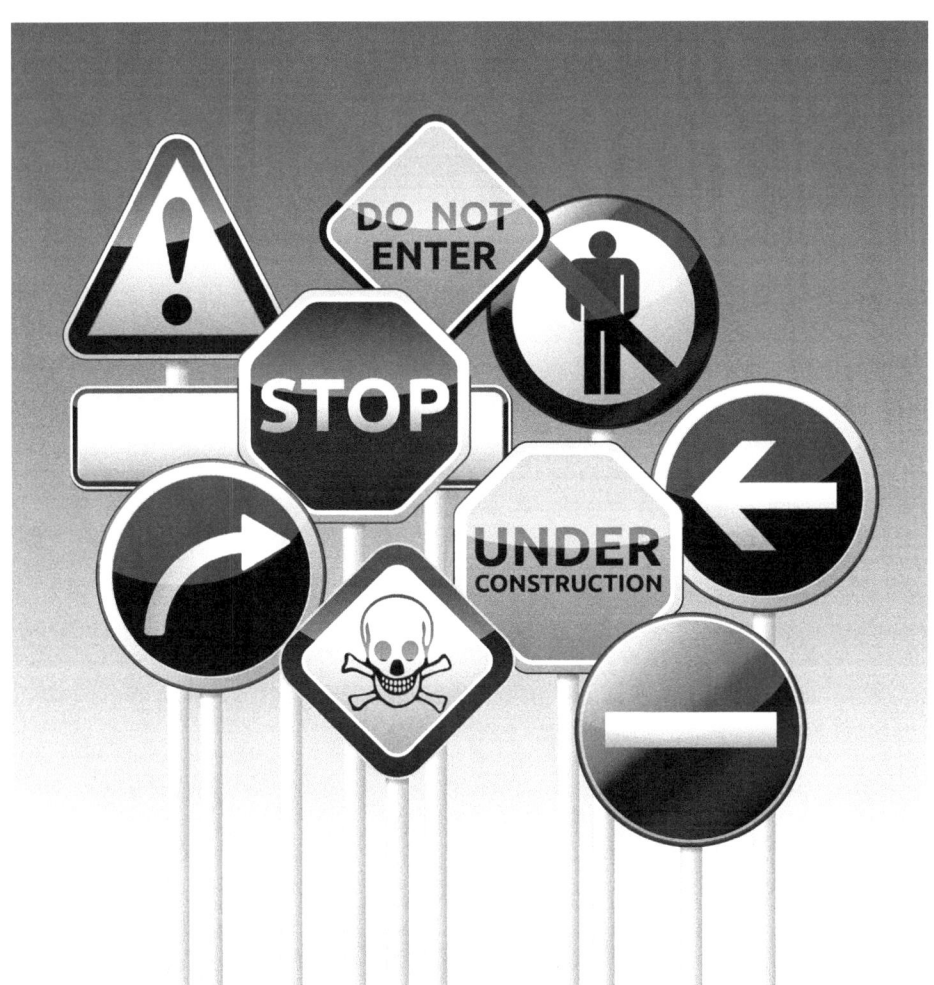

6 Vocabulary for managing and understanding time concepts: Add vocabulary words such as *now, tomorrow, soon, yesterday, today, first, next, then*, and *finally* to your child's communication options. Words that help us manage our time also help us regulate our time. Your child is moving from dependence to supported independence. Time schedules are a part of our world and regulating our daily life. Teaching your child these words by hearing them, seeing them, and using them will support their literacy skills and regulate themselves, understand others' schedules. Add words to support time in space such as, *here*, and *there*.

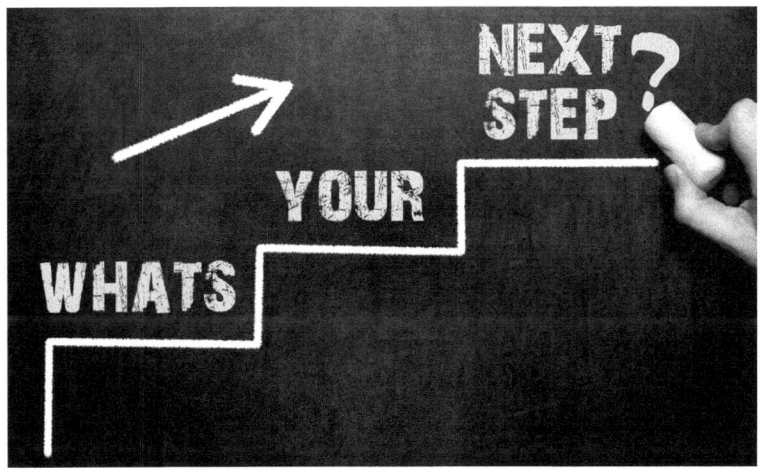

7 Vocabulary for challenging words in English: Speech generating devices have built in vocabulary for an AAC user to access. Working with challenging word changes will likely need to be explicitly taught.

Irregular past tense verbs such as eat and ate, do and did,
Irregular plurals such as foot-feet, tooth-teeth, mouse-mice

8 Vocabulary for slang

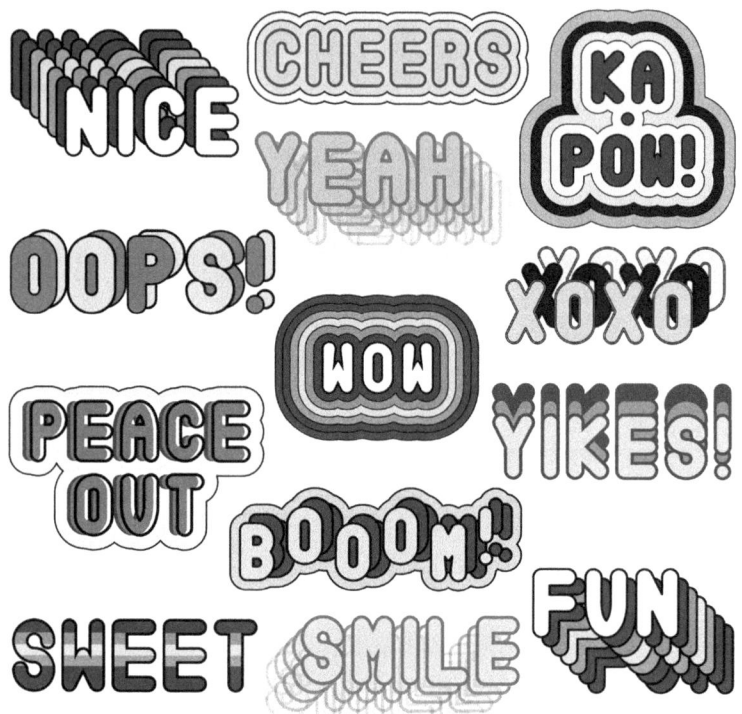

9 Incorporate age appropriate slang and comments into conversation. Slang words can bring conversations to life in a unique way. The words specific to a family, social, or cultural group add richness and connectivity. Sometimes slang words add humor such as. *Duh*, for, of course I understand. Feel free to add slang words to your child's communication board or device to add to the richness of the messages. Decide which language is socially appropriate or is not advised.

Bridging Skills with tools and access

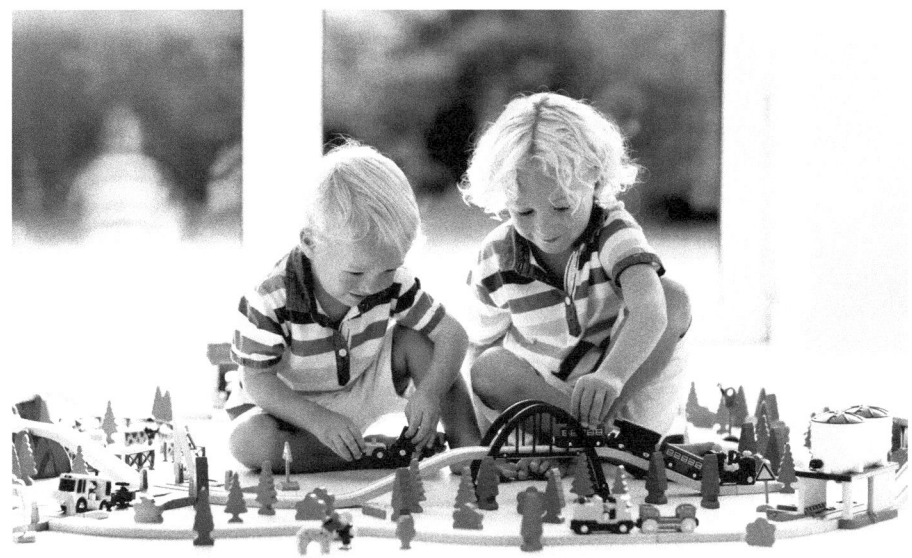

○ My child's multimodal communication plan

It is time for an AAC communications toolkit check. Ask yourself: *What is the status of communication my child is using with the AAC tools and devices including the use of the body? Do the tools work operationally? Do they meet my child's communicative purposes?* Bridging Skills is a great time to get into the habit of completing a regular AAC toolkit check because people change. Children's physical access changes. Their motivation changes. Their program solving skills change. For that matter, technology changes, software, hardware, and interfaces update. New research informs new technology. Revisit your child's completed protocol, *Hear Me into Voice*, and note changes and updates. How is my child using the important smiles, eye contact, silences in communication? What operational skills need support? While you are double checking what is working and what is not, consider trialing other communication tools and access methods. Now is a perfect time to understand what it means to feature match your child's skills with technology.

○ Feature matching children's communication skills with high tech AAC displays

Optimize success in selecting the best high tech AAC device by matching your child's communication skills with the display features the high tech AAC device has to offer. According to Marx and Locast (n.d.) from the Communication Aids & Systems Clinic at the Waisman Center, University of Wisconsin, feature matching is the process in which the team of professionals work with the child and family to optimize the child's present communication skills and future

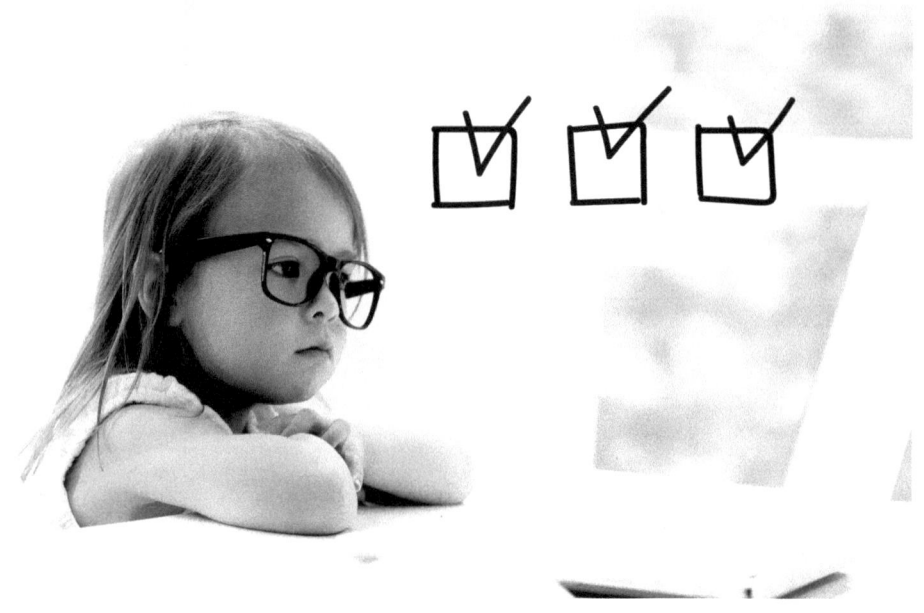

needs with a variety of communication devices and tools. Feature matching informs wise decision making.

Symbols represent language. We all use a combination of symbols every day and so should our children that use AAC. The goal in AAC symbol selection is to *optimize meaningfulness* for the AAC user and in turn for the communication partner. Symbols must be salient, thus meet the communication need with functional objective associations including feelings and emotions. For example, when a child wants to express *friendly*, a symbol for *happy* does not express the correct meaning, but *kind* might. Symbols are everywhere including objects (e.g. mini, partial, and whole), pictures (e.g. photographs, drawings), and in writing that represent single or complex ideas. A *visual scene*, as you recall from *Getting Started* and *Building Fundamentals*, is an image that represents an environment (e.g. classroom, kitchen, park) that may have popup or a sidebar of icons that represent more specific words, objects, or ideas (e.g. requesting a marker at the art table in the classroom visual scene). Factors considered for the organization of the page sets include the AAC user's attention, memory, and receptive and expressive communication skills. Written language is represented around the world through various types of alphabet-based systems. Logographic characters that represent words and phrases such as Chinese and characters that represent not just individual sounds but whole syllables is found in a syllabary language such Korean. Compare and contrast the meaningfulness of the symbols of high tech AAC. Empower the child that uses AAC and communication partners with meaningful symbols that invite participation across the languages.

Display pages and buttons. Displays of icons for the production of verbal messages are preprogrammed on most dynamic display or high-tech speech generating devices. The icons are shown on a variety of *pages* as in a book.

Together they form page sets that may be located in *folders*. Most high-tech devices come pre-programmed with thousands of images with letters, numbers, words, and quick phrases or sentences of a given language. A choice of languages is an option on several devices. The background color of an icon or button, the border of the icon, and the grid spaces between the icons can be programmed for width and color to support your child's visual and attention needs.

Folders. Sometimes an icon represents a *folder* that opens to additional page sets of icons. Many times, folders with page sets have categorical information (e.g. *colors, foods associated with breakfast, lunch, or dinner*). Other times folders are organized linguistically that may include grammatical icons with forms of words (e.g. making an object plural by adding s, turning it into an adjective or verb options of present tense *look, looking*; past tense *looked*, and future tense *will* look). A folder is often differentiated by background color and/or by a different icon border design that makes it look like a paper folder.

Visual scenes. A visual scene is a form of a page set that may have additional popup features or a side navigational bar of additional word, phrase, or sentence choices to see and hear. The display in which an integrated scene (typically a photograph) presents people engaged in shared activities, with 'hotspots' for the concepts embedded within (O'Neill, Wilkinson & Light, 2019). Visual scenes thus offer context that can support users and communication partners in conveying meaning and intentions. Visual scenes can be created from photos as well as vendor supplied static display as well by printing out scenes from a dynamic display.

Icon to grid size and the impact on visual memory. How many icons are typically on a page? Some start with one, move onto two or three, four, and eventually as many as 64 all depending upon the size of the icons. The child's vision status and scanning ability may influence which size of the icons is best. Often the size of the icons is based on grid size and not on vision status (e.g. one icon fills the allotted grid space, two icons split the space, four icons across four quadrants, and etc.). Sometimes, the entire grid may not be in direct view and the user will need to know and physically be required to access one display to scroll to another display of more precise vocabulary. Scrolling requires that the child have the visual memory to recall that they can access more icons by scrolling.

Many high-tech speech generating devices have the option to *hide* icons and their messages to make the selection process easier at first. Hiding buttons means a programmed icon will not be in view until needed yet maintains the location of the remaining icons in view thus making the page less visually complex. Sometimes even the icons that the child knows are temporarily hidden to teach the placement and motor plan of an unknown icon or to teach a specific series of icons to produce a message. Hiding icons does not require that the child re-learn the location of existing vocabulary.

Voice. Speech generating devices have digitized or human voice recordings, synthesized or computer-generated voices, or both. A combination of digitized and synthesized voices can be generated and uploaded to high technology speech generating devices. When possible, record the AAC user's sibling's or peer's voice as a great digitized voice for the child rather than an adult's voice. Explore the synthesized voice options. Let your child choose their favorite synthesized voice.

Audibility. Investigate the audio loudness capacity of the speech generating device. Can the device project messages loudly enough for your child's common communication environments at home, school, and in the community? Does the loudness meet the child's communication partners' listening abilities across environments? If not, is it possible and realistic to attach and use external speakers for special occasions?

Access. There are many ways a child can access or use AAC technology. *Direct selection*, as noted in *Getting Started* and reviewed here, entails using any part of the body to touch a tool or device or activates a device such as fingers, knees, eye gaze, eye blinks, and the promising future of brain interface technology. A *keyguard* provides a raised surface between icon buttons that supports a user with imprecise motor movements with direct selection. As you recall from *Building Fundamentals*, the keyguard is a hard plastic external overlay that fits the grid and button size. *Activation*, as first noted in *Getting Started*, may include touch, degrees of motor movement or pressure by the body or eyes using dwell time and release settings on switches and speech generating devices. *Indirect selection* entails an additional tool or form of technology that a child uses to access AAC. Examples of indirect selection include a child moving across a display by moving a computer mouse, adapted mouse, head pointers, light pointer, head mouse, stylus, joystick, track pad, trackball, and numerous switches. There are many switch options such as a proximity switch that activates when the user gets close to the surface but does not require touch to activate. There is also button, pillow, string, and many, many, more options. *Scanning* occurs when a page set is highlighted in a set pattern that may include item by item linear scanning, row-column scanning, or group scanning. The activation of a scanned icon can be made using a direct modality or using a switch through inverse selection when the switch is held down and released to make a selection. Step scanning requires the person press one switch across each button to navigate to the selection and second switch to activate the message. Automatic scanning can be set by item, row-column, or group and then be activated by a switch. Circular scanning, while used less often, may be an option. *Visual feedback* may during scanning may include highlighted icons, zooming, or outlined borders. *Auditory feedback* supports auditory learners and people with visual impairments by speaking the button name during scanning and then the message upon activation. Both visual and auditory scanning require attending to generating a message that requires additional time, memory, and attention spans.

Programming options. Consider the intuitiveness of the programming options. Learning how to program a device may seem daunting at first but most companies make the ease of editing a priority. With a little practice, programming and editing becomes easier, however, devices that are challenging to program or edit are more likely to be abandoned. Make sure you establish an intuitive way to locate novel folders and pages to locate them as quickly as possible.

Size, aesthetics, weight, and durability. The right size of a device comes down to how well a person can access the vocabulary for receptive and expressive language purposes. Applications on phone technologies may have icons that are too small to access or require scrolling which is potentially both a motor and memory decision. Similarly, tablets and applications are often selected due to the tablet size, price, and pleasing aesthetics with less regard for other features on other speech generating devices such as type of symbols, language organization, accessibility, weight, audibility, and durability. Phones and tablets usually weigh less than more speech generating device in computers that may require back up batteries and with carrying cases come in at three to eight pounds. Feature match to your child's size and strength.

Positioning and transporting devices. Mounts to hold devices come in many formats that allow optimal positioning for selecting messages with pointing, eye gaze, or indirect selection to communicate. Floor and table mounts, as well as wheelchair mounts stabilize devices for access depending upon the user's position, lying in bed, sitting in a wheelchair, standing, moving from place to place. For transporting, some users benefit from having shoulder and waist straps as part of their carrying case that may double as protective cases. Work with occupational and physical therapists to match optimal physical positioning with the eyes, head, neck, torso, hips, knees, ankles, and feet to the positioning of tools and devices supported with mounts, stands, and straps.

Operational considerations. In addition to editing and programing, learn about procedures for the initial set up, backing up software, charging the devices, and creating displays for specific daily events, daily set up, downloading and uploading page sets (e.g. calendars, vision scanning games, page sets for books and math, holidays, etc.).

○ Let's not forget support and funding

Support. Vendor representatives help customers determine the right match between the devices their company offers and the child in addition to providing training and support. Companies usually offer paper-based manuals, internet-based manuals, quick troubleshooting tip handouts in paper or online formats, videos, and live online support for troubleshooting. Investigate warranty, maintenance, and repair procedures including borrowing devices during repair. Call the toll-free numbers of vendors for advice or seek online custom support. Have the device serial number ready. Work or learn alongside of interventionists for support. Enlist the support of friends and other parents for their expertise. You are not alone.

Funding. Insurance companies and other public or private agencies support the funding of communication of speech generating devices. An assessment is required along with a report prepared by a speech-language pathologist as part of the funding process. In addition, physician documentation and other documents are usually required. High tech speech generating device companies often having funding departments with company representatives who work with families, interventionists, and other key stakeholders with the funding process. They are knowledgeable about how to work with insurance companies and government programs. Insurance companies may fund devices as durable medical equipment. Local education agencies often serve as sources for funding when the implementation of augmentative and assistive communication technology serves the child in gaining access to the curriculum that includes communication.

Asking good questions about technology

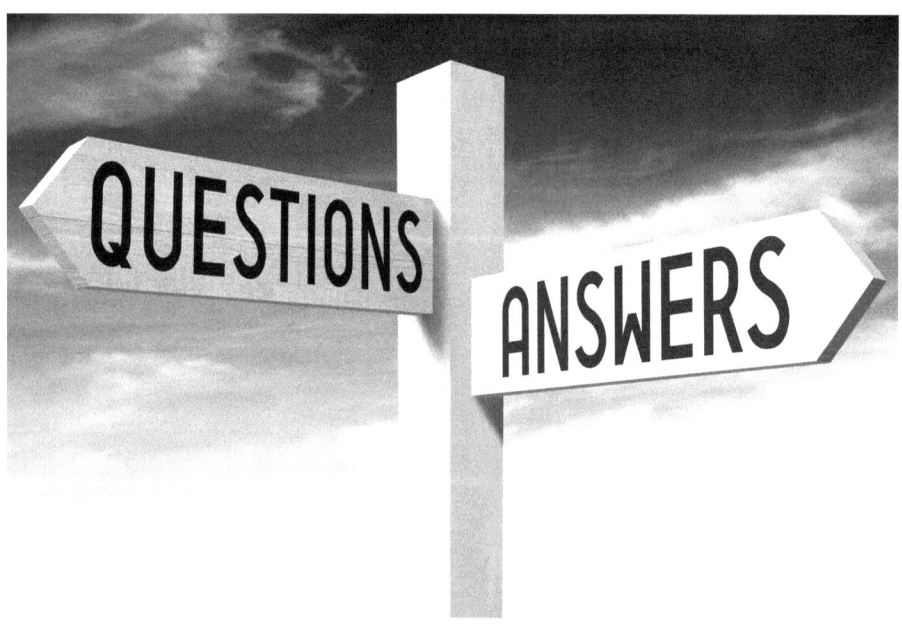

Ask good questions. No one parent, speech-language pathologist, interventionist, or educator has to be an expert on everything about speech generating devices. Vendor representatives know the technology features and they rely on experts who know the child best to feature match technology, support specialists with report writing and funding possibilities. A speech generating device will not match every child perfectly, but the right questions will optimize a good fit. Your child will benefit from your making this a priority. Ask yourself these summary questions.

1 What technologies should be added or replaced to support communication including reading and writing?
2 Is there a need for a different or better access method for my child?
3 Are the symbols appropriate for my child's communication needs? Is my child ready for a greater focus on the words rather than the images? Should we keep the images and build on the complexity and breadth of vocabulary that is available across all of my child's communication modalities?
4 As my child's communication improves, does the present device allow my child to navigate across the modes of communication including reading and writing as efficiently as possible?
5 Is a multimodal communication system in place that includes low tech and high-tech tools?
6 Does my child have non-electronic and electronic modes for quick communication in emergency situations? Have we practiced communication for emergency situations?
7 Which tools and devices are most effective for my child's participation across environments such as the swimming pool, playground, and classroom?

A summary of Bridging Skills

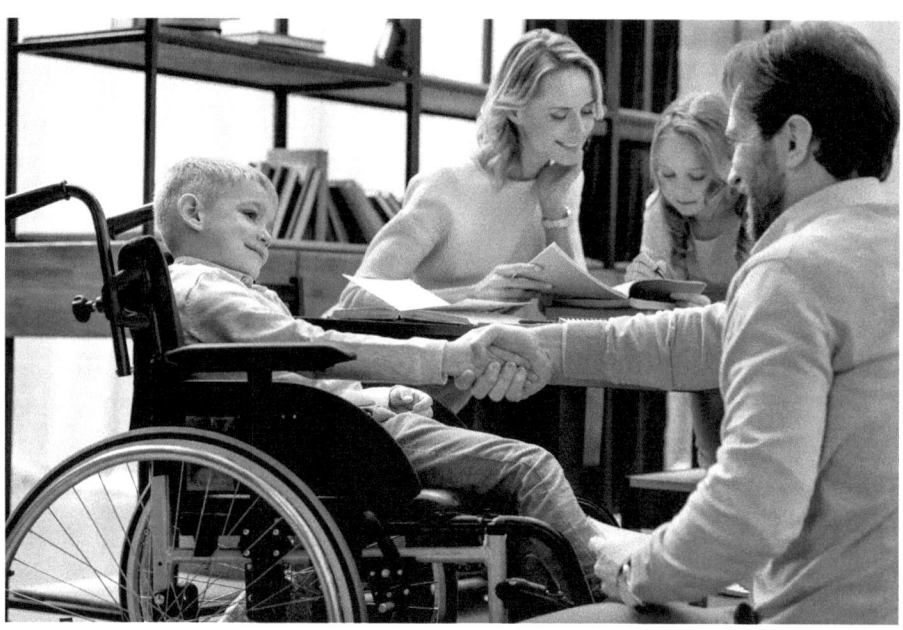

○ Supported independence in inclusive settings

Bridging Skills is a time for your child and you to support independence in inclusive settings. Your child is experiencing success with AAC. Your child requires degrees of support to be successful, not all of the time, but at times to help him or her be a more effective communicator (Beukelman & Mirenda, 2013). Support may be provided in formulating a message, managing the social dynamics of a situation, transferring a communication skill to a new environment, offering the emotional support required to use communication, removing participation barriers, or a combination of all of these needs. As stated in the introduction to *Bridging Skills*, supported independence is creating confidence, self-reliance, self-monitoring, and practice with communication and participation along with a safety net so that when breakdowns occur, guidance will be there to get back on track.

Before we go: a communication wallet

Take a look at the following pages for a template to create a communication wallet (Mayne, 2017). The communication wallet is a low technology AAC tool for users to access to quick messages for social interaction across settings. While the tool is called a communication wallet, feel free to add the information to a communication board, key ring, tip card, or small photo album. The important part is not the wallet itself but the opportunity to have an option for quick messages. The communication wallet may serve as a source for quick social communication, stating needs and intentions, personal identification, and emergency information. Purchase a wallet of the user's choice with a plastic insert with pockets that often hold pictures or credit cards. If the wallet does not have the insert, purchase one separately. Use cardstock or a notecard to type or write out information. Pictures may be used with or without words as appropriate for the user.

○ Wallet insert page ideas

Personal:

- ◉ *My name is _____.*
- ◉ *I may be hard to understand when I speak because I have (disability), I am a person with _____, I had a stroke/traumatic brain injury/other.*

Consider what personal details you wish to include:

- ◉ *I go to (name school, clinic, center, etc.) _____, or I live at (address) _____, or I work at_____, I understand _____ (other languages).*

Best ways to communicate with me:

- ◉ *I understand (e.g. two to three word phrases, short sentences, everything you say _____*
- ◉ *I understand yes/no questions always/usually/sometimes.*
- ◉ *Please find _____ at (phone number/room number/address/other). He or she will understand me best.*
- ◉ *Give me three choices to answer your question.*

- ◉ *I use my _____*
    - ◎ *voice/my head to say (e.g. yes and no).*
    - ◎ *wallet for quick communication.*
    - ◎ *tip cards for extending interaction.*
    - ◎ *(name) device to communicate more complex ideas.*

Social greetings (option: write in cues to the user to look at their communication partner after they say *hi*):

- ◉ *Hi!*
- ◉ *How are you?*
- ◉ *I'm fine.*
- ◉ *See you later.*
- ◉ Other

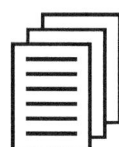

Requesting assistance:

◉ *I need a break.*
◉ *I need help.*
◉ Other

Self-regulation:

◉ Draw a thermometer and color in sections with a range 1–4 or 1–10 as appropriate for the user as a gauge of the range of feelings the person is experiencing from *really well* to *really upset.*
◉ *Relaxation tips that work for me are _____*

Emergency contact information:

◉ Names and phone numbers of family, guardians, caregivers, approved contacts
◉ List of required medicine, pain scale
◉ List of required AAC technologies with pictures of devices, cords and other accessories

Important photo identification:

◉ Driver's license
◉ State issued identification card
◉ School identification card

Other documents:

◉ Daily schedule
◉ School class schedule
◉ Campus map
◉ Bus schedule
◉ Anxiety/emotions/feelings thermometer

Consider color coding areas for context: Personal information, How I Communicate, and Choices with a note to an unfamiliar communication partner such as, *Ask me to point.* Each users' wallet will be different. Use these ideas as a springboard of new or different ideas appropriate for each individual. See the image for an example of a communication wallet. Note the AAC user is literate and therefore does not need picture icons for the messages. However, the thermometer is a helpful visual for the AAC user under times of stress. Note

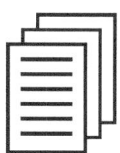

the tab on the second image. Rather than color coding for context, sections of the wallet are tabbed by category nouns, verbs, descriptors, places etc. allowing the user to get to desired sections more efficiently.

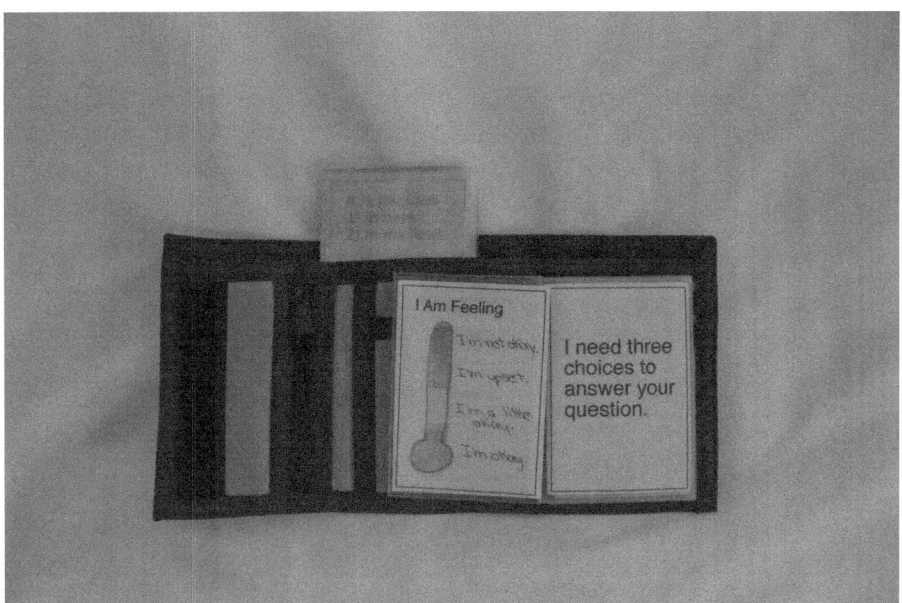

References

Beck, I. L., McKeown, M. G. & Kucan, L. (2013). *Bringing words to life* (2nd ed.). New York, NY: The Guilford Press.

Beukelman, D. & Mirenda, P. (2013). *Augmentative and alternative communication: Supporting children and adults with complex communication needs*. Baltimore, MD: Paul H. Brookes Publishing.

Bookshare. (2020). Retrieved from www.bookshare.org/cms/

Center for Literacy and Disability Studies. (1995). Retrieved from www.med.unc.edu/ahs/clds/

Delpit, L. (1995). *Other people's children: Cultural conflict in the classroom*. New York, NY: New Press.

Federal Communications Commission. (n.d.). Telecommunications relay service – TRS. Retrieved from www.fcc.gov/consumers/guides/telecommunications-relay-service-trs

Geisel, T. (1960). *Green eggs and ham*. New York, NY: Penguin Random House.

Godin, S. (2014, February 6). *If I fail more than you do, I win* [Video file]. Retrieved from www.youtube.com/watch?v=I1Y-usP1mV0&list=PLiYcI981tOLjRmlsnYMXGSNmpaTy-Xz1T&index=9&t=0s

Gray, C. (2015). *The new social story book: Revised & expanded*. Arlington, TX: Future Horizons.

Hawking, S. & Hawking, L. (2013). *George and the big bang*. New York, NY: Simon & Schuster Books for Young Readers.

Klein, C. (2017). Communication and developing relationships for people who use augmentative and alternative communication. *Assistive Technology Outcomes and Benefits, 11*, 58–65.

Light, J. (1989). Toward a definition of communicative competence for individuals using augmentative and alternative communication systems. *Augmentative and Alternative Communication, 4*(5), 137–144.

Light, J. & Kelford-Smith, A. (1993). Home literacy experiences of preschoolers who use AAC systems and of their nondisabled peers. *Augmentative and Alternative Communication, 9*(1), 10–25.

Light, J. & McNaughton, D. (2012). Accessible literacy learning. Retrieved from www.mytobiidynavox.com/#/morestuff/all

Light, J. & McNaughton, D. (2014). Communicative competence for individuals who require augmentative and alternative communication: A new definition for a new era of communication? *Augmentative and Alternative Communication, 30*(1), 1–18.

Light, J., McNaughton, D. & Caron, J. (2019). New and emerging AAC technology supports for children with complex communication needs and their communication partners: State of the science and future directions. *Augmentative and Alternative Communication*, *35*(1), 26–41.

Literacy for Children with Combined Vision and Hearing Loss. (n.d.). Retrieved from http://literacy.nationaldb.org/

Marx, A. & Locast, M. (n.d.). AAC feature matching overview. Retrieved from www.aacpdm.org/UserFiles/file/IC2-Marx-22.pdf

Mayne, L. (2017). *Augmentative and alternative communication: Creation and implementation of an effective AAC plan*. Montclair, CA: California Speech-Language Hearing Association District 10.

Moreau, M. R. (1994). Story grammar marker. Retrieved from https://mindwingconcepts.com/collections/story-grammar-marker

O'Neill, T., Wilkinson, K. M. & Light, J. (2019). Preliminary investigation of visual attention to complex AAC visual scene displays in individuals with and without developmental disabilities. *Augmentative and Alternative Communication*, *35*, 240–250.

Rogers, S. (1999). *Hearing them into voice: The hermeneutics of listening to children who cannot speak: A dynamic approach to assessing and teaching communication* (Unpublished doctoral dissertation). Claremont Graduate University, CA.

Rummel-Hudson, R. (2011). A revolution at their fingertips. *Perspectives on Augmentative and Alternative Communication*, *20*(1), 19–23.

Smith, S. (2020). Expanding expression tool. Retrieved from www.expandingexpression.com/

Super Duper Publications. (2019a). Retrieved from www.superduperinc.com/

Super Duper Publications. (2019b). Compare and contrast fun deck. Retrieved from www.superduperinc.com/products/view.aspx?pid=FD45&s=compare-and-contrast-fun-deck#.XYf19pNKh0s

Super Duper Publications. (2019c). That's silly fun deck. Retrieved from www.superduperinc.com/products/view.aspx?pid=FD29&s=thats-silly-fun-deck&lid=41E46A95#.XXbT4JNKiqA

Tar Heel Reader. (n.d.). Retrieved from https://tarheelreader.org/

Tyler, A. A., Lewis, K. E., Haskill, A. & Tolbert, L. C. (2002). Efficacy, and cross-domain effects of morphosyntax and a phonological intervention. *Language Speech Hearing Services in Schools*, *33*(1), 52–66.

Westby, C. (2019, February 22). *Play and language: The roots of literacy* [Live Webinar]. Retrieved from https://catalog.pesi.com/item/play-language-roots-literacy-35343#tabDescription

Zangari, C. (2012). Call me later: 5 supports for phone communication for persons using AAC. http://prAACticalaac.org/prAACtical/call-me-later

6 Maximizing Participation

Responsive interaction

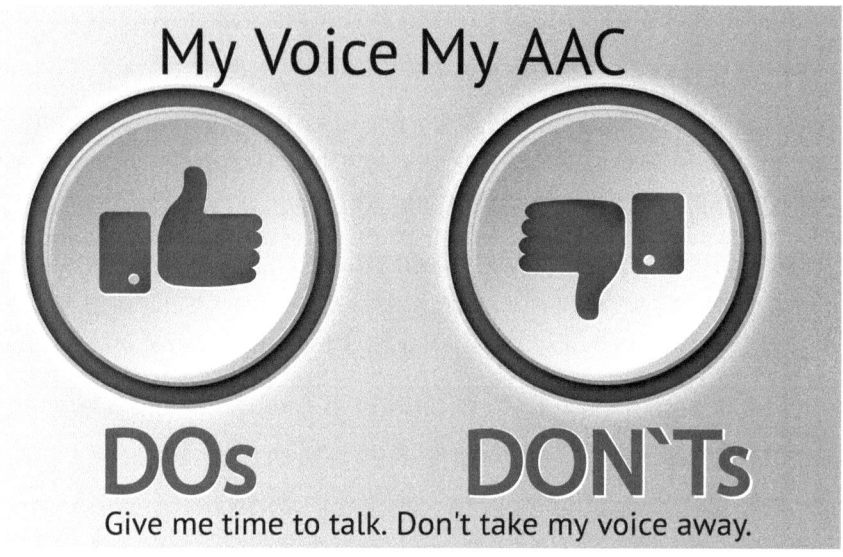

My Voice My AAC

DOs   DON`Ts

Give me time to talk. Don't take my voice away.

I could go around the world six times, take every university course, and still not learn as much about life and God as I have by being with Joy.

-Nurse (Rogers, 1999)

Welcome to *Maximizing Participation*, a spectacular augmentative and assistive communication finale and launching pad all in one. How is *Maximizing Participation* a finale? This chapter brings together the wealth of communication tools your child is using to understand and participate in the world with the expression of ideas he or she has to say for a variety of communication purposes. That is a spectacular finale to celebrate ability in all of its complex forms. How is *Maximizing Participation* a launching pad? Now that your child has an array of tools and strategies, we see the importance of asking the right questions as we continue to build on developing social skills, explore new communication activities, work with facilitators in ways to support successful communication, and dive into more sophisticated levels of literacy and vocabulary for the expression of simple and complex ideas. What is *Maximizing Participation* all about? It is about what your child's communication looks and sounds like now, what communication will look and sound like next, what communication is not quite what you expect it to be, and so … What exactly are you going to do about that? One can argue this model can represent every stage of development. You are right and we encourage any intervention team to proceed accordingly.

The now: Your child is clear on participating using his or her own communication modalities. Familiar communication partners understand, or at a minimum, are aware your child communicates in multiple modalities for many purposes. Less familiar communication partners see inviting tip cards that help them bridge communication with the AAC user.

The next: Ask yourself questions about what skills your child still needs to be developed for the child to maximize communication and participation? We are all life-long learners. Consider what new vocabulary needs to be integrated into your child's life. New vocabulary is required out of necessity or exposure to new experiences both socially and academically. We learn new topics, new technology, and new ways of managing and integrating information. Choose the voice of the tool whether recorded by a peer or chosen from the array of vendor supplied voices. *My child who is Maximizing Participation benefits from The Next functional use of everyday tools by peers and communication partners participating in the community.*

The not quite: As is typical in all of our next steps in learning, we recognize our strengths and areas where we need to improve. Ask the right question for your child: *Where does my child still experience barriers in communication and participation?* Enlist the help of interventionists to determine logical next steps for comprehension, literacy, vocabulary, and forms of expression to maximize your child's potential.

The now what: So, *now what do I do*? You look at the purposes of communication. You look at the status of your child's communication competencies. Decide what skills in each area are successful today and what skills will help your child be a better communicator tomorrow. What is your child's short and long-term goals socially and academically? What does success look like?

We can address *Maximizing Participatio*n by asking and answering three good questions:

#1 Does my child have a way to comprehend and express the purposes of the communication with people that understand and value different modes of communication? To answer this question, verify the modes of communication using the protocol *Hear Me into Voice.* Consider how your child uses each mode of communication (e.g. nonverbal unaided use of the body, vocalizations, word approximations, verbalizations; or aided use of communication boards, wallets, rings, books; vocalizations, word approximations, verbalizations; low tech single message or high-tech speech generating devices). Invest in supporting communication partners with tip cards of how your child communicates and training to support communication and resulting participation.

#2 Does my child, facilitators, and communication partners have ownership of the communication competencies supporting participation? Educators, coaches, and any expert in their field have ownership of their specialty. Most communication partners are not experts in AAC and may not fully understand your child's complex communication profile. Support your child's less familiar communication partners, that may include experts learning other's disciplines and, as promoted throughout this book, learning from parents. Engage experts and observe what successful participation looks like for a child that uses AAC.

Let your child's participation drive language and vocabulary. Vocabulary does not drive participation. Ask communication partners, *How do children play the game? What would be a fun way for my child to play? What do I want my child to learn?* Notice the questions do not say, *What vocabulary will I program?* The questions on participation invite the needed vocabulary. Questions about participation are exciting because they generate possibility for learning, connection, and fun. Selecting words from word lists is daunting. Selecting words for your child to talk about a party or a school project is fun. It is doable because there is a focus. Participation leads you to the core and fringe vocabulary your child needs. The focus on participation first and vocabulary second validates knowledge and learning objectives teachers and interventionists have for children through well designed tasks but may need specific help with incorporating AAC. The focus on participation lends people to think about the child's strengths first, and then addresses the needs such as required vocabulary and the type of tools and devices and access methods. **A focus on participation is ownership for everyone.**

#3 How do I support my child in Maximizing Participation? In addition to the answers from the previous two questions, use these 20 examples to get you started *Maximizing Participation* across environments. You will note that some examples are communication based and some are participation based. Success is success. Decide what success looks like today.

Environments and examples of success

Environment	Success: Learning and Ownership in Participation
1 Home	Expressing to a family member one way he or she communicated that day using any modality
2 School	Playing with a friend; Giving a speech with your speech generating device
3 Community	Going to- or trying a new activity
4 Place of worship	Using a name tag to support communication partners and commenting one-two-three times
5 Art class	Participating in a new craft
6 Physical Education or Team	Getting in the game and cheering for my teammates
7 Music	Using technology to play a personal playset
8 Semantics	Learning a new vocabulary word today
9 Syntax (word order)	Generating a story using simple and complex sentences with conjunctions, clauses and phrases
10 Morphology (word beginnings/endings)	Using prefixes and suffixes to manipulate words
11 Speech sounds	Using a repair or compensatory strategy to improve intelligibility (e.g. holding up four fingers while saying *po*)
12 Talking with friends	Participating with a friend at recess
13 Talking with family	Setting and sharing plans for the weekend
14 Talking with teachers	Answering one question in class
15 Talking with clerks	Paying for an item at the store using quick phrases such as, *Just a minute while I get my money to pay. Thank you.*
16 Talking with less familiar people	Using appropriate social greetings and closures; talking about appropriate topics and comments
17 Birthdays	Going to a birthday party and participating in an activity in which turn taking and choice making occur
18 Family gatherings	Telling a joke that engages family members in telling more jokes, commenting on board game, selecting a movie
19 Community event	Going to a new event and sharing about the experience
20 Holidays	Giving directions to decorate for a holiday, exchanging holiday messages

Learn more about *Maximizing Participation* with your child through the case study about Joy. Learn from her family, friends, educators, and interventionists who support her participation. Learn how Joy and each communication partner's ownership in participation using AAC across environments maximizes everyone.

A case study in Maximizing Participation: meet Joy (In loving memory of Joy's 16 years of maximizing life)

Meet Joy, a Japanese-American 12-year-old middle school tween, a sister and daughter who is *Maximizing Participation* at home, school, and in the community. Joy is outgoing and enjoys dynamic friendships. She participates in general education curriculum and has expectations to go onto college. She was diagnosed at eight months of age with the most severe form of spinal muscular atrophy called Werdnig-Hoffmann syndrome, which degenerates her nerve cells that transmit impulses to her muscles impacting the movement of her arms, legs, speaking, chewing, swallowing, and diaphragm for breathing. Even smiles require time and energy. Her parents know from statistics that 10 percent of children with this diagnosis do not live beyond their fifth year. When Joy turned five, their $1,000,000 health insurance policy was maxed out. Her mother remarked *you have to plan for them to grow up because your child might be that one or two out of a 100 who do, you just don't know*. Her family joyfully adopted Joy at birth and continues to embrace and love her fully.

Joy is an award-winning student. *She is getting all As*, reported Silvia, Joy's licensed vocational nurse who works as an assistant in her classroom where they read stories, create drawings, and share in decision-making. She typed her 5th grade essay on the American colonies using a computer interfaced with Morse code. Her teacher entered her essay in a county essay competition that earned a blue ribbon! Joy navigates from place to place by using a joystick on her electric powered wheelchair. Joy's mother spearheads the coordination of Joy's care while her father uses his technological to support Joy as she accesses tools and devices for learning and communication. *You have got to embrace the illnesses and pain*, her mother affirms, *then you learn and grow*.

○ Section 1 Social interaction: How did Joy expect others to interact with her?

Joy has high expectations for her social interaction as she participates in activities. She appreciates her parents who expose her to everything from watching cartoons to attending a performance of *Les Miserables*, to meeting visitors, and discussing life questions such as her uncle's cancer diagnosis. Together they select themes for her birthday parties and have sleepovers with her friends that, of course, include pedicures. They know in order for Joy to fully participate socially and academically, she needs a way to express her cogent reasons, negotiate, trade and barter, give compliments and defend herself. What they are really instilling in Joy is that she can and must speak for herself!

Joy's outgoing personality aids in breaking down the social barriers. For example, when others look at her wheelchair and withdraw from interacting with Joy or focus on the accompanying medical equipment, Joy waits and looks away. When someone smiles at her she offes an eyebrow lift as a welcoming invitation. During recess, Joy and her friends often cluster together with their paper dolls displayed on her wheelchair tray, each contributing to the action of the story of their play and have fun without exerting too much of Joy's energy. They navigate the school campus, Joy in her wheelchair and her friends walking beside her, on their way to general education classes. They usually are able to interpret her eyebrow movements and glances. They talk about boys and share stories of who likes whom, share opinions and ideas, naturally take turns and then playfully interrupt each other. Joy affirms her agreement or disagreement with her voice and eyes. They all participate in the 6th-grade play Joy writes and directs called, *Six Dancing Princesses*. She arranges for the costumes and casts the roles. The principal arranges for the performance to be premiered for the entire school.

Joy has many ways to communicate with her family, friends, and other communication partners. The easiest way to say *yes* is for Joy to raise both eyebrows. When she wants to say, *You wouldn't believe it!* or when she is disgusted, she rolls her eyes. Anger is also obvious when she, according to her mother, *squishes her eyes, her eyebrows came down*. Joy communicates ideas and answers with her eyes, eyebrows, faint voice, tongue and lips that express far beyond a simple *yes* or *no.* By age nine she was unable to control many of her facial muscles and so lost her outward smile. Yet she teases, tells jokes, and shares beliefs and values using her speech generating device now that it has finally arrived. Joy has a great sense of humor even though her giggle was cut short sometimes by her limited breath supply. Helen, a home health aide states, *Respiration and eating are like running a marathon every day. Each movement she makes requires extraordinary energy. When a typical body burns 100 calories, Joy burns twice as much.* Doctors, along with her parents, decide that having a ventilator for oxygen supply and a stomach tube for feeding will help her reallocate her daily energy. Students and teachers assimilate to the audible inhalation huff and expiratory hiss of the respiratory equipment.

There are daily communication realities Joy confronts. Joy's mother reports, *Unfortunately, some people in the community treat Joy like a 'rock!' She is really just scenery to them. At church, the older people always go over and talk to her. A couple of kids her age go out of their way to talk to her. Then someone else comes and just pulls Joy's friend away from her. It breaks my heart.* Joy becomes reluctant to talk to people when they ignore her or do not talk to her as an intelligent person. They do not understand that Joy has something to say and welcomes friendship.

⊙ Questions for Reflection

Section 1 Social interaction: How did Joy expect others to interact with her?

1   Indicate T=True and F=False.
    a   _____ People learned to expect that Joy would say 'yes' by raising her eyebrows
    b   _____ Communication partners listened, interpreted, and create messages
    c   _____ Joy is reluctant to communicate when people ignore her and treated her like a 'rock'

2   Compete the sentences with the word bank about Joy's strengths and tools for AAC success.

    Word bank: negotiates, embrace, eyes and eyebrows, write and perform

    Joy, a great friend and student, uses her _____ to express quick yes and no answers. She shares information and _____ with her friends using her speech generating device. She likes to _____ plays with her friends as well as go to the mall. Her mother uses the mantra, 'You have got to _____ the illnesses and pain, then you learn and grow.'

Answers

1   Letter a. is True. Joy used her eyebrows and gaze to relay messages. Letter b. is False. Less familiar communication partners did not create messages based on the context of the situation, but familiar partners did. Letter c. is True. Joy was often treated like a rock, a frustration felt by Joy and her family.
2   Joy, a great friend and student uses her <u>eyes and eyebrows</u> to express quick yes and no answers. She shares information and <u>negotiates</u> with her friends using her speech generating device. She likes to <u>write and perform</u> plays with her friends as well as go to the mall. Her mother uses the mantra, 'You have got to <u>embrace</u> the illnesses and pain, then you learn and grow.'

○ Section 2 Communication activities: In what communication activities did Joy participate?

Joy has a rich array of activities to accomplish her personal, academic, and social goals. She loves independent activities such as drawing, imagining stories, solving math problems, writing, and reading, especially mystery books. Joy's mother embraces these goals and activities as well as appreciating the teachers who allow Joy to participate as a whole child. Her mother asked Joy, *How did you just convert that fraction without looking in the math book or writing it down? Joy told me, I think in my head. Joy was so thrilled she got into the 7th-grade algebra class for next year with other 'motivated' kids. Her brain can handle it. You should hear the math stuff she does in her head. I mean she is doing algebra problems and I am writing it down, and she is way ahead of me. Teachers who lower expectations and pass any student out of misplaced sympathy do a disservice to their students.* After school, Joy usually stretches out on her bed and talks with her mother and her home health nurse and recounts stories from the day and prepares for the next day. They scan and download illustrations for history and science assignments. Sometimes Joy accompanies her mother on errands.

Crafts and fashion design are Joy's passions that drive her love to go shopping on the weekends. On a recent trip with friends Joy bought a wild amethyst lip-gloss, two tubes of hair coloring, and hair gel with sparkling flecks. She delighted in sharing these with her friends. With support she strings beads to make colorful jewelry such as bracelets. She creates artwork about her favorite topics, a woman, an angel, and the sunrise. Others ask to purchase her art, but she and her father hate to part with them. They are framed and hang in the hallway close to her room.

Joy has many interests that include watching sports, interior design, and music. She selects sports to watch with her dad and sister. Her mother, let's just say, is less interested. The trio likes basketball and the Olympics, both summer and winter. Joy comments on the beauty of gymnastics, competitors putting everything on the line, a high score being the pinnacle of success, and overcoming failure. She admires the competition, the physicality, and the tempo. With her interior design interests at the forefront, Joy directs her dad and sister in moving furniture and rehang posters in her room. She likes to organize her bedroom and maintain her sense of style while more medical equipment usurps space. This great fun with her dad, however, the fun comes with the unintended consequence of listening to his music playlist. Later the sisters listen to their music together while making new decorations for their rooms.

Joy has dislikes too. Action movies are *too predictable*, but a romance movie now and again is the ticket. She is not a fan of swinging though wheelchair dancing is fun even when the movement taxes her respiratory system. *She can't scratch an itch without someone being willing to give up what they are doing to help her.* She hates having no way to swat the occasional insect that flies around her. Joy has to cope, and she does. Her mother states, *When Joy has her heart set on something and then she can't do it, she shuts down and won't interact. Leave her alone for a while. She will be just fine. She will come back to you.* Around the time that Joy was in 4th grade she said,

I wish I could walk. Her mother replied, *I wish, too. You know what, you can be with your friends, and read and craft; and when you get to heaven, you are going to be the first in line to dance with Jesus.* Joy's mother proclaimed, *Joy is a beacon of light, hope, strength, and courage. She is my sunshine*.

⊙ Questions for Reflection

Section 3 Communication Activities: In what communication activities did Joy participate?

1   Circle 8 of the bulleted activities that Joy enjoyed participating in at home and school.

⊙ Writing   ⊙ Swinging   ⊙ Music   ⊙ Drawing   ⊙ Shopping

⊙ Watching   ⊙ Sleep overs   ⊙ Reading   ⊙ Designing   ⊙ Watching
Sports   with friends   mystery   Fashion   Action
                                      books   movies

2   What did Joy like to do with her friends? Indicate Yes or No on the line.
   a   _____ Joy loves to do all sorts of crafts including making paper dolls at recess
   b   _____ Joy has very narrow obscure interests that do not require interacting with others
   c   _____ Joy talks about age appropriate topics like who likes whom with her friends
   d   _____ Joy is academic and social. She likes going shopping with peers

Answers

1   Activities that Joy enjoys includes writing stories, listening to music, drawing, going shopping, sleep overs, fashion design, watching sports, and reading mystery books. Activities Joy did not enjoy include swinging and watching action movies.
2   Letter a. is Yes. Joy has multifaceted interests with her friends. Letter b. is No. Her interests are not obscure. Letter c. is Yes. Joy loves to engage in age appropriate topics with her friends where she is an active participant is listening and contributing to the conversation. Letter d. is Yes. Joy is both an academic and has diverse social interests.

○ Section 3 Facilitator strategies: Who are Joy's facilitators and communication partners? What strategies do they use to support Joy's communication?

Joy's facilitators start with her mother, father, interventionists, educators, and home health nurses, especially Helen. Jackie and Mai, her friends since kindergarten, are loyal to her and value her as a shining star in their lives. They support Joy in communicating with less familiar communication partners and co-construct messages with her. That means they watch and read Joy's nonverbal language and use her words in the context of the discussion and environmental setting just like a friend who finishes your sentence, or states, *I know what you mean*. A communication tip card attached to Joy's wheelchair is a strategy she uses to communicate quickly with less or unfamiliar communication partners. Her tip card is akin to an *All About Me* page with questions for communication partners. For example, a statement read, *I like mystery books and writing plays. What do you like to do?* Her best facilitators patiently wait for Joy to initiate topics, respond to others with a question or comment, and if necessary, support less familiar communication partners during conversations. Sometimes Joy rephrases messages or looks for objects in the room or words on a page that provide contextual clues or she may be quiet and wait for the arrival of another person who best interprets her intentions. Her mother reports, *At times she gives up, saying oh never mind but she never throws it back at you. Sometimes people just have no idea what to say or do.*

Then there was Mr. Buck, the formidable history teacher. He set clear expectations for the entire class beginning the first week of school. *Mr. Buck was so gruff! If a student took the wrong seat, talked out of turn, came in late to class, he looked them in the eyeball and said, 'We don't do that in this class. The next time you do it, you are out of here. I am not preparing you to get your high school diploma, I am preparing you to go to college!'* Mr. Buck arranged the desk and chairs in the room so Joy could see him plainly and hear the lessons well. He truly believed in and encouraged every student. Mr. Buck states, *Joy teaches me to ask the right questions*. Then he offers choices from multiple-choice answers and she spells out or says the key content words.

With the resources outlined by the school district-wide drill, her mother was prepared to put in additional supplies to complete a go-bag with supplies in the event of a natural disaster or major emergency. She asks important questions like who is responsible for evacuating Joy? Where will she go? How will she communicate if her speech generating device is not available? They met with first responders at the local fire station and listed Joy's contact persons. Together with Joy's home health nurse, they select emergency food supplies, print out extra communication tip cards with her medication needs and schedule as well as her health history. They *update*

AAC software and backed up AAC files. They make copies of pages from her speech generating device and laminate them so she can communicate with unfamiliar partners and use as a back up. All devices and accessories are labeled, duplicate accessories and communication tools are in the emergency go-bag in her wheelchair.

⊙ Questions for Reflection

Section 3 Facilitator strategies: What strategies do Joy's facilitators use to support Joy's communication?

1   Important strategies that work for facilitators include all EXCEPT which choice?
    a   Wait for Joy to compose her answers
    b   Co-construct messages with her
    c   Believe a tip card is too limiting
    d   Ask the right questions of themselves to maximize Joy's potential

2   What steps are considered to plan for emergency situations regarding AAC? Indicate T=True or F=False
    a   _____ Prepare a go-bag with emergency supplies and communication pages
    b   _____ Natural disasters rarely occur so preparation is not necessary
    c   _____ Label all of Joy's communication tools and accessories with her name
    d   _____ Update AAC software and back up AAC files
    e   _____ Write up emergency contact information, medications and her schedule

Answers

1   Letter c. is the exception. Tip cards are quick messages with vital information about Joy. Her facilitators believe the tip cards support less familiar communication partners. Letters a., b., and d. validate facilitator's actions. Facilitators learn to give Joy time to formulate messages and co-construct messages with her. They all learn how to ask better questions and support Joy in maximizing her opportunity to produce quality answers.
2   All but letter b. is True. It is important to have an emergency go-bag prepared with contact information, health needs, and communication needs. Update AAC software and back up AAC software often so it can be downloaded in the event the device is lost or destroyed. While letter b. is true in that natural disasters are rare, they do occur. Planning is a link in safety.

○ Section 4 Literacy: What reading and writing experience did Joy have and need?

Joy's family read books to her from infancy and now talk with her about significant local, cultural, and world issues. Her enrollment in full inclusion from kindergarten onward meant she learned the fundamentals of reading and writing. She checks out books from the library regularly. She has access to the world of reading through electronic formats on her speech generating device with internet. When her eyes are tired, books with digitized or synthesized voices make books audible. Joy reports, *At first the computer voices were terrible but now they are getting a lot better so now I don't mind*. Books for pleasure and school reading are accessible and she can travel the world a thousand times over through their imagery.

Like all muscles in her body, atrophy impacts hand writing and assistive technology is a solution. Using her very limited hand motions, Joy's home health nurse and mom gave Joy a flair felt tip pen in her right hand and clipped a piece of lined paper to a small Styrofoam meat tray for her to write her assignments. She also made drawings with broader tipped colored pens that required little pressure. Now she uses assistive technology for writing that allows Joy to type with her eyes. On-screen keyboards, programs that utilize abbreviations and reduce keystroke demands, graphic organizers, word prediction, and proofreading tools speed up her productivity. The pièce de résistance is that assistive technology gives Joy's writing a voice that her peers, teachers, and anyone willing to listen, can hear and read. Each grade coursework now demands advanced analysis of main ideas, contexts, and inferences across a variety of genres. The demand is the tip of the expectations for an advanced reader including proof reading and Joy is primed for the challenge. She is authoring text such as this excerpt that she wrote from her prize-winning interview with Mala Langholtz, a Holocaust survivor.

> When I was 11 years old and would have been in 6th grade I was sent to Auschwitz. We were lined up and scrutinized as to who would die in the gas chamber and who would be used for work. The women around me would lift me up using their shoulders as to give the appearance of someone taller and older. My name was taken away and, in its place, I was given a number tattooed on the inside of my arm. Each night we said goodbye instead of good night not knowing if we would survive the night. Somehow, I survived. The older women would share their food with me so I could live to tell their stories.

When Joy wrote her application for a position on the yearbook staff, she gave three reasons, *1) to have fun, 2) to use my talents, and 3) to serve my school.* The yearbook adviser and staff accommodated her reduced schedule so she works three times a week and she can rest and keep her lungs clear. They welcomed her as a valued writer on the staff using assistive technology to interview peers, write stories that express her subjects' voice, and print out her stories.

Section 4 Literacy: In which ways and for what purposes does Joy access literacy?

> Word Bank: on-screen keyboard, yearbook, electronic, voice, proofreading
>
> Joy reads traditional books and books in _____ formats. She writes using eye gaze and an _____. She edits her work efficiently with _____ tools. Utilizing her strengths, she writes for the _____. Assistive technology gives Joy's literacy a _____.

Answer

> Joy reads traditional books and books in <u>electronic</u> formats. She writes using eye gaze and an <u>on-screen keyboard</u>. She edits her work efficiently with <u>proofreading</u> tools. Utilizing her strengths, she writes for the <u>yearbook</u>. Assistive technology gives Joy's literacy a <u>voice</u>.

○ Section 5 Vocabulary: What vocabulary maximizes Joy's participation?

Like most teenagers who read, write, listen, and express themselves Joy has acquired many tiers of everyday words, academic, and domain specific vocabulary she uses in social and academic discussions. She uses core and fringe words fluidly on her speech generating device. She learns about prefixes and suffixes that change the meaning of a root word attending to the Latin influences on language in her English class. She examines the origin of the root word to clarify the meaning. Each of these strategies increases her ability to prepare for university reading demands and conversations with her friends as she matures. If she does not understand a word from the context or is unable to think of the definition, she accesses online tools for definitions, antonyms, and synonyms including examples in sentences. Her educational assistant previews her science text and programs fringe words into her device including vocabulary of astronomy, biology, zoology, chemistry, and ecology. Her history vocabulary requires displaying timelines, labeling political conflicts, knowing important places, and identifying leaders across the world. For math Joy uses her technology to formulate algebraic equations and manipulate geometric shapes.

Joy builds increasingly novel, complex sentences with conjunctions, prepositions, adjectives and adverbs, verb tenses, and all types of clauses on her speech generating device. Beyond individual vocabulary words, Joy, her mother, and other classmates have fun suggesting quick phrases with slang words for greetings, agreeing and disagreeing, making comments, cracking jokes, and even letting off steam. Just like her peers, Joy too finds ways to accept an apology or say she is sorry. She uses her device to ask questions about her medical test results and questions about medications. Sometimes she has to access her keyboard to select every letter for words and in turn pays the price for using precious physical energy and time.

Questions for Reflection

Section 5 Vocabulary: What vocabulary does Joy require to maximize participation?

How can Joy and her team be sure they are maximizing vocabulary for Joy?

a   Have displays that focus on core and fringe vocabulary for course work

b   Teach Joy ways to access technology to search word meanings and edit work

c   Include tiered vocabulary to express levels of social and academic concepts

d   All of the above

Answer

Letter d. All of the above is the correct answer. Joy's educational assistant makes sure Joy has access to core and fringe vocabulary. She is learning and accessing editing software for selecting key words on the internet and tools to support writing tasks. Tiered vocabulary supports her academic and social interaction so she can say, *Exceptional!* Instead of *great*.

○ Section 6 Tools and access: What augmentative and assistive communication tools access methods were tried and are now used to maximize Joy's participation?

Joy's communication partners interpret her very rich social communication from her giggles and eyebrow movement, but Joy requires complex language to express the depths of her thoughts without taxing her motor system. Trials, errors, and successes are consistent themes in the acquisition process of her AAC device. Joy's expressive communication with technology started with a small red single message speech generating device exclaiming, *I'm coming through!* as she moved from class to class. A rehabilitation hospital advised Joy's parents use a computer interfaced with Morse code and two switches that would allow her to shift with a track ball and then select dots and dashes.

When the screen on the speech generating device froze and the mount kept her from using her device in bed at home, she had to get help to construct the sentences she chose. Frustrations ensued. She and her parents were ready *to throw it off a cliff*, a sentiment other AAC users expressed (Rackensperger, Krezman, McNaughton, Williams & D' Silva, 2005). But after months of practice sometimes with her friends playing a game, Joy reported that learning to use Morse code *was not that hard.* She was able to write 11 words per minute. That was a far cry from her peers written production of 38–40 words per minute and forget the 120–160 spoken words per minute.

With the loss of motor skills, Joy now accesses technology through eye gaze. One day Joy and her speech-language pathologist spent the two-hour long district-wide earthquake drill personalizing her device. Did Joy like it at first? *No. I don't like it. My eyes get tired*, Joy grumps. However, with correct lighting and practice, fatigue lessens and her fluency increases. She finds that the ability to interface with software to complete internet research, manage citations, organize ideas, and edit her work, validates her effort. Joy creates complex language, posts assignments, sends emails to her friends, and controls her environment. While she humorously dims lights in her room, the light in her eyes shines perpetually brightly.

⊙ Questions for Reflection

Section 6 Tools and access: How do AAC tools maximize Joy's participation?

Circle the 6 AAC intervention tools and strategies that were tried and implemented.

- ⊙ Single message device
- ⊙ Picture exchange communication
- ⊙ Track ball
- ⊙ High tech speech generating device
- ⊙ Eye gaze
- ⊙ Tip cards
- ⊙ Morse code
- ⊙ Icons on a key ring

Answer

Joy reads, writes, learns, and communicates using a <u>high technology speech generating device</u> with <u>eye gaze</u>. Her <u>tip card</u>, while not high tech, aids communication partners in speaking with Joy. Intervention began with a low-tech <u>single message device</u> and advanced to <u>Morse code</u> computer interface <u>track ball</u> until functional speech generating devices were available and access methods supported her degenerating motor system. Icons on a ring and picture exchange communication require a motor system to manipulate and therefore are not included in her multimodal communication plan.

○ Summary

Joy is *Maximizing Participation* using augmentative and assistive communication to contribute ideas, topics, opinions, and information as she lives her life with others. Joy and her team realize that *Maximizing Participation* is not an end game but a jumping off point, a place to ask the right questions to go forward in participation. As Joy moves into high school and prepares for a university experience, topics such as ethics and personal privacy come into play. Joy will need more vocabulary equal to her emotional and intellectual maturity. She and her facilitators will need to recognize barriers and construct new strategies that help her meet those needs. True to the words she wrote in her yearbook application, *I want to have fun, use my talents, and serve my school.* Many people will value her and her unique contributions as she uses AAC. Take a look at Joy's communication plan that details modalities she uses across the purposes of communication.

Purposes	Nonverbal	Vocal	Low Tech	High Tech
Social Etiquette	Uses eye gaze, eyebrows, and wheelchair positioning	Not viable for quick social etiquette; refer to high tech	Tip card: Rely on facial expressions and *SGD	Vocabulary is programmed in SGDs
Share Information	A tip card notifies communication partners to wait for Joy to share a message	Understands but cannot vocally express a complex intent	Attach a fun board with a tip or joke of the day so Joy has easy access	School staff to investigate online discussion forums for Joy to share academic content
Social Closeness	Sustained eye gaze; physically moves closer in wheelchair; uses quick messages and novel phrases	May have a faint sigh or may just be quiet; may vocalize a bit to people who do understand her	Express nonverbally and SGD to display usually inferred from familiar people	Needs expanded vocabulary yet privacy for expressing positive and negative feelings, and emotions
Wants and Needs	Uses her eyebrows and forehead to indicate yes or no	May use vocal sounds	Copies of high tech displays if she is unable to use her SGD	Current technology access. Update emergency kit

*SGD = speech generating device

Joy's multimodal communication plan across the purposes of communication

Joy, with her team, will update plans regularly to reflect her physical, emotional, and cognitive abilities in relation to the effectiveness of the tools and anticipated advancements in technology. Joy has a brilliant voice. She is a remarkable daughter, friend, student, and member of society who makes a difference with every glance, eyebrow raise, academic and social message. Now it is time to consider how we can maximize her participation through *Communication Activities*.

Maximizing Participation with communication activities

Maximizing Participation with *Communication Activities* focuses on your child <u>and</u> communication partners during participation across environments. If in fact, according to Watzlawick, Beavin and Jackson (1967) 'We cannot not communicate,' and that 'all communication has content and a relationship aspect,' and furthermore that 'the nature of a relationship is dependent on punctuation of the parameters of communication procedures' (pp. 48–71), then we naturally must include a skill set for the communication partners of AAC users. We need communication partners engaged in the process of participation. Prutting and Kirchner (1983) describe language as 'action' (p. 29), a dynamic process with participants moving between links of commenting, questioning, referring, repairing misunderstandings, predicting with language. The good news is that *Maximizing Participation* does not mean perfection in every domain

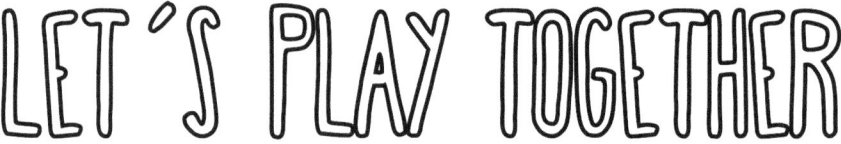

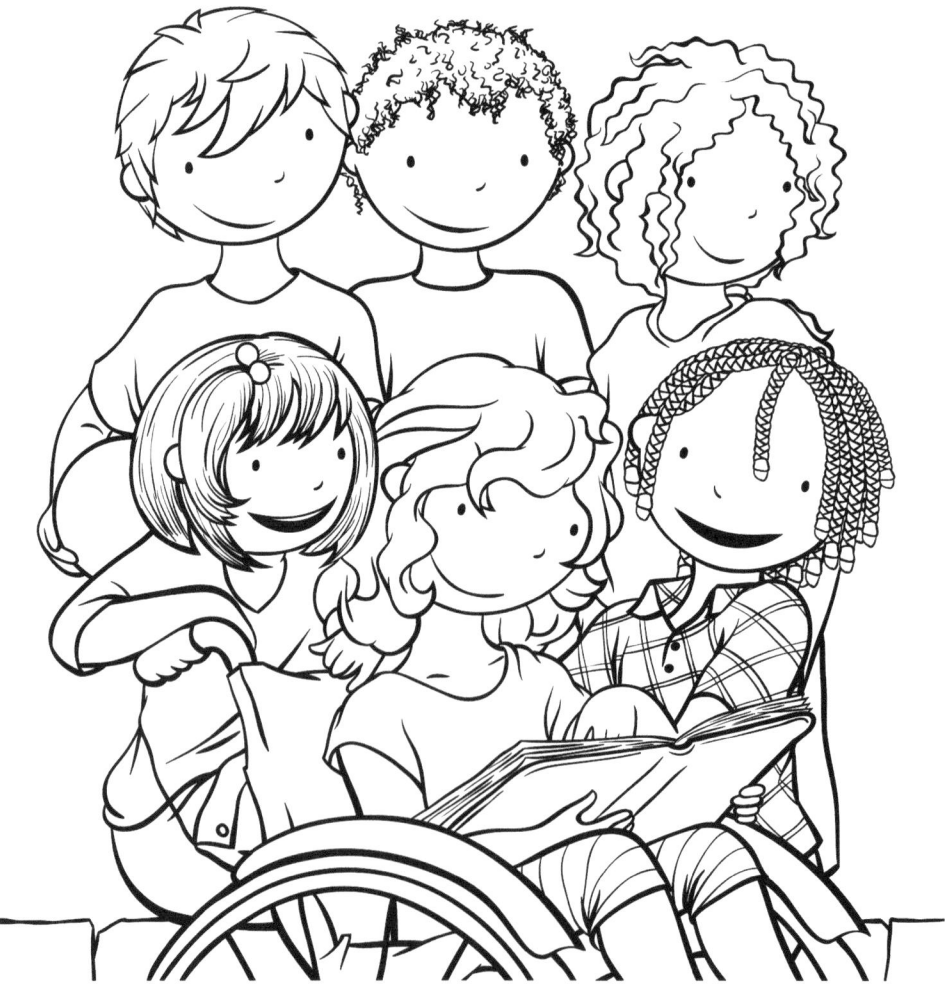

of language today. A message may not be formed with perfect syntax (word order) and morphology (e.g. plural s, past tense -ed) but the intent of a message that may be simple or sophisticated was expressed and understood by others. Language growth, socioemotional growth, academic growth, cognitive growth, sensory growth, behavioral growth, physical growth and more are to be expected, encouraged, and let's not forget … to be celebrated. With the framework in mind that we will support the communication of our AAC user and all partners, let's jump into communication activities for *Maximizing Participation.*

○ Maximizing Participation

Activities Page – Supporting All Communication Partners

1 Break the Ice! Put Yourself Out There with Social Communication
2 Ask for Help: Interacting with Community Helpers
3 I Like Your Hat: The Art of Giving and Receiving Compliments
4 Step into My Office: Barter, Trade, and Negotiate Like a Pro
5 I Did It; I'm Sorry: Fessing Up and Apologizing
6 Emergency Preparedness: A Plan for Communication; A Plan for Action
7 That is Not Okay: Standing Up for Yourself and Others
8 My AAC Book Club

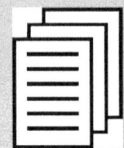

Activity: Break the Ice! Put yourself out there with social communication

A place to start

Ice breakers! Get the ball rolling. Sometimes, or often times, we need to put others at ease in conversation, especially if AAC is involved. Most people do not understand communication devices and your child *Maximizing Participation* does have ways to initiate and break down barriers. The following story is about a man with a physical disability who broke down barriers with two boys. While he did not use AAC, he capitalized on an opportunity to turn a potential failure into success by maximizing his communication.

⊙ Because He Talked to Them

On a grand day at major track and field event, the 1500 meter world record holder in the wheelchair race was navigating the crowds leaving after the day's competition. A few young children were gazing at his impressive competition chair and equally so at his legs that lacked the sinewy upper body tone. Ever the champion, he met their amazed and curious eyes. Undaunted by the familiar stares, the racer engaged the boys with friendly banter, 'Do you like my wheels?' The boys' initial awkwardness melted into giddy joy and conversation with this world class athlete, who did not look like them, and traveled via impressive spheres, made their day because the champion talked to them.

People that use AAC with or without accompanying physical disabilities can make a statement, can ask a question, can initiate or respond to others verbal or verbal engagements to generate interaction. Practicing ice breaker statements gives your child the ability to control communication and interaction. The empowerment of engaging comments and questions will open doors for interaction that may otherwise not occur due to a stranger's lack of knowledge of the unknown in interacting with a person with a communication difference or disability.

Facilitator plan

The facilitator's goal is to generate a list of ice breakers for the child. Think about what makes sense in the environments your child engages in. Think about the correct words that will fit the communication partners. Think about the style of language, formal or informal, that will be used with the communication partner(s) within the environment.

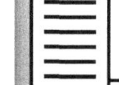

My child's action plan

Practice using the ice breaker statements and question forms.

1 *Hi, I like your … (e.g. backpack, book, soccer ball, hair clip, etc.)*
2 *Do you see my … (AAC device or tool)? This is how I talk to you. I know it sounds different, but that's okay, don't you think?*
3 *Let's talk about your favorite things to do and then I can show you my favorite things to do. I have pictures on my AAC device.*
4 *Isn't my AAC device cool? I can talk to you and you can talk to me. Do you want to try?*
5 *Want to hear my joke of the day?*

My communication partner'(s') plan

Your child can expect some communication partners will engage and others will say nothing at all. Keep encouraging your child. When you try to communicate, you place the proverbial ball in the other person's court. The person can choose to hit the ball, let the ball pass them, or try and swing and miss the ball. Help him- or her understand that trying is success.

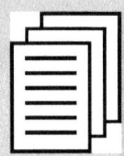

Activity: Ask for help: interacting with community helpers

A place to start

Help your child learn to ask for help with community and school helpers like coaches, clergy, clerks, medical professionals, office personnel, law enforcement professionals, school staff anyone else your child may interact with in the community. Ask your child who she would like to help or to get help from. Once again, bravo! If we are talking about interacting with community helpers, then your child is getting out into the world and experiencing life on a different level. That is success.

Facilitator plan

Learning to ask for help is an important step to successful independence. While it may seem scary to have your child ask questions of others, you will be there to guide success and assure your child's safety until the time is right for complete independence. The need for your child to ask for help from community helpers will vary on the situation. Refer to the list of 24 good reasons why your child should learn to ask questions.

24 Good Reasons Why Your Child Should Learn to Ask Questions

1 Pride in self-reliance	11 Contribute to a conversation
2 Recognize the need for *help*	12 Ask questions others are not asking
3 Know who to ask for *help*	13 Gain a direction
4 Know what to ask	14 Problem-solve
5 Formulate a nonverbal message requesting *help*	15 Demonstrate intellect
	16 Demonstrate a sense of humor
6 Formulate a verbal request for *help*	17 Participate
7 State negation (e.g. *No that is not what I need, let me try to ask a different way.*)	18 Understand another person's perspective
	19 Understand another person's emotions
8 Get an answer to a question a facilitator cannot answer	20 Understand another person's intent
	21 Move towards a solution
9 Gain more information	22 Arrive at a resolution
10 Clarify an answer	23 Initiate a conversation
	24 Satisfy good-old-fashioned curiosity

My child's action plan

Guide your child's action plan by navigating the social intricacies of language including the type of question forms are effective for your child, the organization of the language in the sentence, and the timing of when questions are asked. What forms of assistive technology best support your child in asking questions? Start with questions your child is successful. Then take a multi-pronged approach. Add more question forms, more modalities, more opportunities across people and environments.

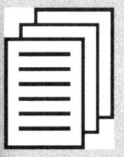

More Question Forms

1	*Where is the...?*	7	*Can you tell me more?*	13	*Who is that?*
2	*Can you help me get...?*	8	*What do you think?*	14	*Can you move my chair?*
3	*Can you help me see the (item) better?*	9	*Can you say that again?*	15	*Can you move that (item) out of the way?*
4	*Which direction is...?*	10	*Wait, what I want to know is ...?*	16	*How do I...?*
5	*Where do I go...?*	11	*Why is that?*	17	*When will...?*
6	*Which is better...?*	12	*What is that?*	18	*Would you please...?*

My communication partner'(s') plan

Communication partners would benefit from knowing that it is okay to give the AAC user time to formulate the question. Time can be tricky in one-on-one situations when silence feels awkward. Help the communication partner know that the time is not awkward for the AAC user in fact, they are working to generate a message, and in this case a question, so silence is golden.

Give the communication partner a language strategy such as, *Okay, I see you have something to say or you have a question to ask, so I will check back in with you.* Then, the communication partner validates your child's communication and continues engagement with activities.

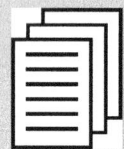

Activity: I Like your Hat: the art of giving and receiving a compliment

A place to start

Who doesn't like a compliment? Who doesn't feel good about themselves after giving a compliment? It is a win-win! Compliments are a topic starter and an ice breaker! Compliments usually get a gracious response and often the giver receives one in return. So, with all of this goodness going on, let's get the art of giving a compliment in your child's AAC repertoire.

Facilitator plan

Have some fun with compliments. Come up with a list of options that make sense for your child. Consider your child's age when putting your list together. Consider the environments in which your child participates. Consider the people your child may give a compliment to in those environments. Think about compliments the child can use that work across people, across contexts, or both. Place compliments on communication boards and in the quick messages section of your child's speech generating device. Then practice giving and receiving compliments with familiar people and then with less familiar people and then acquaintances. This is a good time to remind your child not to talk to strangers.

My child's action plan

Compliments are fun to give and receive! Practice using compliments and see how happy it makes others. Let your child express to you, *See how happy it makes me feel to make others happy.*

Compliment Emotions	Compliment the Person
1 *You are so nice.*	1 *You have a great laugh.*
2 *You make me happy/people feel happy.*	2 *You are so smart.*
3 *You make my day better.*	3 *You are really funny.*
4 *You have a great smile.*	4 *Great! I see it that way too!*
5 *You are a great friend.*	5 *You are wonderful.*
Compliment Actions	**Compliment Things**
1 *You do nice things.*	1 *I like your hat!*
2 *You help me so much.*	2 *I like your car.*
3 *You were amazing at that.*	3 *I like your shirt/dress/shoes.*
4 *That was nice that you let him go first.*	4 *I like your backpack.*
5 *You are so good!*	5 *I like your book.*

My communication partner'(s') plan

Help communication partners know your child is working on giving compliments. Encourage a communication partner to give a compliment to your child and allow your child to formulate a compliment in return using his or her AAC device. Make sure your child has the option to say the quick phrase, *Thank you!*

Activity: Step into my office: barter, trade, and negotiate like a pro

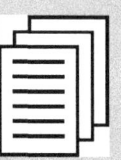

A place to start

Really? Bartering, trading, and negotiating? Yes, really! Children that use AAC need to barter for something they want, make their intentions known and that may include the ability to trade and negotiate! According to *Family Education* (2019; www.familyeducation.com/life/social-emotional-development/teaching-kids-negotiate) teaching children to negotiate enhances confidence, empathy, self-esteem, and social relationship skills. The focus here is stating more than an opinion. It is stating a firm intention with a good rationale and procuring a benefit.

Facilitator plan

Teaching a rationale is simply teaching a good reason for why your child wants to do or obtain something he or she wants. Your child is used to describing things and expanding sentences using language forms. Now, we want to put this great language to work to meet a goal. Work on rationale given the following ideas in your child's action plan. Work with interventionists to help your child with negotiation. 1) Talk about the real reason your child wants something. 2) Then determine the *why*. 3) Set the conditions for what each person will do to accomplish the goal. *If you do this for me, I will do that for you.* We barter, trade, and negotiate by talking about why we want something we want. See the following examples of why we may want to barter, trade, or negotiate for something. You may want to barter, trade, or negotiate to satisfy a feeling or emotion like happiness, calmness, or wakefulness (e.g. *If I get ice cream after school, I will be more awake to do my homework!*). We may negotiate to get support for a school election, to finish a job faster, to complete a project. We also may want to satisfy a want or need like attending special events or adding to a collection (e.g. *I can give you my place in line if you help me...; my turn now, please.)*

My child's action plan

Wouldn't it be fun for me to use my speech generating device to explain to someone why I want to do what I want or why I want what I want? Well that is what it means to barter, trade, and negotiate. We all accomplish our goals by giving reasons. Reasons come from descriptions. Your child has been practicing descriptions for a while. Use your child's ability to describe things to barter, trade, and negotiate! Say to someone, '*Step into My Office*,' and get started with negotiating. Your child may be beginning to see communication from another person's point of view-seeing their eyes looking a certain direction, hearing their voices sound excited, feeling the excitement of formulating a new plan.

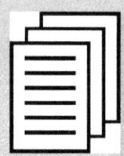

My communication partner'(s') plan

Help communication partners know that your child is working on bartering, trading, and negotiating using a speech generating device or other tools. Show them your child's communication tools and devices so they can see how your child puts messages together. Putting communication partners at ease will allow them to focus on the message and not on the device. Encourage the communication partner to ask questions or comments of your child to keep the negotiation conversation going.

Here is an example of negotiation:

Child: *Let's play.*
Communication partner: *It is time for me to go.*
Child: *One more time?*
Communication partner asks a question or a statement: *One more time and then I will go, okay?*
Child: *Tag, you're it!*

Activity: I did it; I'm sorry: fessing up and apologizing

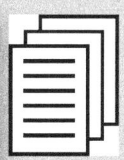

A place to start

We all make mistakes now and again. Likewise, we all need to say *we are sorry* now and again. Sometimes the need for an apology is simple like an accidental bump with a wheelchair. Sometimes an apology can be silly, like apologizing for eating the last of the vanilla ice cream. Sometimes *we are sorry* for others emotional or physical crisis. Sometimes *we are sor*ry because we hurt someone's feelings and whether accidental or not, we need to take responsibility for the pain we cause other people. Giving children who use AAC the language they need to apologize allows them to manage their emotions and behaviors and manage the emotions and behaviors of other. Sometimes people do not accept an apology, and that can be the hard part, or the funny part in the case of the eaten ice cream; but as your child engages in the world of *Maximizing Participation*, the joys, bumps, and bruises of human interaction may require an apology.

Facilitator plan

The vocabulary is easy, *I'm sorry*. Check your child's AAC tools and devices. Locate or add words or quick phrases to communication tools and devices to generate an apology. Some words and phrases may be a simple one-word apology in the word *sorry*. You may want to include *Excuse me*, as a form of *I'm sorry*. Then, use modeling and role-playing activities to teach your child the art of the apology using words on an AAC device, eye contact, and body posture. For example, you can practice accidentally dropping a non-breakable toy and say, *I'm sorry!* Then let your child purposefully make a non-harmful mistake and have him or her use her AAC device(s) to apologize. Apply apologies to real life situations so your child can generalize when an apology is required. Avoid teaching apologies during a climax of a crisis. An apology requires a thoughtful recognition. When a heated circumstance subsides, allow your child to reflect on what happened, and then formulate an apology. Similarly, you do not need to wait until the crisis has completely passed. When the child is aware of his or her mistake the child can say the apology.

My child's action plan

Your child has words to say, *I'm sorry* or *Sorry*, when needed. We say *sorry* to people for different reasons. *Oops*, acknowledges that something went wrong. We say we are *sorry* when someone is sad, hurting for any reason, or we make a mistake, even if it was an accident. We say, *excuse me*, when we bump into someone. We can say forms of apologies with our eyes, body posture, and our words.

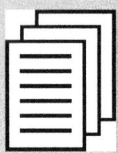

My communication partner'(s') plan

It is likely that the communication partner is the bearer of the insult, the sadness, or prank. The circumstance will greatly influence how you will support the communication partner in understanding your child's wishes to say an apology. It may be best to facilitate the interaction by letting the person know the child has something to say and to give the child a moment to generate the apology using the AAC tool or device.

○ Emergency preparedness: a plan for communication; a plan for action

A place to start

If there is ever a time for essential communication functions, including people that use AAC, it is during an emergency because earthquakes, tornados, hurricanes, and other disasters (e.g. wild fires, flooding, stranger on campus, violence, acts of terror) require action.

Preparation, including using AAC, is key. Most people are reluctant to prepare and thus have not prepared or are prepared minimally for a major emergency to function under the extreme circumstances that natural disasters bring.

Facilitator plan

Let's take a look at options for AAC preparation for an emergency. What is the best prevention? Planning. Collecting. Practicing. Implementing. Address the following statements to prepare for an emergency.

1 The first question in a crisis is: *Is my child safe?*
2 *I have my child's AAC devices backed up. I am checking that automatic backups are occurring.*
3 *I have a tip card prepared with copies in backpacks and a communication wallet that explain how my child communicates.*
4 *My child has a way to communicate with responders (e.g. communication board, AAC device). My child practices, Wait I need my AAC device to talk!*
5 *My child has an identification card available at all times.*
6 *My child has contact information with my name, close friends, and support team members addresses, and phone numbers.*
7 *My child has medical information including extra prescriptions and blood type, contact information, and evacuation plans in a communication wallet or backpack.*
8 *My child has a way to call for help.*
9 *I have a Go-Bag (see the following section, Sources of Information) with supplies including AAC accessories like cords and chargers, a paper copy of AAC boards, food, water, and comfort needs.*
10 *I have spoken with school personnel regarding my child's safety in case of emergency.*

Sources of Information

1 Visit AAC-RERC Emergency Communication, Disaster Preparation, Response and Recovery for People with CCN (n.d.) for information and materials supporting people with limited speech, response personnel, and AAC advocates (http://aac-rerc.psu.edu/index.php/pages/show/id/4).

2 Visit Carole Zangari's (2018) safety advice at PrAACtical AAC (http://praacticalaac.org/praactical/praactical-resources-lockdown-code-red-other-school-safety-drills/) for great resources on school lockdowns and other school safety concerns including verbiage to include in IEPs.
3 For a number of emergency communication tools visit Patient Provider Communication (2018; www.patientprovidercommunication.org/gallery/?Category=Emergency%20Communication).
4 Diane Nelson Bryan (2018) makes communication boards available on the University of Temple Institute on Disabilities (2018; https://disabilities.temple.edu/aacvocabulary/e4all.shtml#index).
5 The National Autism Association (2016) published the following Emergency Personal Profile (http://nationalautismassociation.org/personal-emergency-profile-sheet/) to offer people a unique tool that combines personal information including medical needs, communication bridging information through the child's likes and dislikes, along with tips to communication partners with symbols to support self-regulation of a person with autism.

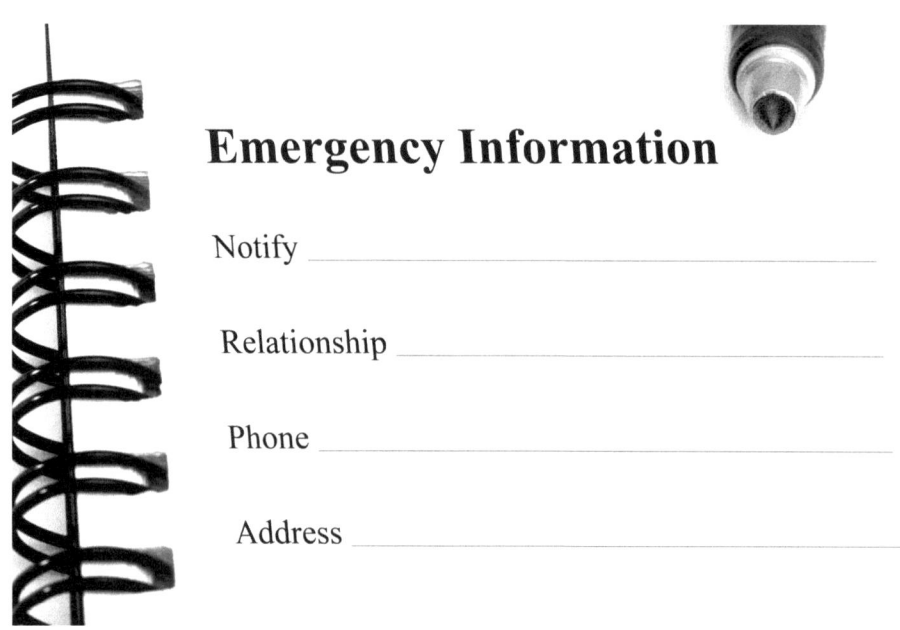

Emergency Information

Notify _____

Relationship _____

Phone _____

Address _____

Blackstone and Goldman (2018) offer the following tips to make an AAC plan for evacuating (leaving the immediate area of danger) or sheltering in place, that means staying where you are. Consider these statements from your child's perspective.

Plan how I will evacuate with my AAC tools, devices, and other assistive technology tools.
Plan how I will communicate if I cannot evacuate with my AAC.
Plan how my device(s) will be replaced if they are lost or destroyed in a disaster.

Prepare a go-kit or go-bag for home, school, bus, and car for each person and pet.

Plan on what I will do if my support providers cannot get to me

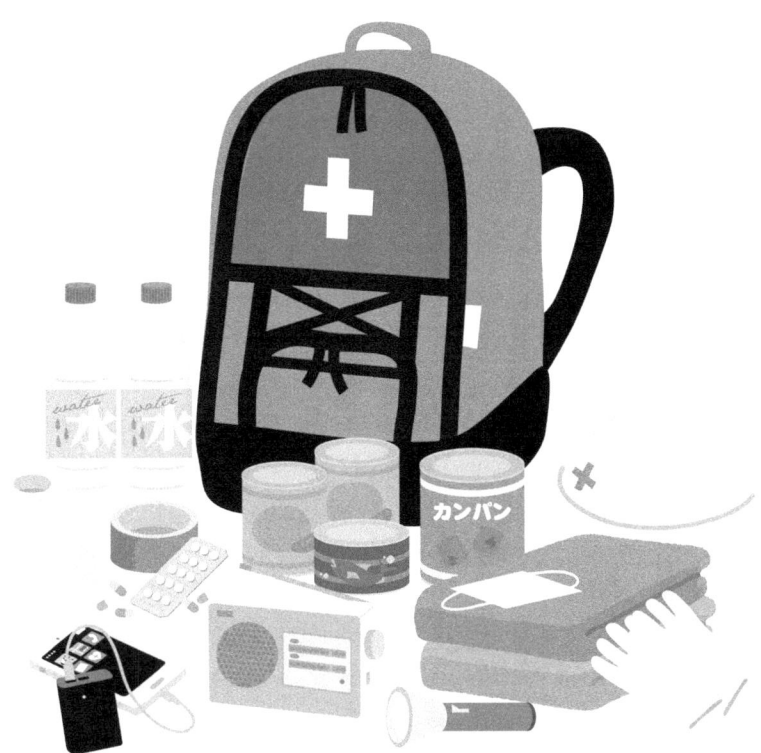

My child's action plan

My child's job in an emergency is to listen and work with first responders who may be people who work in law enforcement, the fire department, the military, the Red Cross, and many other organizations with people trained to help people or could be well-intended untrained volunteers. Make sure vocabulary is available on the main pages of the communication board, book, or device to serve as a form of quick communication with at least one-word, quick phrase, or folder that serves as an emergency message or messages (e.g. help, emergency, My Emergency Plan). Emergencies often cause a state of fearful reaction. Talking about feelings related to emergencies is planning.

- ◉ *I have talked about emergencies with others.*
- ◉ *I know people who may help get me to safety and get medical help during an emergency.*
- ◉ *I will learn about emergency words (e.g. first responder, police, firemen, emergency medical technician or EMT).*
- ◉ *I can use free materials such as matching games to learn vocabulary.* See The Emergency Helpers-Early Childhood Program (2019; www.fire.nsw.gov.au/page.php?id=886) for teacher resources, flashcards, game and activities such as memory match.
- ◉ *I can check out the All About Emergencies from the Autism Helper for great resources for purchase by Long (2016) at http://theautismhelper.com/all-about-emergencies/*
- ◉ *I have read books to learn about what happens during an emergency.*
- ◉ *I talked about my emergency plan at home and school.*
- ◉ *I practice with my AAC emergency board and vocabulary on my tools and devices.*
- ◉ *I will role play, and if I get the chance, practice using my AAC emergency vocabulary board with first responders.*

My communication partner'(s) plan

First responders are communication partners who may or may not have training to support communicate with people that use AAC. Having communication boards and tools like dry erase boards available will help first responders. Explore the tools and resources offered in the Emergency Sources of Information. Your child's AAC emergency planning may save the life of a communication partner too.

○ That is not okay: standing up for yourself and others

A place to start

Do I have the words for self-advocacy? Do I have the words to advocate for someone else? Do I have the confidence to use my words for myself and others? Do I know who to talk to about something when I know something is not okay? Do I know how to and when to say *That is not okay! Something is wrong. I know something is wrong, but I don't know exactly what's wrong. I know exactly what's wrong. I know what I see is wrong* (e.g. forms of written or visual images or media). *I know what I see going on is wrong* (e.g. Actions of others; How others are treated).

Facilitator plan

Teaching your child self-advocacy is important. We spend a lot of time focused on language, communication, fun with participation, and social or pragmatic appropriateness. Equally as necessary is for your child to say, *No, I will call the police/tell my teacher/tell the principal/tell on you, Wait, Hey! It's my turn!* A good place to start is to take an inventory of the current assertive vocabulary available on your child's communication board, wallet, or speech generating devices. Look for single words like, *No, Stop*, and *Wait*. Check for phrases like, *Get away from me*! Decide where words programmed with assertive voices should be located on your child's AAC device so they are highly accessible. Record voices, spoken with authority, for assertive words and phrases and practice using vocabulary that supports your child. Affirm child's ability to be active and independent. Follow up with conversations about rights and responsibilities.

My child's action plan

Incorporate opportunities for your child to use words that allow the child to 'right a wrong,' when a mistake has been made. Words may be required when your child sees someone else hurting others, your child is being swindled, or worse, abused. This means your child needs to be aware that something is wrong. This also means your child knows that he or she can say something with accessible vocabulary. The following ideas are nonverbal and verbal ways to get your child started.

Nonverbal and verbal assertiveness speech act by type and example

Nonverbal	Speech Act Type	Verbal with Assertive Vocal Tone
Head positioning	Command	*No; Wait; Stop*
Firm body posture	Turn Taking	*Wait a minute!* or *It's my turn.*
Body positioning	Trading	*I will trade this for that.*
Sustained eye gaze	Negotiating	*I can give you my place in line if you help me…*
Facial expression	Calling Attention	*That's not right!* or *Hey!*
Pointing or other gesture	Getting Others Involved	*I'm getting my teacher.*

My communication partner'(s') plan

Consider the communication partner, the status the communication partner holds, and the competency the communication partner sees in your child when it comes to the plan needed to support the child and communication partner. Communication partners, or conflict partners in this case, need to be clearly informed that the child holds power through the use of intellect, words, confidence, and the power to seek support. There is a balance of power that may be greater than the conflict partner realizes. Familiar communication partners understand the competency level of my child and need to diligently attend to the nonverbal and verbal message of your child and may need to broker the social dynamic.

○ My AAC book club

A place to start

Maximize Participation by starting a book club! Just think about the opportunities for exchanging ideas, information, and opinions with other kids, those using AAC and peers from the class or rest of the school. Children who communicate with AAC use literacy skills to contribute to the discussion around broad topics of sports, literature, science, people, and actions around them. They are heard and appreciated using their speech generating devices.

Facilitator's plan

Wait a minute! Is my child ready for sharing information about books with others? How can my child prepare to participate during a book club? What are the steps I need to take to start an AAC book club? Join with school and community library personnel to invite participants. Invite peers equally representing children who use AAC and verbal speakers of any literacy level. Establish a book club meeting length schedule (e.g. 1–2 hours on the first Tuesday of the month). Locate and select resources (e.g. pictures, props, a display of books from the library) in the library. Generate topic ideas from the children, educators, and parents. Arrange the meeting room so participants and see and hear each other easily. Create a comfortable space to accommodate wheelchairs. Establish where the available restrooms are located. Plan for and minimize distractions caused by others in a public space. Enlist other participants to take leadership roles in welcoming each member with a nametag, a place to sign in, and a way to welcome each participant at the start of the meeting. Have a member project the names of each participant and what they contributed using an overhead projector. This displayed acknowledgement celebrates their time and efforts to communicate with literacy. One person may guide the discussion, introduce the topic, summarize the contributions, and plan for a social time together. Encourage a child who uses AAC to lead the group. Before coming to the meeting, each child reads a book, article, or internet presentation on the topic at whatever level is most comfortable or finds a resource in the community that focuses on the topic. Your child summarizes the important ideas and sequences, evaluates possible alternatives, and describes the goal and steps leading to the achieving the goal. The child constructs sentences and express most important ideas. Have a blast at the book club meetings seeing your child contribute, react to others, participate, and grow.

My child's action plan

I have a favorite book or question I want to share. I collect the facts and relate my ideas by composing my message on my speech generating device. I reflect on how the book made me feel. I ask questions of others, How is this different and how is it the same as your reading this book? I have comments that say, I agree or disagree with others, who are in the club. Besides when the book club meets, I can talk about these topics and listen to hear how others think about them too. Some use speech generating devices, others share illustrations. I realize I am not alone when peers of all abilities get together and share what matters most to us. We plan before each meeting, so I know what topic to read about next and listen for ways they collect new resources. I organize messages to contribute to the topic planning for the next meeting, suggest changes to be made, and offer other discussion questions.

My communication partner'(s') plan

The communication partners in a book club will be peers using AAC, peers not using AAC, peer mentors, facilitators, family, teachers, and librarians. A quick explanation of the rules of the club and AAC user experiences reduces the strangeness of the first few initial meetings. Post the rules about listening to each other, showing respect for others, and learning how to take another person's perspectives. Support communication partners with a schedule for the book club meeting that includes the topic and a tentative and adaptable schedule. Accept the contributions of each participant and encourage others to ask questions and make comments. Expose them to the resources participants may use during the meeting. Encourage communication partners to become active participants in the meetings by listening, following the discussion, providing equal time for each member to speak. Write up the book club activities and submit the article to the school newsletter, a community website, and/or local organization highlighting the inclusion of persons using AAC and their peers. Contact community business, shop, arts, or athletic leaders to serve as a guest presenter and offer demonstrations. Consider field trips and innovation projects to discuss as a part of the book club experience. Community leaders will find this group meets their goal of community outreach. Participation for children that use AAC is maximized through literacy and interaction with peers.

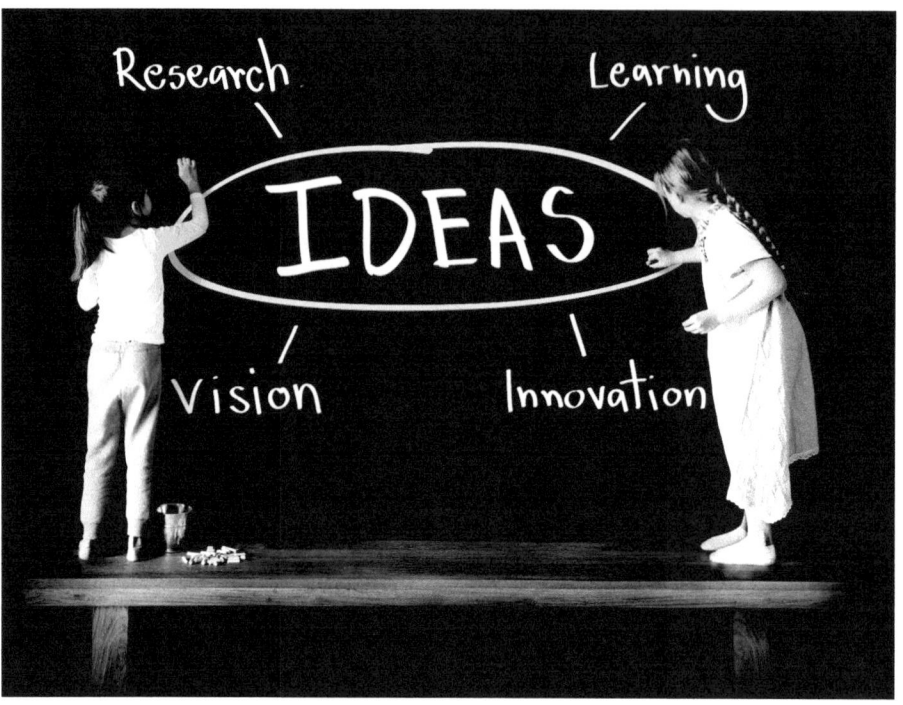

○ Grab and Go Coaches' Corner

Joy teaches me to ask the right questions.

(Middle school educator, Rogers, 1999)

Your plan as a facilitator is to maximize the independence of the child that uses AAC while maintaining safety, quality education, and broad types of opportunities to engage and participate with people, places, ideas, and objects. The right questions to ask focus on the essential meaning of your child's intent and fostering contributions your child makes to interactions. Children that use AAC in *Maximizing Participation* learn to manage situations capably and becoming their own best manager. They recognize, *I may need help, but I am my own #1 manager.* The following *Grab and Go* topics and tips are offered to support facilitators of children that use AAC for *Maximizing Participation.* The tips get to the heart of how to elicit what my child is thinking and learning about a topic. The tips follow both the social theory developed by Vygotsky (1986) and an active learning theory by Feuerstein that integrate the importance of social interaction with a person who has knowledge of language (Vygotsky calls this *the more knowledgeable other*) and the child's *zone of proximal development*, or what my child is ready to learn through a *mediated learning experience* (Feuerstein et al., 1981). A mediated learning experience promotes active engagement addressing needs and rejecting a passive-acceptance approach (Kaniel & Feuerstein, 1989). The concept of focusing on needs through functional goals continues to drive intervention over finding deficits that aim to '*fix something that is wrong*' (Owens, 2014, p. 6).

Look to the topics for steps to support a child Maximizing Participation at home, school, and community.

Grab and Go Topics:

1 You Can Talk to Me: Recognizing Communication Barriers
2 Give Me a Call! I'd Love to Chat
3 I Know … That You Know … What I Have to Say … but I Still Need to Use My Voice!
4 How Do You See This Playing Out? Prediction and Consequence
5 Things I Can Say & Things I Can Do: Managing Conversation
6 Hold On … Fix-It Repair Strategies
7 Tell Me About Your Trip! Memory Books & Binders
8 Authorship
9 Social Boundaries
10 Recognizing Motives
11 That's Funny
12 Email, Text, and Post

○ Facilitator tips for maximizing communication with communication

1 You can talk to me: recognizing communication barriers

Recognize your child's communication barriers and determine solutions to address them. For example, cue new communication partners to speak to my child rather than relay a message through the facilitator. Remind communication partners, including interventionist, that the AAC tool is a bridge for my child to comprehension and a voice to say *hello*, express an idea, to share emotions, have a laugh, make a contribution, and so much more.

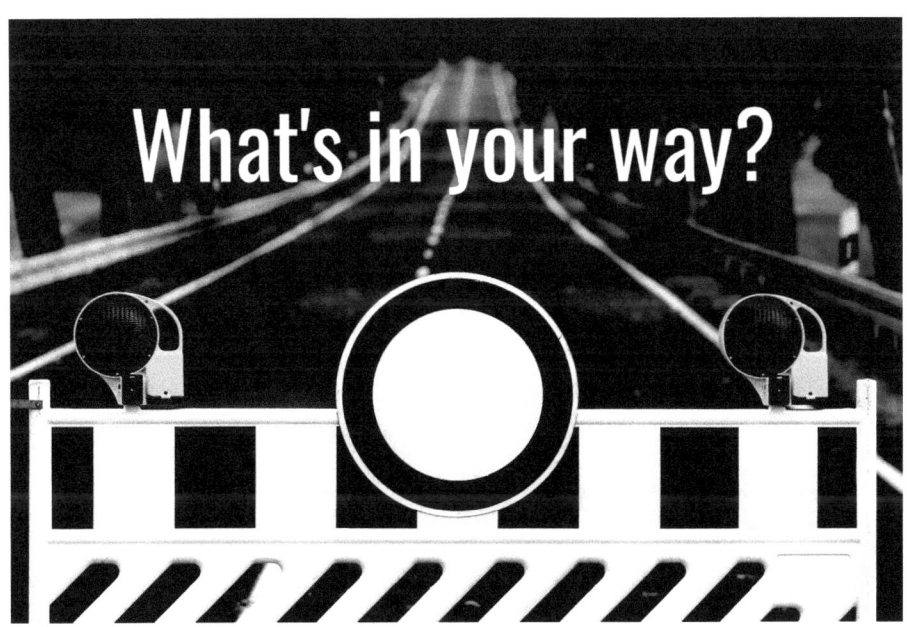

2 Give me a call! I'd love to chat

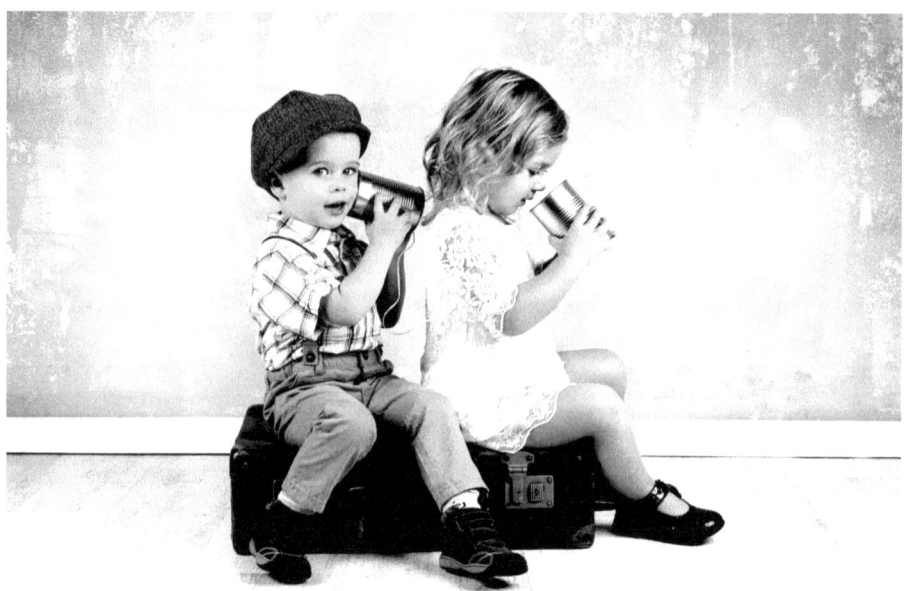

Carole Zangari, an ASHA Fellow, offers five tips for talking on the phone for AAC users titled, *Call Me Later* (2012; https://prAACticalAAC.org/prAACtical/call-me-later-5-supports-for-phone-communication-by-people-who-use-aac/). In addition to practice ideas Zangari offers a tip for a phone app called *Unus Tactus* that allows people to make a one touch photo dialing system and geofencing capabilities to monitor the location of a person. Text to voice, speech-to-speech, and internet-based telephone services are just a few options to be explored at Federal Communications Commission (n.d.; www.fcc.gov/consumers/guides/telecommunications-relay-service-trs). Telecommunications Relay Service webpage.

3 I know . . . that you know . . . what I have to say . . . but I still need to use my voice

I smile. You smile.
I use AAC... so do you.
I hear your voice.
Hear my voice.

It is always great when we understand what someone wants to say or do without their saying a word to you. It may be a particular glance or a body position and you know exactly what to do. However, we want our children who use AAC to have the opportunity to express their messages, even though communication partners may think they know your child's intentions. Let the child voice an introduction to a topic, start a conversation, stand up for him- or herself, crack a joke, disagree, or register an opposing opinion.

4 *How do you see this playing out? Prediction and consequences*

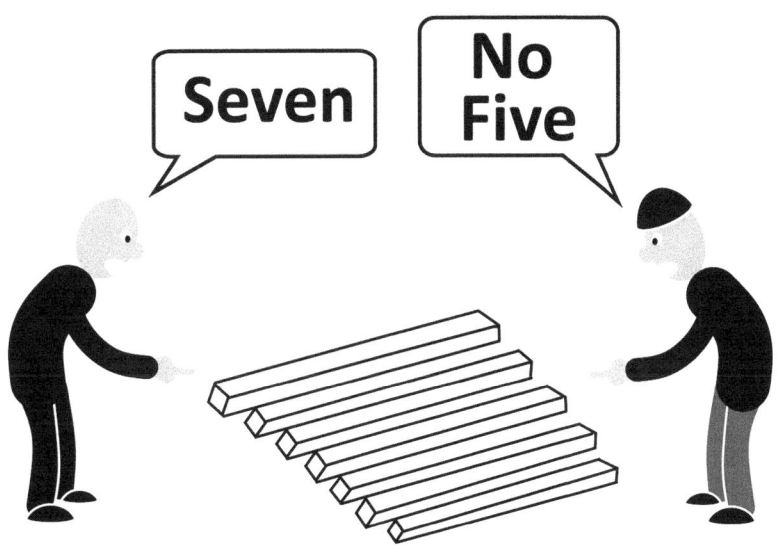

Predicting outcomes and observing consequences of other's behavior is a required academic task. Stories are helpful because you can talk about the characters and discuss what characters are experiencing, why they are feeling the way they do, discuss whether the characters perceptions of the situation are correct or not, consider how others feel, and then talk about the consequences of the actions and what should or could be done. To get you started with any book look at the following examples and build your perspective taking repertoire from here.

Prediction: prompt questions

- *What do you think will happen next?*
- *Do you think that . . . (e.g. . . . the noise is a cat? . . . they can resolve the problem?)*
- *How do you think he will feel . . . (e.g. tomorrow, after he hears the news)*
- *What should they try to do?*
- *Where will they go next?*
- *When do you think they will go/finish/try to...*

Consequences: prompt questions

- *Daniel helped his friend so what do you think the friend will do the next time Daniel needs help?*
- *The girl did not finish her homework so now what will the consequence be when she wants to go to the birthday party?*

5 Things I can say and things I can do: managing conversation

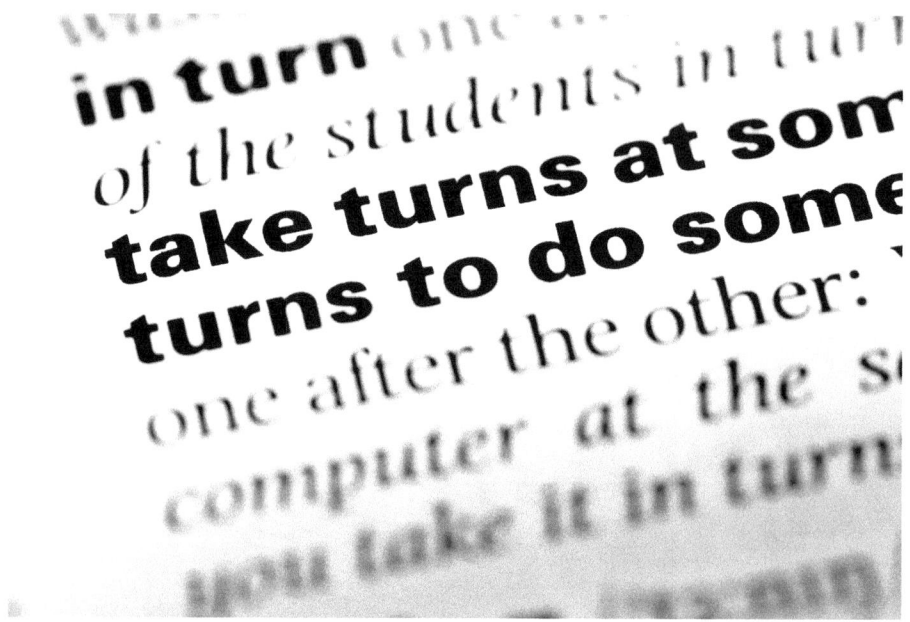

Suggest appropriate ways and times to introduce, manage, change the topic, and end a conversation. See the phrases highlighted in bold for vocabulary recommendations in the left column under the heading *Things I Can Say* and nonverbal communication in the right column under the heading *Things I Can Do*.

Things I Can Say & Things I Can Do

Things I Can Say	Things I Can Do
Excuse me is a socially acceptable quick phrase that is polite and gets the point across that I have something to say.	Location matters. *I make my presence known by **placing myself** physically into the area where communication partners are talking.*
I have something to say. I let my communication partners know I have a topic to introduce or contribute to an existing conversation.	**Eye contact.** *I use eye contact and an icon on my speech generating device that makes a tapping sound as in calling a meeting to order. It's fun, funny, and attention getting.*
Give me a minute to put my message together. This phrase allows communication partners to keep the topic going and to anticipate my upcoming message.	Equally as important is knowing that *I **may need to wait** a minute to be addressed by the intended communication partner(s) to state my message.*
I need to go. Thank you for talking with me. See you later! Any combination of phrases appropriate to my age, language, culture, and environment are great ways to finish up a conversation.	**Be persistent** and use **multiple ways** to gain attention. *If one way does not work like eye gaze or a tap, a combination of a verbal message using a speech generating device and a nonverbal cue may do the trick.*

6 Hold on . . . fix-it repair strategies

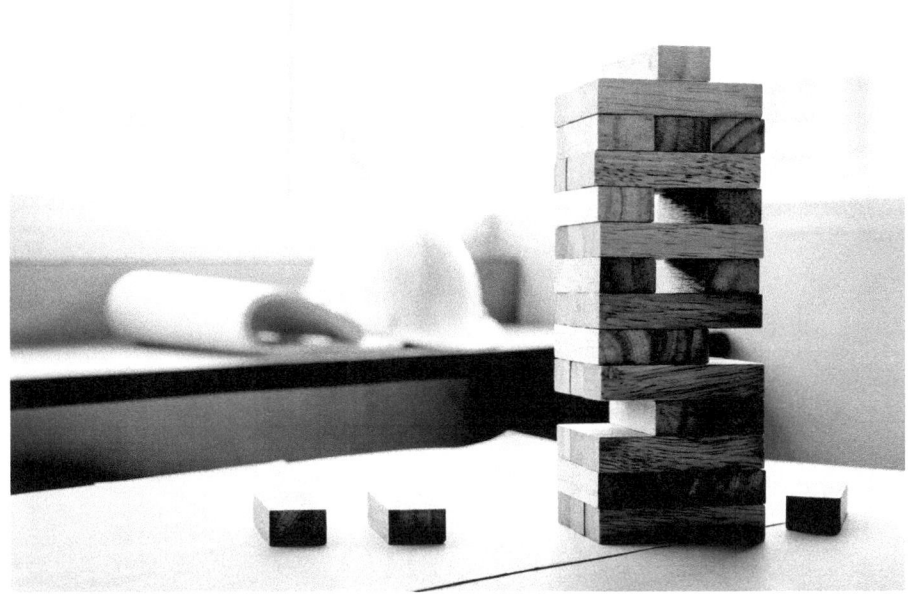

Plan out your repair strategies. A repair strategy is generally seen as *fixing* an error in word choice or grammar. This *fix-it* strategy is certainly true and important. Consider broadening the idea of a repair strategy to include elaboration. If my child does not understand a comment, or a communication partner does not understand my child, use the opportunity to facilitate a message using a phrase such as the following: *Please give me an example of what you mean? Can you show me a picture? Tell me that again, I am not sure I understand. I am not sure I heard you correctly. Tell me more about your idea.*

7 Tell me about your trip! Memory books and binders

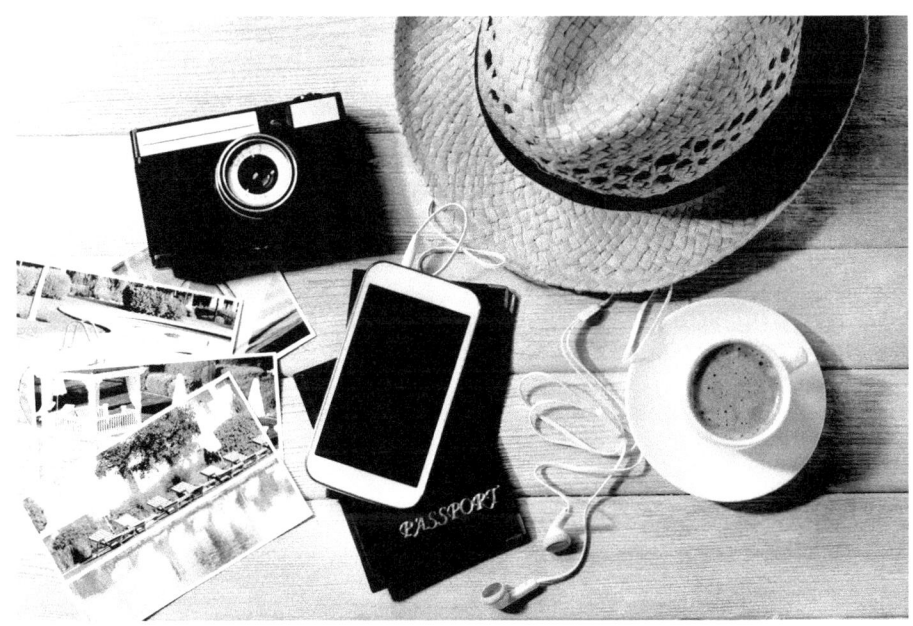

Photos, brochures, stickers, flyers, maps, tickets and any fun collection of items from events make for a great way to share experiences with friends and family. Memory sharing makes for fun conversation. Make communication pages to discuss new memories of family trips, school field trips, birthdays, special events, and other stories. Put memorabilia into sheet protectors or zip lock bags. Copy a few pictures to add to book, binder, or bag.

8 Authorship

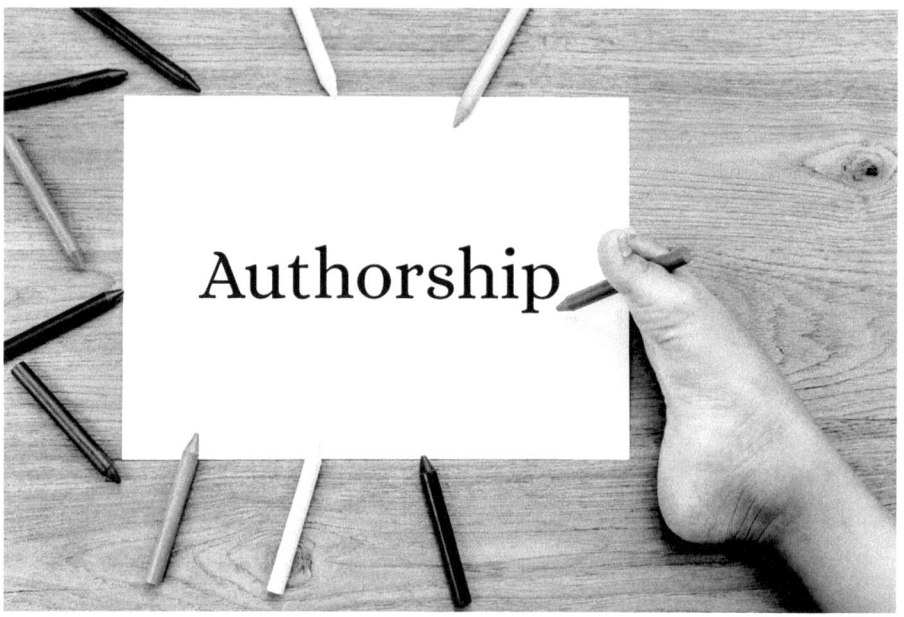

Authorship is a fact that a person created art or writing. Children with motor disorders may benefit from levels of prompting during authorship such as touch cues or support at the wrist, elbow, shoulder, or foot! Peter Tran (2019), a child with the diagnosis of autism and severe dyspraxia types with facilitator support. When authorship is questioned Peter states, *It is a lot more than holding up someone's wrist. It is a partnership, a trust that the facilitator accepts the AAC user has ideas and 'brain glitches' with attention, word-finding, anxiety, eye-hand coordination, or like me obsessive-compulsive disorder. The goal is autonomy. Support is an expeditious, efficient, and respectful way to express what the AAC user has to say.* Keep authorship alive with writing and drawing including degrees of support on the path to independence.

9 Social boundaries

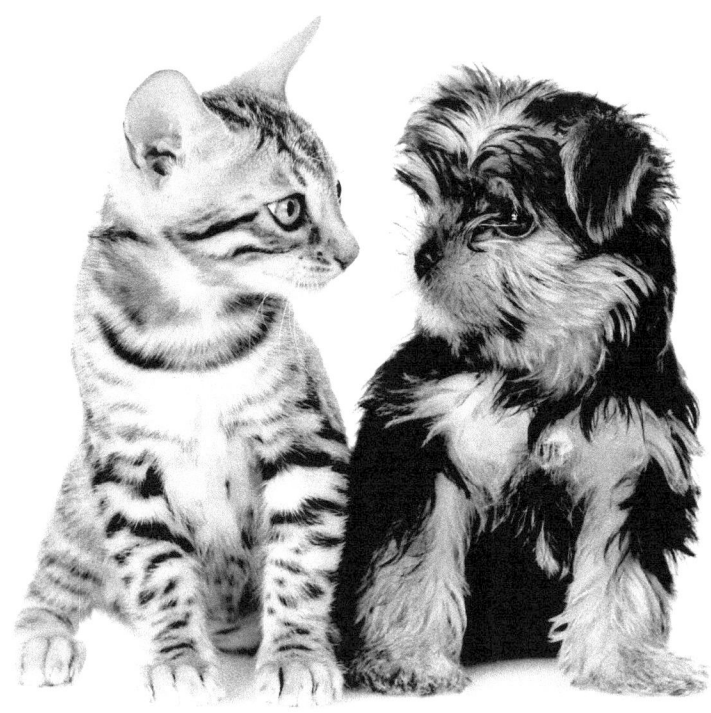

Have you ever been greeted by the best hug on the planet by a loving, outgoing middle schooler with a complex communication profile? It's a gift. Unfortunately, it can also be a safety concern if the recipient of the hug is a stranger. Children need to recognize that not every person may want a hug. They also need to learn when it is socially acceptable to give a person a hug. Children can also learn how close in proximity they may be to familiar, less familiar, and unknown communication partners. Offer explicit training in how to recognize social boundaries such as personal space. Teach the child how to give a handshake or a wave as a great alternative.

10 Recognizing motives

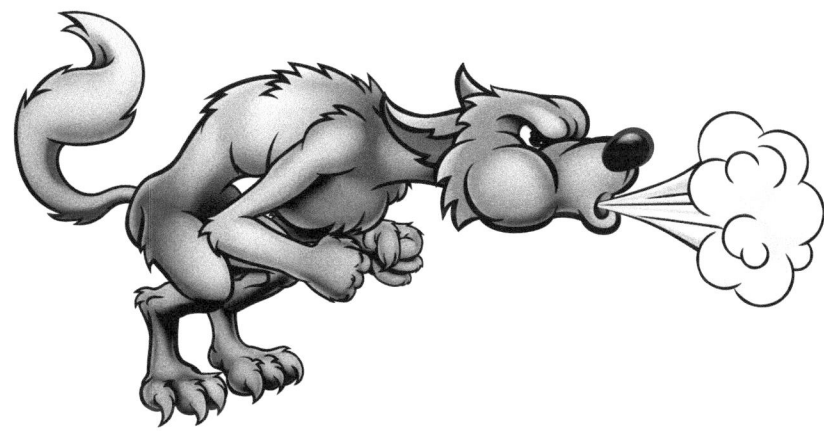

We use reading for so many purposes. Teach your child to recognize other's motives. Draw experiences from stories such as *The Three Little Pigs* (Halliwell-Phillipps, 1890) and *The Wonderful Wizard of Oz* (Baum, 1900) that teach the difference between empathizing and recognizing motives in others. The idea of motives can be spun into other topics such as understanding motivations and then perspective taking. The idea is looking beyond what people are doing and ask why they are doing what they are doing. Motive is often associated with negative actions but they do not have to be negative. Develop healthy perspectives. Given your child's age, you easily could use a storybook with illustrations. For older children tie concepts to current events in the news.

11 *That's funny*

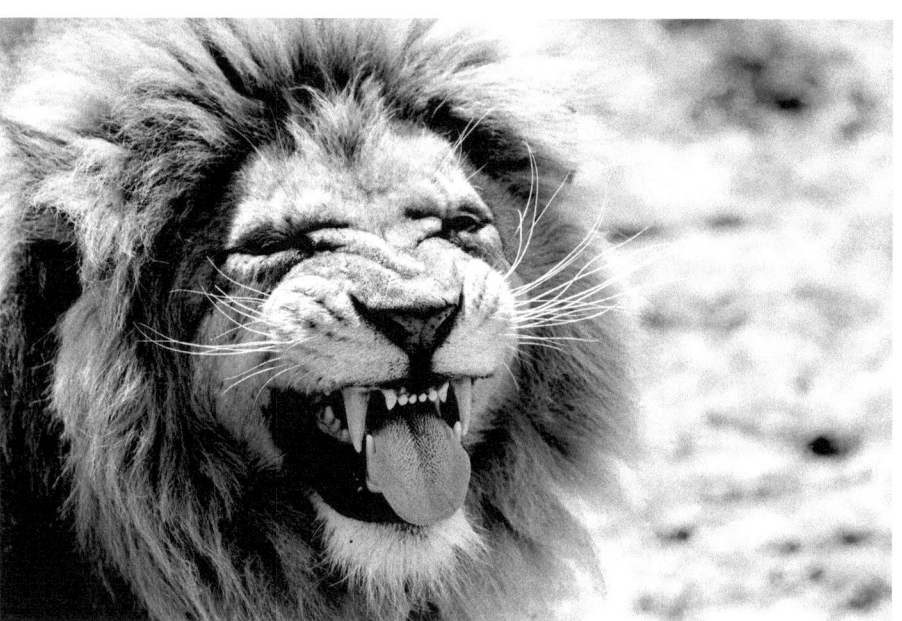

You know your friend who sends you every funny cat, dog, alligator, or prank video possible? Put some of those videos and sources to work. Expose your child to humor in comics from books, cartoons in the newspaper, or videos from media sources. Humor is fun and a great way to connect people and to enjoy forms of media. Make a page of funny pictures to include in your child's binder of memories discussed in, *Before We Go: Making Connections A Topic Book*.

12 *Email, text, & post*

Kids experience grownups and other children writing emails, texts, and posting information all of the time! Writing a message to a parent or sibling using parentally approved technology can be a very motivating way to build

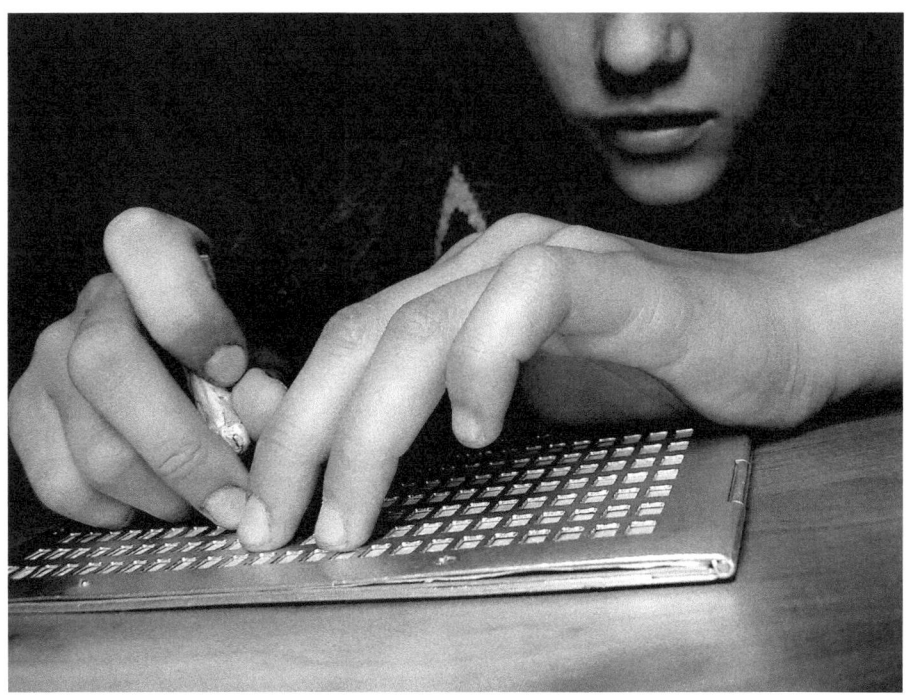

literacy skills. You do not have to run out and buy your child a phone. Decide what you think is the most appropriate form of technology for your child to communicate electronically. Many schools have email addresses and internet safety contracts that must be signed by the parents making it easier for the child to email in a safe environment. Email from school to home. From home email grandparents and close friends.

Maximizing Participation with language literacy

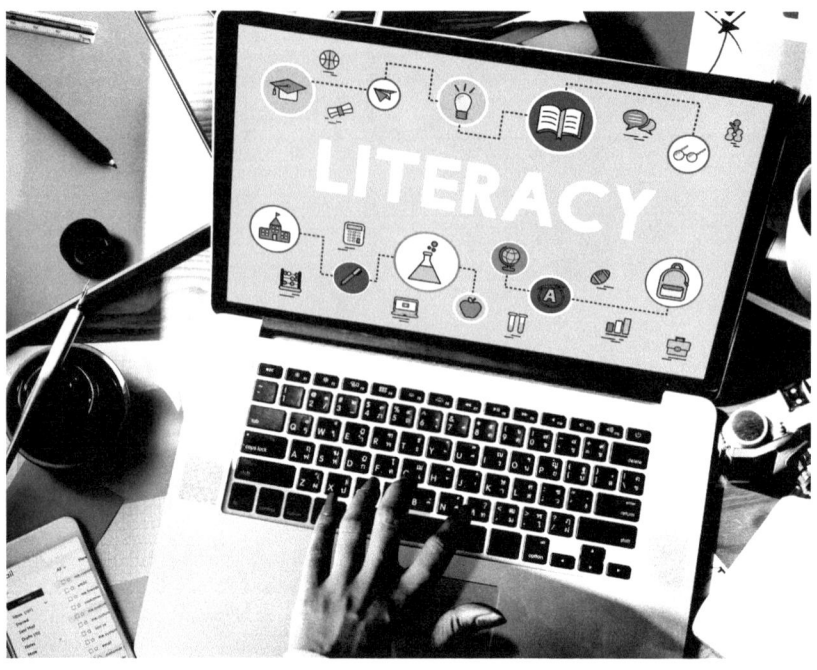

○ **Language is never out of the picture** *(Ehren, 2018)*

Language literacy is critical to *Maximizing Participation* for children that use AAC. Reading icons are a part of your child's AAC language skill, however the ability to access icons does not equate to literacy (Benedek-Wood, McNaughton & Light, 2016; Light & Kent-Walsh, 2003, May 27; McNaughton & Lindsay, 1995). Literacy employs sounds and letters, organized as words on icons. Ehren, Lenz and Deshler (2016) highlight the need for children to read a variety of texts in multimodal settings across all academic disciplines including science, technology, engineering, and mathematics (STEM) disciplines. The authors go on to state that children need literacy skills to be developed at a young age with a solid infrastructure that is explicitly taught. Language impacts every level of thinking, literacy, and learning from skills, to strategies, to subject matter and higher-order thinking (Ehren et al., 2016). Literacy skills give us access to understanding cultures and influences how we engage in social situations. Ehren (2018) states that literacy is more than just reading and writing words; it is the combination of words into phrases, sentences, paragraphs and the comprehension of the concepts at each level that contribute to a person being literate. She goes on to say that language is a foundational skill for all levels of literacy and success in academic and post academic settings. Literacy has a reciprocal relationship with language, communication, and participation. Literacy is a powerful form of independence and a way to share interests and stories. Children that use AAC have literacy skills that need to be learned, motivation to be driven, and success to be had. One translation of literacy skills is successful participation. Children using AAC need to have literacy that is accessible, inclusive, innovative, and socially interactive with enough repetitions and visual representatives that make reading an engaging and ongoing worthwhile experience!

Opportunities for language literacy and what we do

1 Preparation: The child is organized and ready to learn (e.g. materials, environment, physically and emotionally stable, with access to technology). The child understands the purpose of reading different materials for pleasure, information sharing, opinion forming, fiction, imaginative, persuasive. The child understands where to begin, the breadth of thinking, (e.g. what tasks to do, how many tasks to do, the complexity), and what finished looks like (e.g. *Finished* means, *I completed 10 math word problems, finished my essay diagram, and finished part two of three parts of my word study*.)

2 Word study: Phonics work or phonemic awareness tasks may be very relevant for a child *Maximizing Participation*. Work with children on understanding syllables including prefixes and suffixes, root words that help children understand higher level words. Make learning vocabulary fun. Roll the dice: 1=Use the context, 2=Go to the glossary, 3=Search the internet, 4=Find in the dictionary, 5=Hear or read the word in a different sentence, 6=Tell Me for Free!

3 Genres and platforms: Grade level or interest level genres read across traditional paper-based books and electronic platforms.

4 Fluency: Read for accuracy, rate, and expression (Hasbrouck & Glaser, 2012). Read a chapter, a set number of pages, or minutes a day. Build incentive by seeing a movie based on the book or visiting a museum to see artifacts related to the book genre.

5 Publish ideas: Children may publish their ideas by writing using utensils and paper or typing. The writing process includes prewriting, drafting, revising, and editing for the purpose of producing narrative, persuasive, expository, and descriptive text.

6 Observe modeled reading and writing: Observe people around you. What are they reading? How much time do they read and write? What do they recommend you read?

7 Shared reading and writing: Read books with family and peers. Take turns reading a paragraph or page at a time. Share writing by taking turns adding to a story.

8 Guided reading activities to support text comprehension (Musselwhite, Erickson, Stemach & Odom, 2005): Before reading: Build and/or activate background knowledge of similar experiences the children have had and set a purpose for reading. During reading: Read and/or listen to the text. After reading: Complete a task and provide informative feedback.

9 Independent reading and writing: Let children choose their own book to read. Monitor how realistic the choice is and offer a similar genre or the same book at a different reading level. Write a book review and submit it to the library or bookstore. Learn to annotate and highlight key information in the book. Draw or create a craft associated with an aspect of the book. Act out a play based on the book given a script the children write.

10 Literature study: Discuss elements of the story (e.g. character analysis, setting, feelings, plot, conflict, resolution, themes, genre, etc.). Compare and

contrast elements within the story and then to other stories. Create new endings, develop new knowledge, and test predictions. Form an AAC book club and meet regularly for group discussions.

○ Literacy comprehension strategies

Now that we have many ways to build language literacy what can we do to specifically target comprehension? The following list contains 10 ready to go ideas. As you read the comprehension strategies think about how they apply to your child as an AAC user.

Literacy comprehension strategies, description, and my plan

1 Connecting prior knowledge: *I will help my child connect prior and existing knowledge to the text by pointing out similarities and differences to life experience.*

2 Questioning: *I will ask questions that check for comprehension of the text (e.g. engaged with the story, invested in learning what happens).*

3 Monitoring comprehension level: Level 1 Literal: Understanding of the story elements (e.g. character, plot, setting, conflict, emotions, resolution). Level 2 Inferential & Evaluative (e.g. understanding implications, prediction, the greater whole, current events)

4 Capturing intent: Visualize scenes and events and talk about the illustrations, key words, and concepts. Draw an interpretation. Write an outline of the story elements. Sequence events by time and place from newspaper comic strips or books.

5 Analyzing: *Who are the characters? What do we know about the relationship between the characters and events? What do we know about the developing plot, conflict, and resolution?*

6 Inferring: *What do you know about the character/setting/plot based on the information stated in the story? What do you think the author wants you to know, think, or believe?*

7 Determining important ideas: *What are main ideas of the story? If your child could rank the most important ideas how would they be ranked? Let's determine the important ideas based on categories such as from the perspective of each character, lesson learned, emotions and feelings, or impact on other people, places, or things.*

8 Synthesizing: *How does the behavior of this character impact that character? How can we compare and contrast what we know based on the evidence? What conclusions can be made?*

9 Summarizing: Based on the conclusions stated we now know that … Make a list, order events, chart sequences and intensity of emotions, narrate a summary of ideas

10 Evaluating: *My perspective is…, My interpretation is…, I feel that…, I agree with…, I disagree with…, My recommendation is…*

○ The moving parts of writing

Any stage your child has achieved with writing is a great stage. The important part of understanding writing at this level is that there are many moving parts to the definition of writing. As your child grows, so will his or her writing skills. Think of writing skills and *Maximizing Participation* in the multidimensional way it is. See that writing can mean many things. You see **knowledge-based** skills that focus on building vocabulary and grammar and experience. You see **ideology-based** skills that types of writing including expository, persuasion, descriptive, and narrative skills. You see **practice-based** skills such as putting in the time to gain experience with writing skills and writing conventions (e.g. capitalization, organization, punctuation, and spelling – often referred to as COPS), and improving penmanship. You see **technology-based** skills that include access to general technology and assistive technology.

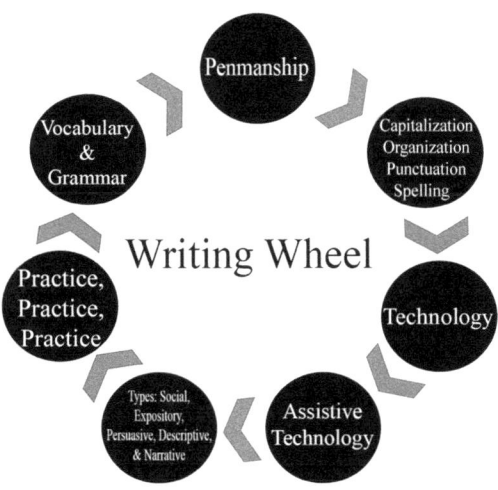

Start with determining your child's present level of writing across knowledge, ideology, practice, and technology. Ask yourself the following questions.

1 *What do I know about my child's present writing skills including generating a signature, writing one word, phrase, sentence or short answer responses, writing expository, persuasive, narrative, and descriptive types? If I do not understand my child's writing skill level, what team member(s) can I talk to who will explain to me more thoroughly my child's skills?*

2 *What are the barriers my child faces with writing (e.g. motor access, anxiety, sensory, attention, memory, motivation, self-regulation, depression, interfering physical motor skills or planning (i.e. tremor, spastic coordination), and other co-occurring conditions)?*

3 *What assistive technology provides optimal physical access for my child to write or publish a written document (e.g. easier to manipulate pens than pencils, larger keyboard, on-screen keyboard, switch scanning, eye gaze)?*

4 *How much time is dedicated to practicing writing? Is the time sufficient to accomplish the task? How soon does fatigue become counterproductive?*

5 *What types and amounts of prompting are used (e.g. verbal, physical, visual, time)? What is my plan to reduce or eliminate prompting?*

6 *Does penmanship matter now or will it matter in the future?*

7 *Are writing conventions like capitalization, organization, punctuation, and spelling a priority now? Will they be important in the future?*

Reading, writing, thinking, and speaking about the written text and drawn images bring richness to our understanding of each other and the world. Language literacy is a vital skill for a child that uses AAC. Language literacy is critical for *Maximizing Participation*.

Maximizing Participation with vocabulary

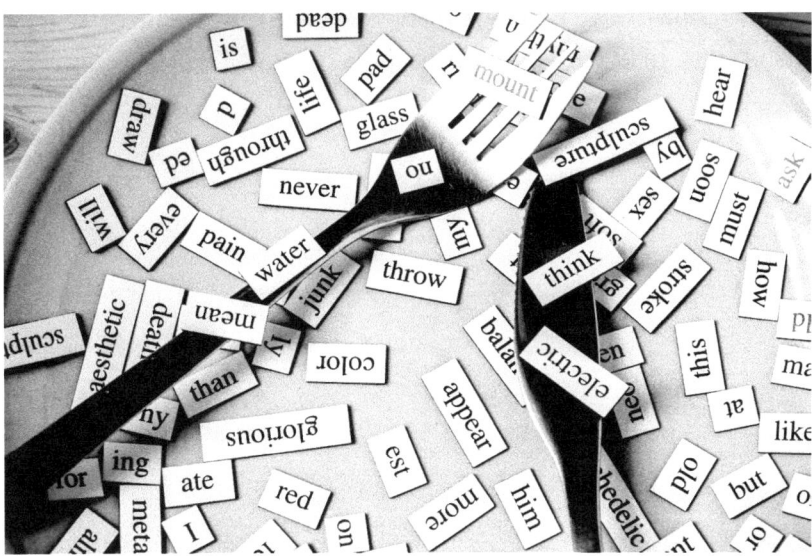

In *Maximizing Participation*, the needs of the communication partners are now equal to the needs of the AAC user. Is this a bold statement? No, we need our children that use AAC to be an equal member of any conversation. The child needs to initiate, comment, summarize, retell, or any other communicative act expected in the social situation. Therefore, the needs of the communication partners must be recognized and supported. This may be a shift in thinking, but it is a necessary shift because our communication partners must know the effective and efficient ways to communicate with my child. In *Maximizing Participation*, we place the focus of vocabulary on how to use the meaning of words to meet social and academic requirements for interaction with others and participating in the world. However, there will be more people rather than fewer who will require support in how to communicate with the child that uses AAC. Explore options for expressing vocabulary through experiences for *Maximizing Participation.*

1 Vocabulary to speak and write with rich language

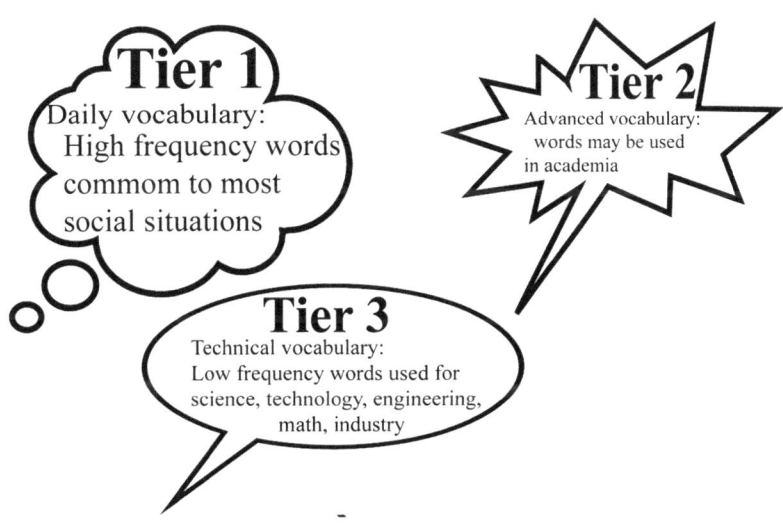

We want our children to express ideas that match their ideas that may require complex language. People want rich language that entices vivid imagery creating a multisensory connection between words and the intent of the message. Descriptive words bring ideas to life.

2 Vocabulary that states, *Yes, I Research*!

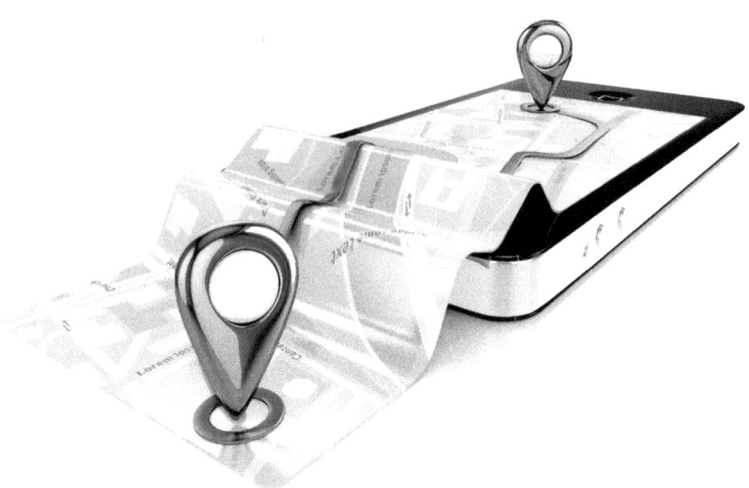

Research skills will be required for academic purposes requiring students to be able to navigate and organize ideas, materials, and technology. Encouraging research helps children understand themselves within the context of the world around them. Take a wonderful ride into history as current as the daily news to the beginning of time. Before heading out on a ride through history, learn the vocabulary you need to know to accomplish your purpose.

Vocabulary examples: *key words, research, report, review, abstract, introduce, summarize, effect, analyze, interpret*

3 Vocabulary for what's on your bookshelf these days?

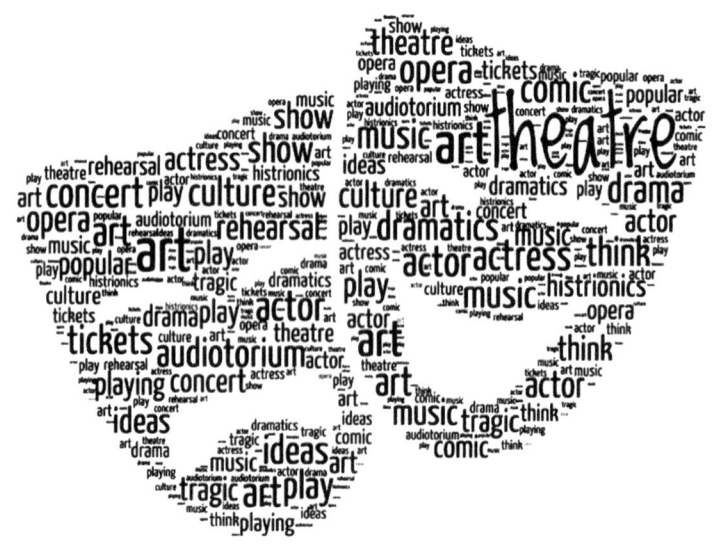

Reading level and interest level varies person to person regardless of AAC use. Expose your child to reading for fun about topics of interest while building the nuts and bolts skills at your child's instructional level. Respect each child's choice of books and authors. Learning the parts or elements of a story help readers capture meaning from their choices in book authors, and genres.

Vocabulary Examples: *genre, setting, plot, characters, conflict, action, resolution, consequence, alternative, implication*

4 Vocabulary for, 'I'm feeling it'

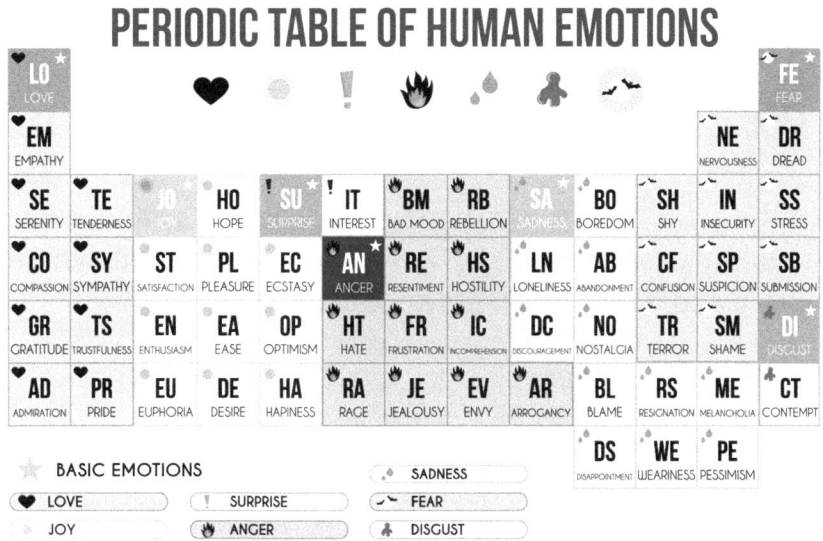

A periodic table of emotions is a great way to convey that humans have a full spectrum of emotions. Words expressing feelings and emotions have tiers or levels of complexity too (Hutton, 2008; Spivey, 2013). Include vocabulary that gets to the heart of the feelings and emotions of the characters in a story. If a character is feeling *blah*, maybe they are feeling *lackadaisical*. Another character may feel *apprehension* or *panic*. Start with the basics and then explore how *happiness* can represent *contentment*. Or, is *sadness, depression, embarrassment, grief*, or maybe a combination of all of them. Additionally, if you are starting with the basics of *happiness, sadness, anger, disgust, fear, and surprise*, then bravo because expressing emotions is a part of a healthy mind and body.

5 Vocabulary for telling jokes, 'Wait, Have You Heard the One About...?'

Jokes are a fun way to connect with friends or serve as an ice breaker. While many speech generating devices have some pre-programmed jokes, it would be fun to program novel age appropriate jokes. Types of quick phrase starters include examples like: *Did you hear the one about...; Knock, knock ... What do you call ... How do you know when ...* Include responses to jokes on speech generating devices. Examples of jokes can be a play on double word meanings,

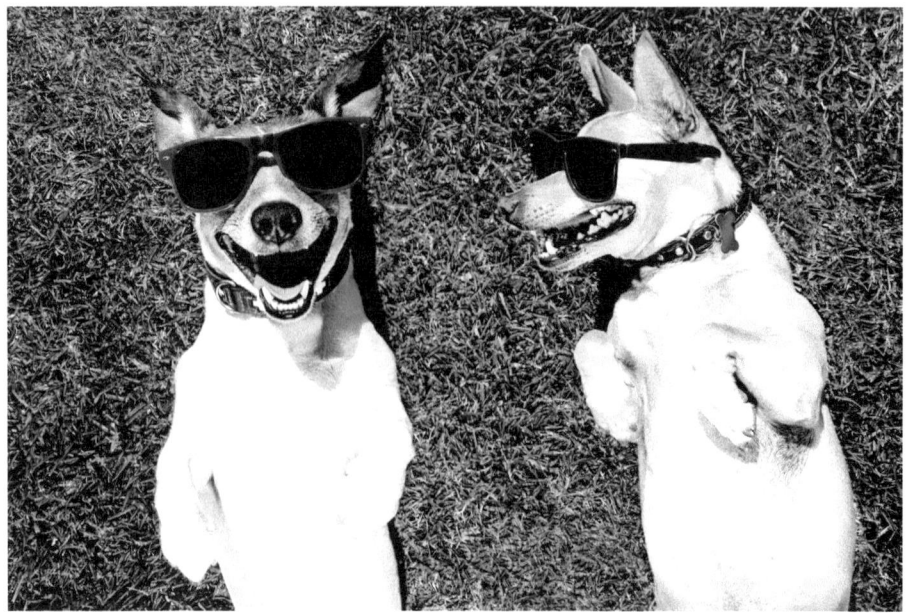

substituting sounds in words, surprise endings, and even playing on role reversals. Children *Maximizing Participation* anticipate the flexibility of their vocabulary and enjoy these plays on words.

Vocabulary Examples: *joke, crack up, burst out loud laughing, I don't get it. Just kidding; I'm teasing. No joke. Not a laughing matter.*

6 Vocabulary for … Get the duct tape! … and other useful repair strategies

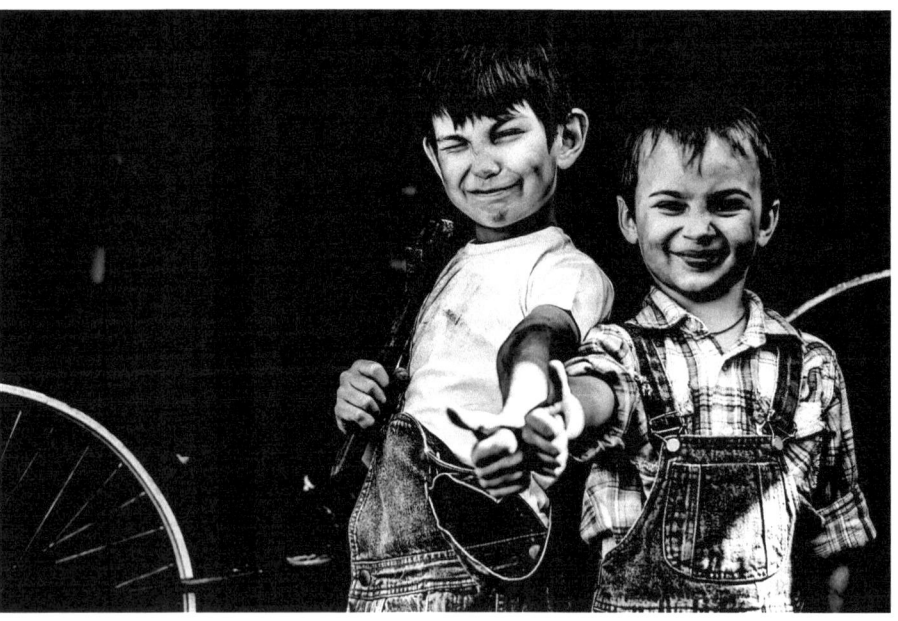

Yes, this title is a bit tongue and cheek, but a solid selection of vocabulary for repair strategies is not. Have repair strategies and phrases that are easily accessible for the child on a speech generating device or communication board. If humor suits your child, coming up with a fun quip could be a great way for your child to connect with a communication partner.

Vocabulary Examples: *Let me duct tape that message! That is not what I meant to say. Wait a minute while I complete my thought. Hold on, I need the duct tape!*

7 Vocabulary for *I changed my mind*

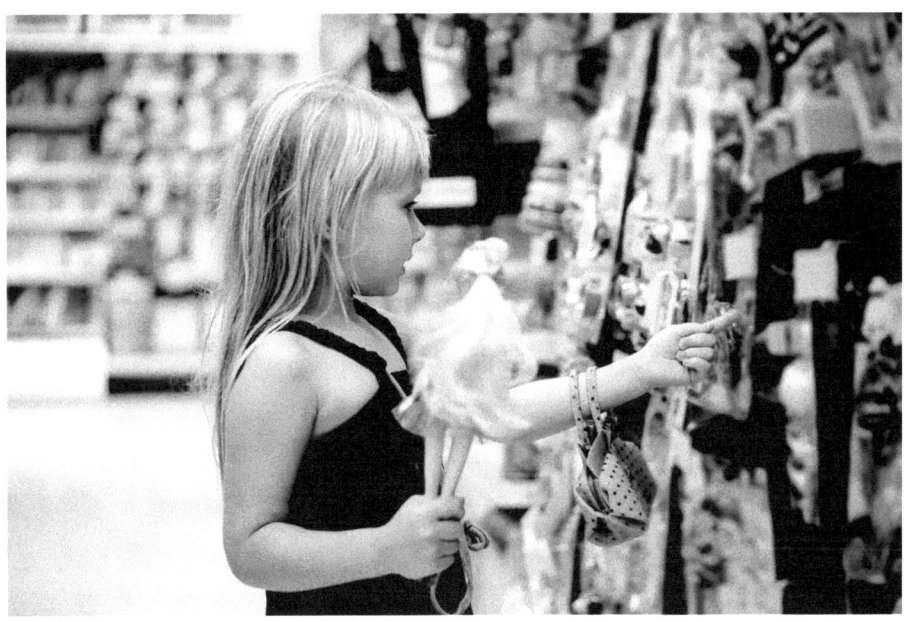

Sooo, you changed your mind or have a change of heart. A message repair does not always have to be due to an error. Have words and phrases programmed to support this type of intent.

Vocabulary Examples: *I changed my mind. Retract, adjust, instead, different*

8 Vocabulary for ... *I had another thought*

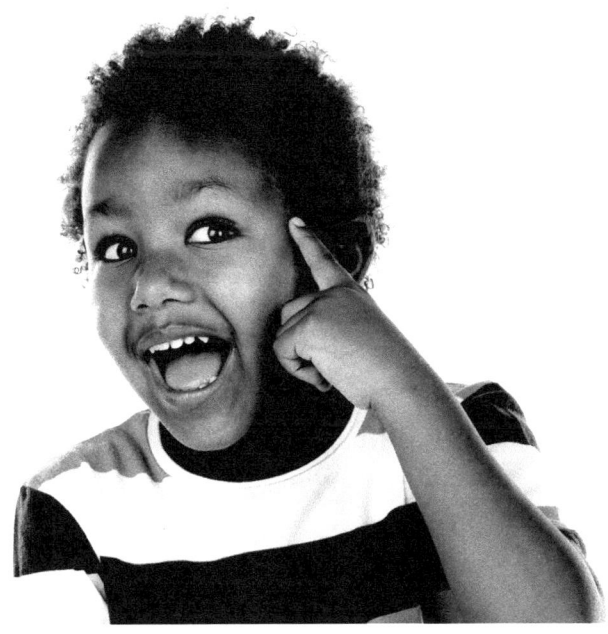

Have you ever had that great idea after a conversation moved on to another person or maybe to another topic? Well kids can have this same experience, so let's give our kids that use AAC the option to be able to express additional ideas whenever they come to mind. Sometimes composing an opinion takes more time using a speech generating device and your child needs to make a contribution even when the topic may have changed.

Vocabulary example: *I have an additional thought/another idea/one more thing I want to say; I have a contribution; Do you have any other thoughts?*

Maximizing Participation with tools and access

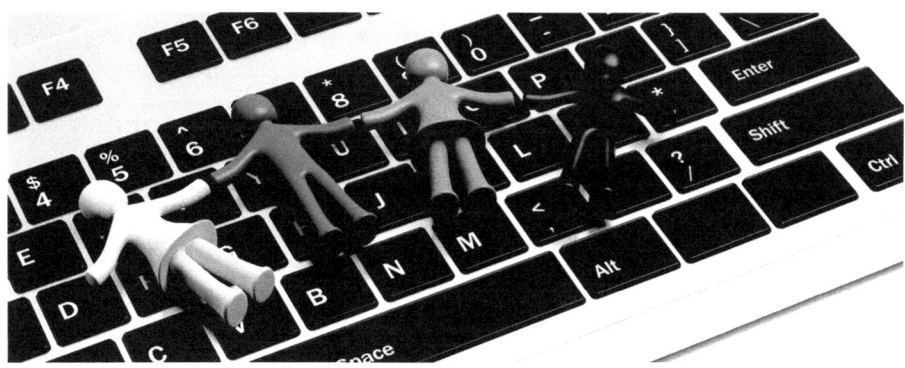

○ My multimodal AAC plan

Maximizing Participation means your child has **multimodal** tools and the necessary access methods that meets the **just-in-time** standards meaning the fastest and most efficient nonverbal, low or high technology is employed to express a message in the timeliest manner. It means the user can **communicate any message, for any purpose, at any time**. *Maximizing Participation* does not mean that your child has completely mature language skills to understand everything, produce grammatically extensive messages, and demonstrate perfect literacy skills every time. It does mean that your child may need help with programming and other strategies to succeed in establishing and participating in communication opportunities and getting around barriers to participation. Choosing the right emotional, physical, and cognitive support continues to influence success.

Technology advances quickly. You know that fact. The same holds true for advancements in AAC. Complete a regular back up of your child's AAC device. Devices connected to the internet will likely receive announcements of software updates from AAC companies. Explore innovations in hardware, software, and accessibility tools to see how the advancements facilitate your child's communication and participation. Ask experts about advancements and the benefits of software and hardware along with a cost benefit analysis that may warrant a new device. Work with the AAC company funding department to determine the purchase options.

Your child's physical abilities may change resulting in an increased or decreased need for accessibility. Work with interventionists and keep a keen eye out frequently to address the following questions: *What are the optimal ways my child uses his or her body to communicate? Have there been physical changes such as growth or improved motor planning skills that require new access methods? What are the optimal ways my child uses low technology tools to communicate? What are other low technology options to consider that would satisfy a new or developing need? What are different low technology tools that may meet an existing need more effectively or efficiently? What are the optimal ways my child uses high technology tools and devices to communicate?* Revisit *Feature Matching* in the chapter titled *Bridging Skills* to optimize technology choices and your child's physical and communication status. Throughout this book the idea of connecting with communication partners is discussed using low technology and high tech tools and devices. Guidelines for making a communication wallet are offered in Bridging Skills. An example of a tip card titled, *Let's Chat*, is also offered. Use the *Let's Chat* page or create one that best matches the communication topics for your child. In some cases the topics on the *Let's Chat* page are fine but you may need more space. Personalize the *Let's Chat* page for your AAC superstar.

A summary of Maximizing Participation

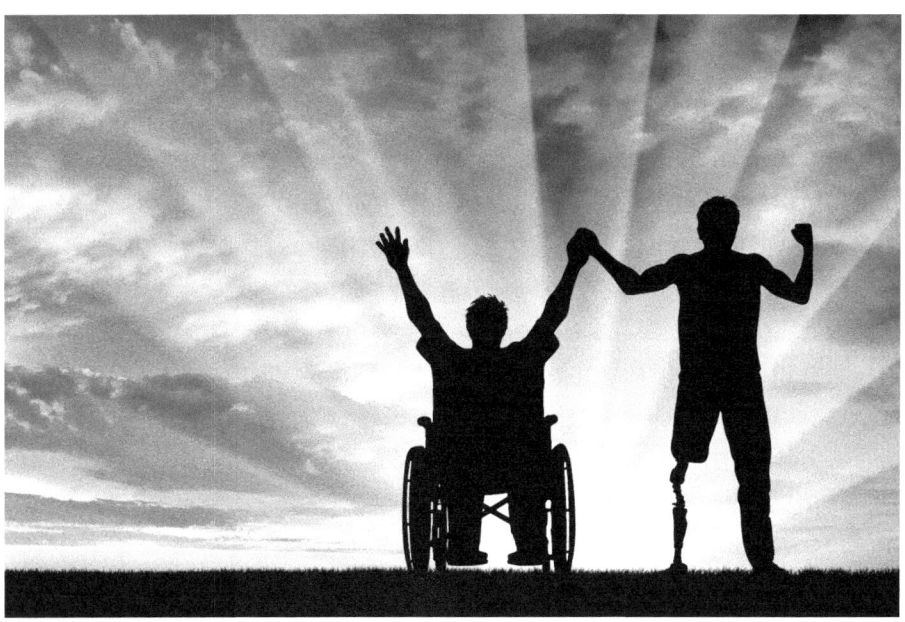

○ Ideas in action

Maximizing Participation, a finale and a launching pad, is a grounding perspective. If we are *Maximizing Participation* for a child who uses AAC at any stage of development, from *Getting Started* to the highest levels of independence then you have your finale, your pat on the back, success, a job well done. Your child's participation is growing because your child has access to the necessary tools, strategies, and language. Then, you look at the next possibility, a new experience, a different communication partner, a novel problem to solve, and you see your new launching pad. Therefore, we have our *Ideas in Action* that means we are asking the right questions (ideas) and are executing an effective plan (in action) for *Maximizing Participation* for the child that uses AAC.

Before we go: *Let's Chat: An easy way to talk with me*

How fitting that the finale of this book ends with a tool that promotes a launching of communication through a tool titled, *Let's Chat*. Engage communication partners with this tool that allows the child who is an AAC user to share information with others and offer questions to communication partners. *Let's Chat: An Easy Way to Talk with Me* (Murtha & Mayne, 2019) is designed to accomplish the goal of engagement with peers and adults. Complete the page with interesting facts and ideas. Add pictures to the back of the page to provide a visual of favorite experiences, people, or things. Laminate or place the page in a sheet protector. Keep the tool in a place communication partners can access it quickly. Use *Let's Chat* for *Getting Started* with conversation, for *Building Fundamentals* of connection, for *Making Connections* with others, for *Bridging Skills* of independence, and *Maximizing Participation* because . . . in your child's words . . . *Hear Me into Voice*.

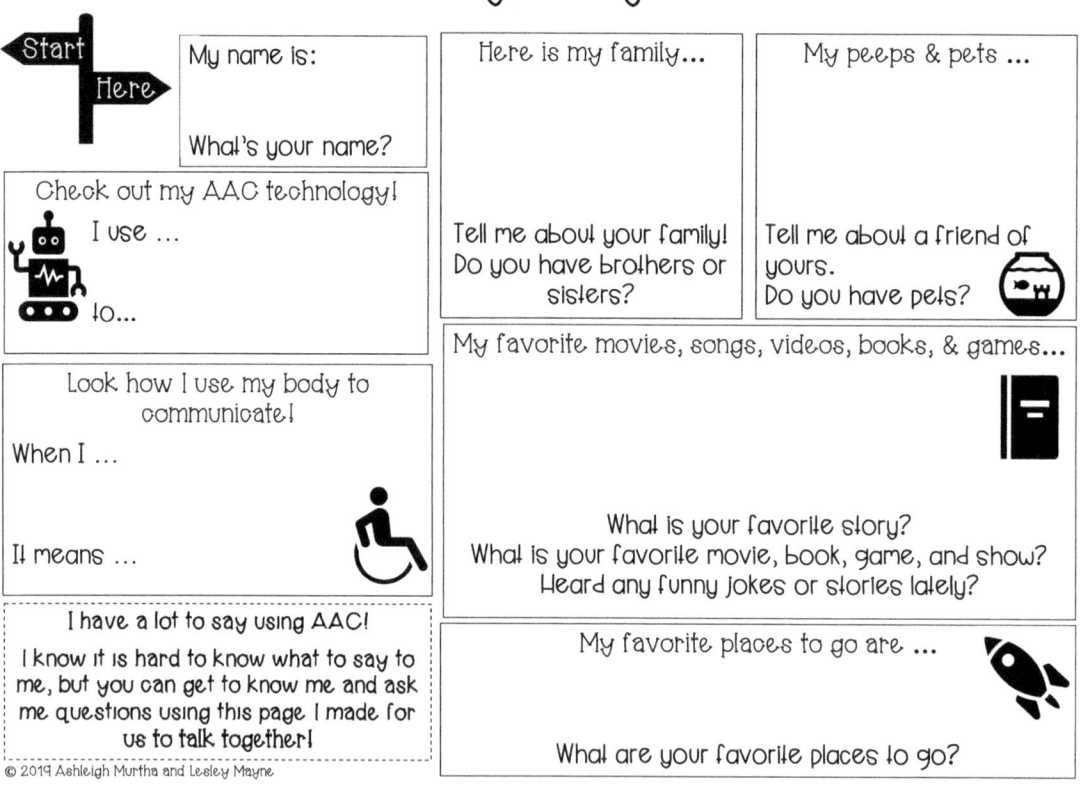

Figure 6.31   Let's Chat: An Easy Way to Talk with Me

References

AAC-RERC. (2010). Emergency communication: Disaster preparation, response and recovery for people with CCN. Retrieved from http://aac-rerc.psu.edu/index.php/pages/show/id/4

Baum, L. F. (1900). *The Wonderful Wizard of Oz*. Chicago, IL: Geo M. Hill Company.

Benedek-Wood, E., McNaughton, D. & Light, J. (2016). Instruction in letter sound correspondence for children with autism and limited speech. *Topics in Early Childhood Special Education*, *36*(1), 43–54.

Blackstone, S. & Goldman, A. S. (2018, June 5). People who use AAC in emergencies and disasters: Tales from the trenches [Webinar]. In *USAAC Webinars*. Retrieved from www.isaac-online.org/wordpress/wp-content/uploads/2018-USSAAC-eprep-June-2018-FINAL.pdf

Bryan, D. N. (2018). Emergency communication4all. Retrieved from https://disabilities.temple.edu/aacvocabulary/e4all.shtml#index

Ehren, B. J. (2018, September–October). Why SLP services are essential to adolescents, and why we can't go it alone [Webinar]. In *American Speech-Language-Hearing Association Online Conference, Spoken and Written Language in Adolescents: Fresh Solutions*. Retrieved from www.asha.org/Events/lang-conf/Sessions/.

Ehren, B. J., Lenz, K. B. H. & Deshler, D. (2016). Adolescents who struggle and 21st-century literacy. In C. A. Stone, E. R. Silliman, B. J. Ehren & G. P. Wallach (Eds.), *Handbook of language and literacy: Development and disorders* (2nd ed., pp. 619–636). New York, NY: Gulliford Press.

The Emergency Helpers Program Memory Match. (n.d.). Retrieved from www.fire.nsw.gov.au/gallery/files/pdf/emergency_helpers/memory_game.pdf

Family Education. (2019). Teaching kids to negotiate. Retrieved from www.familyeducation.com/life/social-emotional-development/teaching-kids-negotiate

Federal Communications Commission. (n.d.). Telecommunications relay service – TRS. Retrieved from www.fcc.gov/consumers/guides/telecommunications-relay-service-trs

Feuerstein, R., Miller, R., Hoffman, M. B., Rand, Y., Mintzker, Y. & Jensen, M. R. (1981). Cognitive modifiability in adolescence: Cognitive structure and the effects of intervention. *Journal of Special Education*, *15*(2), 269–287.

Fire and Rescue. (2018). Emergency helpers: Early childhood emergency program. Retrieved from www.fire.nsw.gov.au/page.php?id=886.

Halliwell-Phillipps, J. O. (1890). The three little pigs. In *The nursery rhymes of England*, London, UK: Frederick Warne & Co. 37–41 Retrieved from https://archive.org/stream/nurseryrhymesofe00hall#page/15/mode/1up

Hasbrouck, J. & Glaser, D. R. (2012). *Reading fluency: Understanding and teaching this complex skill*. Austin, TX: Gibson Hasbrouck & Associates.

Hutton, T. (2008). *Three tiers of vocabulary and education*. Retrieved from www.super-duperinc.com/handouts/pdf/182_VocabularyTiers.pdf.

Institute on Disabilities at Temple University. (2018). Technology: Augmentative and alternative communication (AAC). Retrieved from https://disabilities.temple.edu/aacvocabulary/e4all.shtml#index.

Kaniel, S. & Feuerstein, R. (1989). Special needs of children with learning difficulties. *Oxford Review of Education*, *15*(2), 165–179. Retrieved from: www.jstor.org/stable/1049971

Light, J. & Kent-Walsh, J. (2003, May 27). Fostering emergent literacy for children who require AAC. *ASHA Leader*, *8*, 4–29.

Long, S. (2016, April 6). All about emergencies. Retrieved from http://theautismhelper.com/all-about-emergencies/

McNaughton, S. & Lindsay, P. (1995). Approaching literacy with AAC graphics. *Augmentative and Alternative Communication*, *11*(4), 222–228.

Murtha, A. & Mayne, L. (2019). *Let's chat: An easy way to talk with me*. [Unpublished document]. Riverside, CA.

Musselwhite, C., Erickson, K., Stemach, J. & Odom, J. (2005). Start-to-finish literacy starters and core language. Retrieved from www.crsd.org/cms/lib5/PA01000188/Centricity/Domain/13/Shared%20%20Guided%20Reading.pdf

The National Autism Association. (2016). Personal emergency profile sheet. Retrieved from http://nationalautismassociation.org/personal-emergency-profile-sheet/

Owens, R. E. (2014). *Language disorders: A functional approach to assessment and intervention*. New York, NY: Pearson.

Patient Provider Communication. (2018). Emergency communication. Retrieved from www.patientprovidercommunication.org/gallery/?Category=Emergency%20Communication

Prutting, C. & Kirchner, D. (1983). Applied pragmatics. In T. Gallagher & C. Prutting (Eds.), *Pragmatic assessment and intervention issues in language* (pp. 29–64). San Diego, CA: College Hill Press.

Rackensperger, T., Krezman, C., McNaughton, D., Williams, M. B. & D' Silva, K. (2005). "When I first got it, I wanted to throw it off a cliff": The challenges and benefits of learning AAC technologies as described by adults who use AAC. *Augmentative and Alternative Communication*, *21*(3), 165–186.

Rogers, S. (1999). *Hearing them into voice: The hermeneutics of listening to children who cannot speak: A dynamic approach to assessing and teaching communication* (Unpublished doctoral dissertation). Claremont Graduate University, CA.

Spivey, B. L. (2013). Super duper handy handouts: Helping children understand and deal with emotions. Retrieved from chrome-extension://oemmndcbldboiebfnladdacbdfmadadm/www.superduperinc.com/handouts/pdf/390_UnderstandFeelings.pdf

Tran, P. (2019, May 29). Fighting for the right to communicate at Cal-Tash 2019 [Blog post]. Retrieved from https://highschool.latimes.com/la-canada-high-school/fighting-for-the-right-to-communicate-at-cal-tash-2019/

Vygotsky, L. (1986). *Thought and language* (A. Kozulin, Ed.). Cambridge, MA: MIT Press.

Watzlawick, P., Beavin, J. H. & Jackson, D. D. (1967). *Pragmatics of human communication: A study of interactional patterns, pathologies, and paradoxes* (pp. 48–71). New York, NY: W. & W. & Norton Company.

Zangari, C. (2012, June 20). "Call me later:" 5 supports for phone communication by people who use AAC [Blog post]. Retrieved from https://praacticalaac.org/praactical/call-me-later-5-supports-for-phone-communication-by-people-who-use-aac/

Zangari, C. (2018, May 14). PrAACtical resources: Lockdown, code-red, and other school safety drills [Blog post]. Retrieved from https://praacticalaac.org/praactical/praactical-resources-lockdown-code-red-other-school-safety-drills/

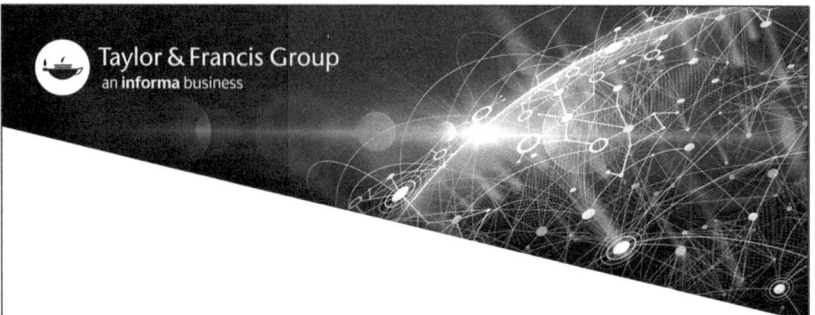
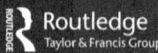
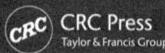